Midwifery: Best Practice Volume 4

D1581616

For Elsevier:

Commissioning Editor: Mary Seager
Development Editor: Rebecca Nelemans
Project Manager: Jess Thompson
Designer: Andy Chapman

Midwifery: Best Practice Volume 4

Edited by

Sara Wickham RM MA BA(Hons) PGCert
Independent Midwifery Lecturer and Consultant, Wickford, UK

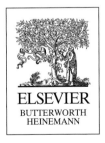

ELSEVIER
BUTTERWORTH
HEINEMANN

EDINBURGH LONDON NEW YORK OXFORD PHILADELPHIA ST LOUIS SYDNEY TORONTO 2006

BUTTERWORTH
HEINEMANN
ELSEVIER

© 2006 Elsevier Limited. All rights reserved.
First published 2006

Cover image courtesy of www.JohnBirdsall.co.uk.

No part of this publication may be reproduced, stored in a retrieval
system, or transmitted in any form or by any means, electronic,
mechanical, photocopying, recording or otherwise, without the prior
permission of the Publishers. Permissions may be sought directly
from Elsevier's Health Sciences Rights Department,
1600 John F. Kennedy Boulevard, Suite 1800, Philadelphia,
PA 19103-2899, USA: phone: (+1) 215 239 3804; fax: (+1) 215 239 3805;
or, e-mail: *healthpermissions@elsevier.com*. You may also complete your
request on-line via the Elsevier homepage (http://www.elsevier.com),
by selecting 'Support and contact' and then 'Copyright and
Permission'.

ISBN-13: 978 0 7506 8895 6
ISBN-10: 0 7506 8895 5

British Library Cataloguing in Publication Data
A catalogue record for this book is available from the British Library

Library of Congress Cataloging in Publication Data
A catalog record for this book is available from the Library of Congress

Knowledge and best practice in this field are constantly changing.
As new research and experience broaden our knowledge, changes
in practice, treatment and drug therapy may become necessary or
appropriate. Readers are advised to check the most current
information provided (i) on procedures featured or (ii) by the
manufacturer of each product to be administered, to verify the
recommended dose or formula, the method and duration of
administration, and contraindications. It is the responsibility of the
practitioner, relying on their own experience and knowledge of the
patient, to make diagnoses, to determine dosages and the best
treatment for each individual patient, and to take all appropriate
safety precautions.
To the fullest extent of the law, neither the publisher nor the editors
assumes any liability for any injury and/or damage.

The Publisher

Printed in Spain.

The
Publisher's
policy is to use
**paper manufactured
from sustainable forests**

Contents

Introduction

Hello, and thank you for deciding to have a look at *Midwifery: Best Practice Volume 4*! The articles republished in (and commissioned for) these volumes have all been hand-picked as those which most effectively represent the spirit of our collective search for 'best practice' in midwifery. We have always made practice the main focus of these books, and, with this in mind, articles from *The Practising Midwife* form the backbone of the contents. In Volumes 2 and 3, we added in a few original research articles from *Midwifery* as well as some original articles commissioned especially for these books. In Volume 4, we have continued to include all of those things, and have additionally included a few articles from another journal – *The Journal of Midwifery and Women's Health* – in the hope of offering an even broader perspective on the topic of best practice.

There are nine sections in this book – four of them are the 'key' sections which we have included in every volume of *Midwifery: Best Practice* – 'Women and Midwives', 'Pregnancy', 'Labour and Birth' and 'Life After Birth'. Interspersed with these are four 'Focus On...' sections, which include a range of articles looking at current hot topics. This time, we have two sections on 'Diversity', one on 'Building Communities of Women' and one on 'Birth Centres'. As ever, the last section of the book includes personal stories, experiences and reflection upon practice.

In the first three volumes, each of the key sections began with an introduction and ended with a section listing questions for reflection, the idea being that midwives could use these for PREP activities. This time, things are a little different; I have tried to come up with some new and interesting slants on some of the issues covered, and generated some more creative questions for anyone who would like to use the book in this way. This time, the questions are raised before the articles in each of the key sections, and you are invited to think about the questions before reading the articles, as each one relates to one or more of the articles in that section. There are a few brief follow-on questions at the end of each of the main sections and you can, as ever, use these questions as triggers for PREP or other continuing education activities. Each of the 'Focus On ...' sections concludes with one or more 'Questions for debate', which can also be used for personal reflection, or for group discussion and debate.

I must admit that I often think it would be nice to be able to talk with the midwives who use these questions in their own practice and education, and have a chat about the answers, perhaps even turning some into a follow-on article, and we have finally come up with a way of doing just that. In the name of entertainment, curiosity and ongoing debate about midwifery practice, we are inviting responses to the question in Section 5 of this book (Labour and Birth) – on a postcard, email or letter! There are, by the way, no right or wrong answers; we are simply inviting you to answer it in your own words, from your own experience (and that of colleagues if you like, though please check with them first, or make their comments anonymous).

As an extra incentive to put pen to paper (or fingers to keyboard), Elsevier have donated £500 worth of vouchers which can be spent on their books; we will take good care of all the responses which come in and, on 31 December 2006, we will pull five responses out of a birth pool and send each of those people a £100 book voucher! Please make sure that you include your contact details (partly so that we can send you a voucher if you win, but also because, if we get enough responses to think about including something in another book or article, we wouldn't use anything unless we could get in touch with you and get your permission first). More details and the all-important small print which goes along with any competition can be found at the back of this book.

Most importantly of all, I would like to extend a very warm thank you to all of the authors of the articles which have been republished here, and to the editors of the journals who worked to publish them in the first place: Jenny Hall, Clinical Editor and Viv Riddoch, Managing Editor of *The Practising Midwife*; Ann Thomson, Editor-in-Chief of *Midwifery*; and Tekoa King, Editor-in-Chief of *The Journal of Midwifery and Women's Health*. Thanks also to the authors of the articles which have been written especially for this book: Sarah Buckley, Penny Champion, Lorna Davies, Mindy Levy and the women of the Birth Resource Centre – Nadine Edwards, Jane Crewe, Lyssa Clayton, Andrea St Clair, Fiona Armstrong and Lee Seekings-Norman – who all worked against the clock and

in spite of a communal tummy bug to get their article ready in time! As ever, huge thanks also go to everyone at Elsevier; Mary Seager and Rebecca Nelemans who, as the editing team, are the 'face' of the *Midwifery: Best Practice* series, but also to the people who work behind the scenes. Extra thanks this time to Natalie Friend, who helped organise the 'competition' and who will be taking good care of the postcards, emails and letters till the winners are drawn!

Sara Wickham

Acknowledgements

We would like to thank all those who have contributed to this volume of *Midwifery: Best Practice*:

Anne Adamson, Jo Alexander, Tricia Anderson, Fiona Armstrong, Penny Armstrong, Denise Austin, Kirsten Baker, Simone Baker, Maria Barrell, Catherine Bassom, Cheryl Tatano Beck, Claire Beckinsale, Jane Bowler, Diane B Boyer, Sarah J Buckley, Natasha Carr, Penny Champion, Lyssa Clayton, Suzanne Colson, Margaret Cooke, Jane Crewe, Esther Culpin, Lorna Davies, Morwenna Davies, Stephanie Day, Corinne Diroff, Jeanne Watson Driscoll, Nadine Edwards, Gillian Fletcher, Diane M Fraser, Jenny Fraser, Elizabeth Fulton-Breathat, Ina May Gaskin, Mandy Grant, Barbara Hammes, Virginia Howes, Vanora Hundley, Sally Inch, Dawn Jackson, Judith Jennrich, Rosie Kacary, Holly Powell Kennedy, Mavis Kirkham, Carrie Klima, Susan Law, Beverley A Lawrence Beech, Mindy Levy, Heather Lirette, Rona McCandlish, Laura McCully, Shirley McDonald, Judith S Mercer, Candace Mooney-Hescott, Fehmidah Munir, Mary Newburn, Michel Odent, Myra Parsons, Katherine Pollard, Nicki Pusey, Becky Reed, Yana Richens, Jill Sanghera, Virginia Schmied, Lee Seekings-Norman, Athena Sheehan, Rachel Simpkins, Katja Stahl, Andrea St Clair, Vicky Tinsley, Victoria Vest, Lynn Walcott, Deborah S Walker, Louise Wallace, Gill Walton, Kim Watts, Andrea Wolahan, Julie Wray.

SECTION 1

Women and Midwives

SECTION CONTENTS

1.1 The impact of the establishment of a midwife managed unit on women in a rural setting in England 2

1.2 Culture, control and the birth environment 9

1.3 Drawing the line: caesarean sections on demand 15

1.4 Searching for autonomy 18

1.5 The risky business of normal birth 29

Where might we go from here? 32

Exploring the issues...

Before you read the articles in this section, you might like to make a note of what you think are the five most important issues facing women and midwives today – that is, any issues which create problems or tension and which you feel should be changed. I realise that most people, in response to this, will think, 'but the issues will be different for everyone!' Indeed they will, but imagine, if you like, that you are a contestant on a game show where lots of women and midwives have been polled for their responses to this question, and you are trying to come up with the top five answers. More after the articles!

The impact of the establishment of a midwife managed unit on women in a rural setting in England

Kim Watts, Diane M Fraser, Fehmidah Munir

Objective: to determine what impact the changes from consultant-led care to midwife-led care in a local maternity service have had on women using that service.

Design: case study – data were collected by postal questionnaire, semi-structured, tape-recorded interviews, observations and scrutiny of records.

Setting: a small town in rural England.

Participants: all pregnant women eligible for a midwife-managed unit (MMU) birth in a small rural town in England.

Findings: the women using the MMU were satisfied with the care they received and the MMU style of care. Women giving birth at the MMU and at home required less pain relief and were more likely to have an intact perineum than a similar group of women giving birth in hospital. Continuity of carer did not appear to be an issue for women as long as they felt supported by a known team of midwives. Transfer for complications during the birthing process was a cause for anxiety and stress for women and their partners. Women, whilst satisfied with the MMU, would prefer the consultant-led maternity hospital to be re-established in the town. The home-birth rate rose by 28% when the consultant unit closed.

Implications for practice: while the establishment of a midwife-managed unit has provided increased choice for a minority of women, the removal of the consultant unit in the town has disadvantaged the majority of pregnant women. While guidelines are needed when establishing these units, the application of restrictive inclusion and exclusion criteria can sometimes force women to make less appropriate birth choices.

Introduction

The establishment of midwife-managed units (MMUs), or birthing centres in many cases, has been in addition to the consultant-led care already in place (e.g. see Zadoroznyj, 2000; Hodnett, 2001; Clow & Christie, 2002). This was not, however, the case for a town in rural England. The closure of the local obstetric-led maternity services in August 1998 had resulted from the unavoidable loss of the inpatient paediatric services at the small general hospital in the town. The subsequent establishment of the MMU followed consultation with both the local population and key stakeholders. Included in this consultation was the consultant-led obstetric unit 25 miles away, along small country roads. This unit, in the nearest city, assumed the role of 'host unit' for women needing transfer from the MMU or surrounding community. Women at high obstetric risk were still able to access antenatal care in the town but intrapartum care was provided at the consultant-led obstetric host unit. In the five years prior to the closure of the local maternity hospital, home-births averaged only 1% per annum as compared to the national average of 2% (Macfarlane et al., 2000).

Underpinning the reorganisation of maternity services was an assessment of women's chances of developing complications during the childbirth process. This led to the development of risk categories.

Applying categories of risk to women has resulted in its own unique problems, as debated by Wilson (1996) and Campbell (1999). Wilson (1996) suggests that risk categories can vary greatly between units and the validity of using population-based statistics to develop risk categories has been questioned. Indeed, the introduction of 'risk categories' can sometimes lead to the perception of inequity of choice rather than increasing the choice for women' (Wilson, 1996; Campbell, 1999). In this particular unit strict criteria were applied for women when choices of place of birth were discussed with them (Box 1.1.1). Women fitting the criteria of 'low risk' were offered either giving birth at the MMU, at home or at the consultant-led maternity hospital. Women in the 'high risk' category, which included primigravid women, were only offered consultant-led care in maternity hospitals with 24-hour paediatric and anaesthetic services.

The model of offering women whose pregnancies are considered to be low risk a choice of having their babies in a local setting with minimal intervention is in line with UK Government policy (DoH, 1993) and a subsequent Audit Commission Report on Maternity Services (1997). Furthermore, there has been a wealth of evidence, from studies designed to elicit the views of childbearing women, that mothers were dissatisfied with the medicalisation of childbirth and had positive psychological outcomes when they felt they had more choice and control of their childbirth experiences (Jacoby & Cartwright, 1990; House of Commons, 1992; Bramadat & Driedger, 1993; Hutton, 1995; Garcia, 1995; Gready et al., 1995; McCourt & Page, 1996; Green et al., 1998; Fraser, 1999).

However, one of the complications of isolated birthing centres is that of transfer. Identifying which women are likely to remain in or move between high- and low-risk categories can create difficulties when planning maternity services. The transfer rate from previous evidence has varied between 14% and 29% (Davies et al., 1996) and may result in increased anxiety levels in women (Walker, 2000) if not adequately prepared for transfer (Creasy, 1997).

Against this background the evaluation of the new maternity services in this rural community was commissioned. The commissioners of the study wished to explore what effect the establishment of the MMU had on women, their families, health professionals directly providing the service and those indirectly linked to the service. Although suggestions had been made to locate the MMU in purpose-built accommodation, a decision was taken to refurbish the labour ward of the previous consultant unit to provide five birthing rooms, one of which housed the 'pool'. The MMU was self-contained and no hospital medical staff were expected to provide services unless an emergency (e.g. cardiac arrest) arose. In keeping with the current philosophy of a health service geared to the needs of the consumer, the health authority was required to establish how well women's needs were being met by this new service. The evaluation of the service from the user's perspective is discussed in this paper.

Box 1.1.1 Criteria for admission to the MMU

Multigravida
Gestation between 37 and 42 weeks inclusive
Cephalic presentation
No past medical problems
Normal pregnancy to date
No previous significant obstetric complications
Personal choice

Methods

In order to achieve the project aims in the six-month time period specified (March–August 2000), mixed methods were adopted to capture the complexity of the context surrounding changes in the maternity service. Cronbach (1982) argued that a case study evaluation is able to capture the complex process of evaluating effectiveness in a specific context and within a specified budget. The use of multiple methods in a case study increases validity and robustness (Stufflebeam, 1991; Murphy et al., 1998). This was achieved in the current study by undertaking surveys, interviews, making observations and scrutinising documents. Much of the research design was of a qualitative nature. Triangulation was used not so much as a test of validity but more, as proposed by Denzin and Lincoln (1994), as an alternative to it. This was considered necessary as it was anticipated that different data sources would reveal varied perceptions of and solutions to maternity services in the area rather than confirming one another unproblematically.

The sample

The study sample drawn from users of the maternity services had two components. Firstly, different cohorts of women who would be surveyed by postal questionnaire and, secondly, a small sample of women who would be invited to be interviewed in their homes. It was at this stage that it became evident that the percentage of home-births in the town and surrounding rural area had risen to above the national average following the closure of the consultant-led unit. During the study period 61 women gave birth at home and received care from MMU midwives. This equated to 28% of births attended by MMU midwives. As a result it was important to include this group of women in the sample for data collection. For the postal survey, women who had given birth between April 1999 and the end of March 2000 (first full year of the MMU in operation) were identified from the following groups:

- All women who had given birth at the MMU
- All women who had given birth at home and received care from MMU-employed midwives
- All women transferred from the MMU or home to the host unit
- All women eligible for the MMU but had chosen the host unit.

Women eligible for the in-depth, face-to-face interviews were drawn from those who had given birth after April 2000 and before the end of June 2000. The intention was to select a random sample from the following groups:

- Women who had given birth at the MMU
- Women transferred from the MMU or home to the host unit
- Women with a postcode for the town who fitted the criteria for MMU birth but had chosen the host unit.

However, given the timescale of the project, the first 10 women who had given birth since April 2000 were asked whether they would participate in the study. Eight of these women agreed to be interviewed in their homes.

The women's questionnaires were adapted from those already used nationally for clinical and midwifery practice audit purposes (Lamping & Rowe, 1996). The questionnaires incorporated both open and closed questions to enable the surveyed populations to convey their own perceptions, beliefs and value judgements. The questionnaire was divided into sections covering demographic details, antenatal, intrapartum and postnatal care. The women were asked to complete and return a consent form enclosed with the questionnaire. Four separate women's questionnaires were developed, one for each place-of-birth scenario. In addition, a scrutiny of women's records was undertaken (using a data collection form for consistency) to identify the outcomes recorded by health professionals; these were then used for comparative purposes with questionnaire data. The interview schedule was unstructured, women being given the opportunity to talk about whatever was important to them about their pregnancy and childbirth experiences.

Access and ethical considerations

Two different Local Research Ethics Committees (LRECs) were approached for this study. Permission was obtained to survey, interview and access records for women using the MMU facility. The LREC for the host unit would only permit women to be contacted via a third party, employed by the Trust. The CESDI (Confidential Enquiry into Stillbirths and Deaths in Infancy – a triennial dataset to inform the maternity services) co-ordinator at the local health authority was contacted prior to postings of

questionnaires to ensure no adverse outcomes had occurred before contact was made by the research team. LREC restriction on access made it impossible to identify non-responders and compare with those who had responded.

Data analysis

An overall response rate of 66.4% was obtained from the postal questionnaire survey (see Table 1.1.1). The survey data were coded and entered into a database using the Statistical Package for Social Sciences (SPSS Windows version 9.0). After primary analysis of the open-ended questions, responses from women were recorded and themes identified which were categorised. Data were analysed using descriptive statistics and where appropriate inferential statistics were applied.

Interviews were transcribed in full and then coded as issues emerged, as well as utilising broad pre-specified codes to reflect the questions asked. From these codes, themes were identified and agreed by the research team from their individual reading of the interview data. Once these provisional themes had been identified, the interview transcripts were re-scrutinised to search for contradictory themes or opposing views that might have been missed on first reading.

The observational element of the study was restricted to the physical environment and to the MMU staff.

Findings

Limitations to the study

The intention of this study had been to include all women attended by MMU-employed midwives or who would have been eligible for an MMU birth. Unfortunately, the requirement by the LREC to use a third party to send out host unit questionnaires on behalf of the research team resulted in a flawed sample being identified.

Table 1.1.1 Response rates for women's questionnaires

Questionnaire category (according to place of birth)	Total population (n) meeting criteria	Response	Percentage return (%)
MMU birth	91	59	65
Home birth	61	41	67
Host unit birth – women who were eligible for MMU	107*	54*	51
Transfer birth	12	10	83

*Flawed data set; not all those returning questionnaires would have been eligible for MMU birth.

Of the 107 women originally identified by the host unit staff as fitting the criteria stated for inclusion in the study and subsequently sent a survey, on further examination only 46 met the inclusion criteria for MMU birth. Of these 46, only 12 returned questionnaires with completed consent forms and could be used for analysis. Comparisons between groups must therefore be interpreted with caution.

Choice of place of birth

As the issue of choice appears to have a positive psychological effect on pregnancy, the question of choice of birthing place was included in the survey. Only 18 (44%) from the home-birth group and five from the eligible host unit group who returned questionnaires ($n = 12$) were offered the choice of giving birth at the MMU. It was found that 59% of these women were offered the choice by a midwife who was providing their care. The remaining women were offered their birth choices by the general practitioner (GP) or the consultant overseeing their care. Women who gave birth at the MMU were more likely to be registered with a GP linked to the midwifery team based in the town, in comparison to the home-birth group ($\chi^2 = 22.01$, DF = 4, $p < 0.0001$), who were more likely to be registered with a GP practice outside the town. This was also the case for women from the host unit group. The most important factor for MMU women when deciding where to give birth was closeness to home ($\chi^2 = 52.31$, DF = 3, $p < 0.0001$). Women then stated that 'knowing the midwife', 'a smaller unit' and 'a familiar hospital' were additional important factors when choosing the MMU. When comparing this with the women giving birth at the host unit, the majority ($n = 10$) wanted to birth at a unit that had full support services available and the remainder ($n = 2$) stated that the host unit was slightly closer to their home than the MMU. Women from the home-birth group gave a range of reasons illustrated in Table 1.1.2, of which unplanned home-birth ($n = 9$) was the most frequently cited. There were multiple reasons for unplanned home-births; some

Table 1.1.2 Reasons given for home birth ($n = 38$; % rounded up)

Reasons given for place of birth	n	%
Booked for MMU/hospital but baby arrived too early	9	24
Didn't want to go to host unit	6	16
Being in control	6	16
More relaxed	6	16
Don't like hospital service	5	13
Other children at home	3	8
Discussed with midwife	3	8

called the midwife too late for the lengthy journey to hospital, others were given the option by the midwife of remaining at home or transferring to the MMU in advanced labour, and others were not eligible for the MMU and did not want to go to a hospital they did not know.

Continuity of care

The majority of women from the three groups ($n = 105$, 97%) received antenatal care at their GP surgery and this was mainly provided by a midwife ($n = 97$, 89%). When asked how many different midwives were seen during their pregnancy the MMU group saw significantly more midwives than the home-birth group ($\chi^2 = 13.57$, DF = 3, $p = 0.004$) and the host unit group. Women in the MMU group and home-birth group had seen all members of the team providing their care during the antenatal period. All 12 women from the host unit group received their consultant antenatal care in the satellite antenatal clinic held in the town. Although there was no significant difference between the groups in the number of different midwives seen postnatally, the home-birth group were more likely to be visited regularly by the midwife present at birth than the MMU group ($\chi^2 = 14.02$, DF = 2, $p = 0.001$). Host unit women were unlikely to see this midwife postnatally.

Intrapartum differences

Women in the MMU, home and host unit groups were asked about the methods of pain relief they had used during the birthing process. Epidural analgesia was only available in the host unit and a waterbirth was only available at the MMU (or at home if privately hired). 'Entonox' was the most commonly used form of pain relief and was the only method for 53% ($n = 31$) of MMU births, 42% ($n = 16$) of home-births and four host unit births. Pethidine was only used by four of the 59 MMU women, one of the 38 home-birth women and three of the 12 host unit women. Eight women at the MMU used the pool for pain relief but this was not available for the other two groups of women. These questionnaire responses were comparable to the data extracted from all of the available MMU maternity records ($n = 91$). Further scrutiny of the maternity records found that women giving birth at the MMU or at home were more likely to have an intact perineum ($n = 35$, 60% and $n = 39$, 64%, respectively) than the host unit group ($n = 3$, 25%). The small sample size from the host unit made the application of statistical tests of significance inappropriate.

Satisfaction with care

In response to a Yes/No question regarding satisfaction with care, the majority of women from all three groups who returned questionnaires were satisfied with all aspects of their care (see Table 1.1.3).

Women interviewed who had delivered at the MMU were very pleased that they had had the opportunity to have their baby there and were very satisfied with their care. In particular they liked the one-to-one care that the midwives provided during the birthing process and the homely, relaxed atmosphere of the MMU. The opportunity of giving birth at the MMU allowed greater choice for some women and removed anxiety:

... at home (in labour) I was a bit scared ... the funny thing was once I got under the roof, once I knew I was there (the MMU) I lost the fear ... I can't even explain it as there's nothing there ... except the midwives ... I have got so much faith in them ... that once I knew they were about I just, that's it I wasn't frightened any more ... (MMU 1)

The majority of the women appeared to have been satisfied with their choice of birth place (MMU: $n = 39$, 66.1%; home-birth: $n = 32$, 84.3%; host: $n = 7$, 58%). However, concerns were expressed by a few women regarding certain aspects of their care. For example, a woman booked for MMU birth would have preferred to have seen the consultant during the pregnancy:

I only saw the consultant once during pregnancy at eight weeks due to shortage of facilities and staffing at the hospital (MMU) ... this caused me some anxiety during my last weeks of pregnancy as I knew I had 25 miles each way to reach a fully staffed hospital if I had problems. (MMU 2)

When women were asked if they would recommend their place of birth to a friend, a high percentage of women said 'yes' (MMU: $n = 56$, 95%; home-birth: $n = 37$, 97%; host: $n = 9$, 75%). Some women expressed mixed feelings about this aspect, as illustrated in the following quote:

the care I received from the midwives was really good ... but if there had been better facilities (more effective pain relief) I may have possibly had an easier time. (MMU 7)

Reasons given for not recommending the MMU had more to do with the anger that the consultant unit had closed than dissatisfaction with the MMU:

I don't think the service (maternity services provided by this Health Authority) is up to standard for the area which it covers and the tax I pay for such amenities. (MMU 5)

I feel that it is unsafe, because if you or the baby was to suffer difficulties during or after birth there is no adequate facilities, so therefore you would have to endure a very distressful journey to the host unit. (MMU 6)

Additional comments on areas of satisfaction/ dissatisfaction with the new services included:

- the midwives were very friendly and professional ($n = 24$, 39%)
- the obstetric and paediatric services should be reinstated in the town ($n = 20$, 33%)
- all women should be offered the option of 'giving birth' at the MMU ($n = 9$, 15%)
- the choice should be made by the women and not by those caring for them as they have to live with the consequences ($n = 3$, 5%).

This last point was well illustrated by one of the women interviewed:

I think they should give the woman the choice; like you say the choice is yours, if you know that there is no consultant there and no pain relief, big pain relief, and you choose to go there (the MMU) and you end up in an ambulance going to XXXX on a blue light then its all your own fault ... you could sign a form ... if anything goes wrong then the women take it on themselves. (MMU 5)

Table 1.1.3 Level of satisfaction with aspects of care (% rounded up)

	MMU ($n = 59$)		Home births ($n = 38$)		Host unit ($n = 12$)	
	n	%	n	%	n	%
Satisfied with care in pregnancy						
Yes	56	95	36	95	12	100
No	2	3	2	5	0	0
Missing	1	2	0	0	0	0
Satisfied with care in labour						
Yes	57	97	36	95	11	92
No	2	3	1	3	1	8
Missing	0	0	1	3	0	0
Satisfied with care after birth						
Yes	59	100	37	97	11	92
No	0	0	1	3	1	8

The issue of transfer

The transfer group was treated separately as the women originated from both MMU and home-birth groups. On analysing the questionnaires from the transfer group it was found that nine women were assessed at home by an MMU midwife and the tenth woman was transferred for induction of labour, postdates. Five of these women were subsequently admitted to the MMU before being transferred to the host unit. None of them were transferred back to the MMU postnatally. Case records were not available for this group to verify the following reasons given by the women for their transfer:

- required assisted delivery ($n = 4$)
- retained placenta ($n = 3$)
- excess blood loss after delivery ($n = 1$).

Four women reported that their family and friends found it difficult to travel to the host unit to visit during their stay.

The transfer group of women were not as satisfied even though there had been a safe outcome for them and their babies. The following comments illustrate these feelings:

We waited 20 minutes for an ambulance when the birth started to go wrong. (T2)

It was very traumatic. I was trying to push my baby out all the way, whilst trying to hold onto the stretcher and the midwife. I thought I was going to die along with my baby. (T1)

Although one woman said the midwives were great, she still felt insecure having so far to travel by ambulance. Women from the transfer group were also asked whether they would recommend the MMU as a place of birth and they were divided in their responses, with five being negative. Various reasons were given:

- lack of 'life-saving equipment' (women's comments as they were aware that no doctors were on the premises)
- distance to travel to host unit
- the uncertainty of things going wrong
- a feeling of insecurity.

The majority of women from the transfer group ($n = 8$) would like to see obstetric, consultant-led services return to the town so that any complications could be dealt with in the same location as the MMU.

Discussion

The closure of small community-based hospitals in rural areas, or the maternity component of them, can create difficulties in providing an integrated maternity service for women in rural communities. This has not been the case in the services evaluated by this study. The service

integration was improved and women overall were satisfied with the care they received.

For women at low obstetric risk a local birth centre reduced anxiety in relation to not getting to 'hospital' in time and avoided unnecessary time in hospital because of 'false alarms'. Being able to birth in a local setting reduced travel time and costs for partner, friends and relatives. For women in the high-risk group, and those changing category from low to high risk, the advantages were not so great as they had further to travel for intrapartum care. The issue around risk found in this study mirrors the findings of Wilson (1996) and Campbell (1999) in that the application of risk categories may cause inequity.

The homely atmosphere of the MMU and the success in achieving one-to-one care in labour enabled women to feel more relaxed, confident in their carers, less likely to need as much pain relief and less likely to sustain perineal trauma. These findings concur with those of other researchers (Bramadat & Driedger, 1993; Garcia, 1995; Saunders et al., 2000).

However, the issue of not having consultant-led obstetric and paediatric services at the site still caused concern for many women. They felt that they were disadvantaged by not having everything at hand as they did when the obstetric unit was there. The concern over transfer was similar to that of the Edgware Birth Centre evaluation (Saunders et al., 2000).

The importance of continuity of carer, as described in *Changing Childbirth* (DoH, 1993) did not appear to be as much of an issue for women in this study. The fact that women felt supported and in control of their experiences was more important to them than continuity. A known team of midwives in the town reassured women and made it less important to have their 'own' midwife for the birth. The women felt it was important that the team knew about them and were all nice, confident and professional.

Women were aware that the number of home-births had risen dramatically following the closure of the consultant-led service. This was in part due to restrictions of the catchment area and the exclusion of primigravida from MMU birth. While guidelines are needed when establishing these units, the application of restrictive inclusion and exclusion criteria can force women to sometimes make less appropriate birth choices. These findings reiterate those of Wilson (1996) and Campbell (1999) in the credibility of using risk categories for women.

Conclusions

Overall, the women in the town appreciated the establishment of the MMU and the professionalism and support of the midwives providing the care. However, a percentage of those women would prefer to see a consultant-led maternity hospital back in the town, with the MMU running alongside it. This would reduce the anxiety caused by transfer over a considerable distance for women who develop complications. It is evident from the comments made by women in this study that they viewed the option of giving birth at the MMU as being very different to giving birth at home, even though they knew there were no extra facilities available at the MMU over home. The woman's perception of being in a separate environment other than home appeared to allay anxiety and fear.

It is clear from the findings of this study that the removal of the obstetric, consultant-led services in the town has not provided the type of service that women want and believe they should be allowed access to. However, the establishment of the MMU as an added choice rather than a replacement of the consultant-led service has been important for some women and has improved the maternity services for them. The women surveyed would like changes to the admission criteria so that it is more inclusive than exclusive.

REFERENCES

Audit Commission Report. 1997. First Class Delivery: Improving Maternity Services in England and Wales. Audit Commission, London

Bramadat D, Driedger M. 1993. Satisfaction with childbirth: theories and methods of measurement. Birth, 20: 22–29

Campbell R. 1999. Review and assessment of selection criteria used when booking pregnant women at different places of birth. British Journal of Obstetrics and Gynaecology, 106: 550–556

Clow SE, Christie K. 2002. Birthing a birthing unit. Abstract 163, ICM 26th Triennial Congress Programme, Vienna

Creasy J. 1997. Women's experiences of transfer from community-based to consultant-based maternity care. Midwifery, 13: 32–39

Cronbach LJ. 1982. Designing Evaluations of Educational and Social Programs. Jossey-Bass, San Francisco

Davies J, Hey E, Reid W et al. 1996. Prospective regional study of planned home-births. British Medical Journal, 313: 1302–1306

Denzin NK, Lincoln YS. 1994. Handbook of Qualitative Research. Sage, California

Department of Health (DoH). 1993. Changing Childbirth – Report of the Expert Committee. HMSO, London

Fraser DM. 1999. Women's perceptions of midwifery care: a longitudinal study to shape curriculum development. Birth, 26: 99–107

Garcia J. 1995. Continuity of carer in context: what matters to women? In: Page L (ed.), Effective Group Practice in Midwifery: Working with Women. Blackwell Science, Oxford

Gready M, Newburn M, Dodds R et al. 1995. Birth Choices: Women's Expectations and Experiences. National Childbirth Trust, London

Green JM, Coupland VA, Kitzenger JV. 1998. Great Expectations: A Prospective Study of Women's Expectations and Experiences of Childbirth. Books for Midwives Press, Hale

Hodnett ED. 2001. Home-like versus conventional institutional settings for birth. Cochrane Database of Systematic Reviews, Issue 2, 2002

House of Commons Health Committee. 1992. Second Report of Maternity Services, Vol. 1. HMSO, London

Hutton E. 1995. What women want from the maternity services. British Journal of Midwifery, 4: 576–580

Jacoby A, Cartwright A. 1990. Finding Out About the Views and Experiences of Maternity Service Users. Clarendon Press, Oxford

Lamping DL, Rowe P. 1996. Survey of Women's Experiences of Maternity Services (short form). London School of Hygiene and Tropical Medicine, London

Macfarlane A, Mugford M, Henderson J et al. 2000. Birth Counts Statistics of Pregnancy & Childbirth. The Stationery Office, London

McCourt C, Page L. 1996. Report on the Evaluation of One-to-one Midwifery. Thames Valley University, London

Murphy E, Dingwall R, Greatbatch D et al. 1998. Qualitative Research Methods in Health Technology Assessment: a Review of the Literature. National Coordinating Centre for Health Technology Assessment, Core Research. Available at http://www.soton.ac.uk/~hta

Saunders D, Boulton M, Chapple J et al. 2000. Evaluation of the Edgware Birth Centre. North Thames Perinatal Public Health, Harrow

Stufflebeam DL. 1991. Professional standards and ethics for evaluation. In: McLaughlin MW, Phillips DC (eds), Evaluation and Education: A Quarter Century. University of Chicago Press, Chicago

Walker J. 2000. Women's experiences of transfer from a midwife-led unit to a consultant-led maternity unit in the UK during late pregnancy and labor. Journal of Midwifery and Women's Health, 45(2): 161–168

Wilson J. 1996. Antenatal risk assessment. In: Alexander J, Levy V, Roch S (eds), Midwifery Practice: Core Topics 1. Macmillan, Basingstoke

Zadoroznyj M. 2000. Midwife-led maternity services and consumer "choice" in an Australian metropolitan region. Midwifery, 16(3): 177–185. Doi.10.1054/midw.1999.0207

Midwifery 2003; 19(2): 106–112

Culture, control and the birth environment

Mary Newburn

In 2003, the House of Commons Health Select Committee conducted an inquiry into its maternity services. This was last done in 1991, when a landmark report turned around the trend of government and parliamentary reports by including a sociological perspective. The Winterton Report suggested that there was such a thing as a medical model of care, and questioned whether this was clinically beneficial and what women wanted (House of Commons Health Committee, 1992). This report led the Government of the day to set up the Expert Maternity Group, and *Changing Childbirth* became official policy in 1993, emphasising the importance of women having choice, control and continuity of care and carer (Department of Health, 1993a, b).

The cornerstone of these reports was that the interests of women should be at the centre of how the maternity services are planned and how care is given to individual women and families. There seemed to be a widespread belief, spanning political parties, that if women had one-to-one care from a known midwife or other health care professionals and the opportunity to make informed choices, this would change the pattern of provision. More women would have home births, have access to a birth pool in labour, and be able to avoid medical interventions that they found intrusive.

Have things improved?

In the 12 years since the last Health Select Committee inquiry, and in the decade since *Changing Childbirth* was published, there have been many changes. It is difficult to assess the range and extent of these as evidence is patchy and incomplete. However, we do have some indicators.

Home births

The proportion of home births seems to have doubled overall and, in some areas of England, to have increased to around one in 10 of all births (National Childbirth Trust, 2000; Birth Statistics, 2003b). Heads of midwifery in Wales have set themselves a target of increasing the rate for the whole country to 10% over 10 years (Welsh Assembly Government, 2002).

However, across England as a whole, the home birth rate is still only around 2% (Department of Health, 2003), and even lower rates in Scotland suggest that in many areas arranging a home birth is as difficult as it ever was (Scottish Executive, 2001).

The latest Health Select Committee Report emphasises that women are still not being informed about home birth or offered a full range of birth choices, despite Department of Health assurances two years ago that the Government intended to make home births more widely available (House of Commons Health Committee, 2003a).

Use of birth pools

It is very difficult to get a clear picture of the proportion of women who have access to a birth pool in labour as there are no official figures. However, there has been a slow but steady growth in the number of midwife-led units and birth centres specialising explicitly in supporting birth as a physiological process (Saunders et al., 2000; Newburn & Singh, 2003). In these units, access to a birth pool and use of water for pain relief has come to be expected and arranged as normal day-to-day practice. The Department of Health is now funding research on ways of increasing 'out-of-hospital' births in the areas of Southampton and Portsmouth, where there are several small units with birth pools.

Some positive developments...

While there is therefore some evidence of developments outside the medical model, on the whole it is not yet the case that women manage to avoid interventions that they find intrusive. There have been some positive developments. For example, the National Sentinel Caesarean Section Audit and the associated surveys of obstetricians and women have demonstrated that there is widespread support for the belief that birth is a normal process that should not be interfered with unless there is good reason (Thomas et al., 2001).

Following publication of NICE guidelines, there are many anecdotal reports of a reduction in the use of admission traces for healthy women with a normal pregnancy giving birth in hospital (National Institute for Clinical Excellence, 2001). Furthermore, joint initiatives involving the Royal College of Midwives, the Royal College of Obstetrics and Gynaecologists, the National Childbirth Trust (NCT), and other professional and voluntary organisations have highlighted the obstacles to physiological birth (National Childbirth Trust et al., 2000; Tyler, 2001; Royal College of Obstetricians et al., 2001, 2002). They have suggested actions to reduce interventions and facilitate normality, with enthusiastic participation by clinical managers and practising midwives.

Perhaps the pace of positive change is quickening. In the last year or so, a normal birth care pathway has been developed for Wales, and early reports suggest that this is having a positive measurable impact on birth outcomes.

... But interventions still increasing

Despite this, however, there is no escaping the stark truth that since the last Health Select Committee inquiry the caesarean section rate has doubled (Department of Health, 2003; House of Commons Health Committee, 2003b). This is the single most telling indicator of the state of maternity care in the UK. In addition, routine induction for post-term pregnancy seems to be increasing since publication of RCOG/NICE guidelines (Royal College of Obstetricians and Gynaecologists Clinical Effectiveness Support Unit, 2001). Epidural use has increased, while the number of normal births with a spontaneous onset, progress and birth has diminished (Birth Choice UK, 2003).

Sadly, many of the conclusions of the 1992 report are just as relevant today as they were then.

The latest Commons report

The Health Select Committee report refers to Jo Green's study on women's attitudes to pain in labour (House of Commons Health Committee, 2003a). Since her earlier survey, *Great Expectations*, was published, the number of pregnant women who are very worried about labour pain had grown from 16% to 26% (Green et al., 1998). It is

not clear why that might be; perhaps it is a contributory cause or one of the effects of the increasing use of technology to start, monitor, augment and birth babies. This raises questions about the birth culture within the maternity services and across the UK in general. What factors are influencing attitudes and practices? What do pregnant women and their partners believe and aspire to? How are health care professionals behaving and how has this changed?

A vital qualitative study on attitudes to childbirth and caesarean sections is due to be published by Jane Weaver and colleagues in Cambridge. In the meantime, evidence from Canada suggests that the culture within provider units is highly influential. A study by Ellen Hodnett of units with a lower caesarean section rate found that they shared particular characteristics, including close teamworking and mutual respect, a belief that birth is primarily a physiological process and a pride in a low caesarean section rate (Biringer et al., 2000). Hodnett, having recently carried out a randomised controlled trial of continuous support during labour in highly medicalised settings, has concluded that the context of care, including the usual beliefs and practices in maternity units, can be more influential than a single social intervention intended to support physiological birth, despite this being effective in less medicalised environments (Hodnett et al., 2003). This confirms an observation made by Johanson and colleagues (2002).

The NCT 'Better Birth Environment' Survey

In 2002, a group at the NCT used a strategic planning tool to tease out obstacles that prevent women in the UK from having straightforward vaginal births. We identified many factors, including education of children, prospective parents and health professionals; cultural factors, such as the changing roles of women; the growth in use and reliance on complex technology; an increase in litigious behaviour; and the birth environment in hospital. We then considered the kinds of changes that might be necessary to overcome these barriers.

As the potential agenda was so vast, a manageable place to start was identified. We set out to raise awareness of the physical environment, both in hospital and other places of birth, from a woman's perspective.

We designed a survey (Newburn and Singh, forthcoming) with the purpose of finding out:

- what women considered important in terms of the physical environment and use of space; and
- to what extent women had a sense of control over their immediate environment during labour.

At the same time, we invited women to nominate their local unit if, on the basis of their experience, they felt it was eligible for an award for providing a good environment in which to give birth.

Probably the most important factor of all affecting women's experience of labour is the interaction that they have with the people around them. As there have already been studies on patterns of midwifery care and support but little on the physical environment and the contribution it can make to an easier or more difficult birth, we concentrated on the availability of facilities and opportunities for control of the birth environment.

Full details of the methodology and results are available to heads of midwifery from the NCT Policy Research Department in a toolkit, together with the opportunity to use the questionnaire locally to assess women's experiences and views (priced at £50 – see Box 1.2.1).

The remainder of this article highlights some of the key findings, particularly in relation to aspects of care highlighted by the Select Committee: place of birth, access to a birth pool and rates of intervention.

Methodology

Altogether, 40,000 questionnaires were distributed via *New Generation* and *Practical Parenting* magazines, and an NCT online version was also available. Women were eligible if they had given birth since 1998 and experienced labour. Almost 2000 valid responses ($n = 1944$) were returned from all parts of the UK by the deadline.

Eighty-five per cent of women had had a vaginal birth and 15% an emergency caesarean section. Women were asked to indicate whether they had had an emergency caesarean section as this is a major intervention, with significant consequences for women's health as well as additional financial costs to the health service. Women were not asked for any further specific details about their labour or clinical care.

Altogether, 12% of women had had a home birth, 25% used a midwife-led unit and 61% gave birth in a conventional hospital unit jointly run by midwives and obstetricians. Of those using midwife-led units, 2% of the total said that the unit was freestanding and 23% said that it was on the same site as a hospital. A small number were unsure how to describe the place where they gave birth.

What do women find helpful?

Nearly all the women (94%) said that their surroundings could affect how they gave birth, with as many as half agreeing strongly that the physical environment can affect the extent to which birth is easy or difficult. Given their very clear views on this point, it seems likely that women may hold the key to increasing normal births through improving the environment.

Box 1.2.1 Creating a better birth environment toolkit

The toolkit is available from NCT Maternity Sales (0870 112 1120). Priced at £50, it includes content and guidelines, the full report, an audit checklist, CD, evaluation network certificate and straightforward birth information sheet. The report can also be purchased separately (£50) or with an hour-long consultation with Mary Newburn (£200).

We asked the women what physical aspects of the room in which they spent most of their labour were either helpful or unhelpful in helping them to achieve the kind of birth that they wanted. Many aspects were put forward as having made a difference and these are all published in the full report. Those referred to most frequently are listed below.

Helpful aspects

Aspects of the room that women found helpful for encouraging the type of birth they wanted included, starting with the factor mentioned most frequently:

- space for walking and moving around
- a birthing pool or a large bath
- en-suite toilet/bathroom
- a comfortable, adjustable bed
- low lights or adjustable lighting
- privacy and quiet.

Unhelpful aspects

Aspects of the room that women found unhelpful for encouraging the type of birth they wanted included, starting with the factor mentioned most frequently:

- a clinical 'hospital room' atmosphere
- a small room with little space to move around
- a hard, uncomfortable bed that was not adjustable or was incorrectly positioned
- lack of privacy, such as having the door open or being able to be heard by others
- toilet outside the room
- a room that was too hot, too cold or where it was not possible to control the temperature.

Place of birth

Women who gave birth at home or in a midwife-led unit were more likely than those in a conventional hospital unit to say that they had access to facilities and opportunities for control (see Table 1.2.1). The environment for women who gave birth at home included most of the features that the sample found helpful in labour.

Table 1.2.1 Experiences during last labour by place of birth

	Home birth	Freestanding midwife-led unit	Midwife-led unit alongside hospital	Hospital unit	All women
Clean room*	96	98	89	88	89
Not in sight of others	85	82	84	84	84
Able to walk around*	98	87	75	61	69
Able to stay in the same room*	96	91	78	73	76
Comfortable chair for partner*	87	67	62	57	61
Easy access to a toilet*	86	84	64	63	66
Control who came into room*	92	56	41	29	40
Beanbags, pillows and mats*	89	72	45	31	42
Unable to hear other women*	92	56	54	53	58
Could control brightness of light*	96	66	50	41	50
Easy access to snacks/drinks*	95	68	40	30	41
Room looked homely*	96	78	40	22	37
Able to control temperature*	94	44	28	25	35
Easy access to a bath*	94	73	66	50	60
Sure others could not hear me*	60	43	38	34	39
Access to pleasant place to walk*	93	60	32	21	34
Easy access to a shower*	89	69	56	46	54
Easy access to a birth pool*	48	76	56	39	46
Able to move the furniture to suit*	95	51	42	28	40
Nicely decorated room*	97	89	59	51	59
Clock easily in view	69	79	72	73	72
Comfortable bed*	87	84	73	62	68
Could see resuscitation equipment*	20	41	66	75	66

Note: The proportions above are women who agreed that they had access to the facilities listed. Chi-squared tests were applied and differences marked with an asterisk are statistically significant ($p < 0.05$). Factors are listed in order of importance to women.

Home births

Women who had had a home birth were overwhelmingly positive about their birth experience, as these quotes illustrate:

I had a home birth and, although I have nothing to compare the experience with, I felt relaxed and in control in my own environment, which in turn made labour easier to bear and ensured I had the experience I wanted. I know that in hospital I would have felt less at ease and been less likely to cope with the labour.

It was home – my private space. Other people there were visitors invited in, so I controlled the physical space. There was space for everything I needed without being cramped.

Midwife-led units

The facilities and opportunities for control in midwife-led units also tended to be high. In particular, there was greater access to a birth pool, which was seen as a real priority by many women:

Both my babies were water babies. I cannot stress enough how much I thought it helped me.

It was important to have a pool. I wanted a water birth but this was just not available or possible at my nearest hospital.

As with home births, there was usually a range of factors working together to enhance the woman's sense of feeling positive and able to cope:

The only way I managed to have such a positive birth experience was by being totally focused on what I was doing (i.e. managing pain through breathing, etc.). If anything distracts you (e.g. other external factors) this is less achievable. The room was large and spacious, so I was able to move about freely and change positions. There were various different seating, squatting and lying options available (e.g. beanbags, mats, chairs, tables and beds). There was calm music playing, calm colours and calm lighting. The midwives had a very personal, flexible approach – I led, the midwives followed.

There was an exercise ball which I found invaluable for support, plenty of floor space and mats to move around easily as I laboured on the floor. There was an en-suite toilet and shower which was great as I spent some time during second stage on the loo.

Hospital

Facilities in conventional hospital units, where most women give birth, were the most limited. In particular, there was often too little space to move around freely and seldom a pleasant place to walk. Women had significantly less control over who came into the room, the brightness of the light or the temperature, and few felt able to move the furniture around to suit their preferences:

I laboured all day in a room with three other women and had almost no privacy. The delivery room was too small to walk around, and claustrophobic with six doctors and midwives messing around. The toilet was shared with the next room and the baths and showers were down the corridor.

There were too many people walking in and out. The staff were unfriendly and I was given no control or choice. The room was not clean. I felt my birth room was too small and made me nervous because it was so full of people and equipment.

It would have been nice to walk around some gardens or even a quiet car park with a few flowers, but there was nowhere but the busy wards to walk. I felt in the way, but my room was so small, I could only do three paces back and forth.

Half as many women had access to a birth pool (39%) compared with those using a freestanding, midwife-led unit (76%).

In some cases facilities were designed with woman's needs in mind:

The environment makes you relax if it is right, stops you feeling relaxed if it is wrong. In the later stages I was in a room with a birthing pool, which was nice and dark.

However, there were too few birth pools to meet the demand from women, and sometimes rigid protocols limited their spontaneity and choices:

There is only one birthing pool in the hospital so it was a case of first come, first served. It was down to luck whether you got a water birth or not.

After being in the bath for 2+ hours I wanted to push. But the hospital has a policy of not allowing babies to be born in the bath so I had to get out and walk back to my room. This was awful, probably the worst part [of labour].

One woman commented that she would not have known what the options were locally and how her choice of place of birth might affect her labour had she not been part of the local NCT network:

For my first child in 2000, I was due to give birth in hospital A. I only found out through my NCT antenatal class that I could elect to go elsewhere. And after a visit to hospital A, which was clearly only geared up for lying on your back on a high bed, I decided to change to hospital B.

Access to facilities and labour outcome

Women reported that certain aspects of their environment made their labour easier or more difficult, and this was born out by the findings on access to facilities and feelings of control in relation to labour outcomes. Women who had emergency caesarean sections were significantly less likely than those having a vaginal birth to have had access to a good range of valued facilities. For example, three-quarters of the women who had a vaginal birth had been able to move around as much as they liked, compared with less than half of those who had an emergency caesarean (74% versus 45%). And twice as many women who had a vaginal birth (39% versus 20%) said that they had a room that looked homely. (Full details are included in the main report.)

There is widespread concern about the current level of caesarean section rates and a consensus that many factors have contributed to the rise (Thomas et al., 2001; House of Commons Health Committee, 2003a). While it may be both expensive and time-consuming to tackle some of these factors, such as increasing recruitment and retention of midwives or reducing litigation, the findings from this survey indicate that significant improvements could be made to birth rooms, and women's control over their birth environment, fairly easily. A checklist of recommendations for change is included in the NCT Better Birth Environment Toolkit.

Summary and conclusions

These findings illustrate that women's needs are not being adequately met in many hospital birth units. Women, particularly those expecting their first baby, often know little about how the culture of hospitals varies, or the helpfulness of facilities and opportunities for control and one-to-one support that are more readily available at home or in a midwife-led unit. Nor do they know how much their opportunities for comfort and control may be compromised in a conventional hospital setting. If they are feeling anxious about whether they will be able to cope with the pain of labour and whether their baby will be born safely, it is perhaps not surprising that a significant proportion feel it is important to have access to an epidural service and a special care baby unit (House of Commons Health Committee, 2003a).

However, these facilities are not in themselves more likely to make labour straightforward and manageable. Midwives and organisations such as the NCT have a key role to play in sharing knowledge about what women actually find useful – or disruptive and unhelpful – during labour, so that all pregnant women can make choices that are informed by the full range of relevant information.

The recommendations from the early 1990s, that women should have care from a known midwife, has not been realised consistently, although in environments that are highly medicalised neither knowing your midwife nor one-to-one support seem sufficient to affect labour outcomes substantially (Johanson et al., 2002). Where there is strong midwifery leadership, a clear philosophy of normality and one-to-one support, outcomes are different (Biringer et al., 2000).

Women appear to be offered more choices than a decade ago, but the range of options available still tends to be dominated by a medical model of care. Women still do not receive adequate information on the significance of alternatives as good-quality, evidence-based information is not consistently available, nor are they given the support to choose freely from the full range of options (Singh &

Newburn, 2000). However, evidence-based information leaflets alone are known to be inadequate to overcome a range of cultural barriers (O'Cathain et al., 2002; Stapleton et al., 2002).

A small and growing proportion of women are having home births and have access to a midwife-led unit. Use of a birthpool in labour has become more accepted in all birth settings, although access to suitable facilities and protocols for use in hospital units are sometimes restrictive. Further change is needed to provide care during labour as part of a midwifery model, so that the kinds of medical interventions women find intrusive can be limited as far as possible without compromising safety.

REFERENCES

Biringer A, Davies B, Nimrod C et al. 2000. Attaining and Maintaining Best Practice in the Use of Cesarean Sections: An Analysis of Four Ontario Hospitals. Report of the Cesarean Section Working Party of the Ontario Women's Health Council. Ontario Women's Health Council

Birth Choice UK. 2003. Available from: http://www.birthchoiceUK.com

Birth Statistics. 2003. Office of National Statistics, London

Department of Health. 1993a. Changing Childbirth: Part 1. Report of the Expert Maternity Group. HMSO, London

Department of Health. 1993b. Changing Childbirth: Part 2. Survey of Good Communication Practice in Maternity Services. HMSO, London

Department of Health. 2003. NHS Maternity Statistics, England: 2001–02. Office of National Statistics, London

Green JM, Coupland VA, Kitzinger JV. 1998. Great Expectations: A Prospective Study of Women's Expectations and Experiences of Childbirth. Books for Midwives, Hale

Hodnett ED, Gates S, Hofmeyr GJ, Sakala C. 2003. Continuous support for women during childbirth (Cochrane Review). The Cochrane Library, 3. Update Software, Oxford. Available from: http://www.update-software.com/clibng/cliblogon.htm

House of Commons Health Committee. 1992. Maternity Services: Health Committee, Second Report (chairman Nicholas Winterton), Vol. 1. Report together with appendices and the proceedings of the committee. HMSO, London

House of Commons Health Committee. 2003a. Choice in Maternity Services. Ninth Report of Session 2002–03, Vol. I. Report and formal minutes. Available from: http://www.parliament.the-stationery-office.co.uk/pa/cm200203/cmselect/cmhealth/796/796.pdf

House of Commons Health Committee. 2003b. Provision of Maternity Services. Fourth Report of Session 2002–03, Vol. I. Report, together with formal minutes. Available from: http://www.parliament.the-stationery-office.co.uk/pa/cm200203/cmselect/cmhealth/464/46402.htm

Johanson R, Newburn M, Macfarlane A. 2002. Has the medicalisation of childbirth gone too far? BMJ, 324(7342): 892–895

National Childbirth Trust. 2001. Home Birth in the United Kingdom. National Childbirth Trust, London

National Childbirth Trust, Royal College of Midwives, and Royal College of Obstetricians and Gynaecologists. 2000. The Rising Caesarean Section Rate – A Public Health Issue. Report of a national conference organised by the National Childbirth Trust, the Royal College of Midwives, and the Royal College of Obstetricians and Gynaecologists, London, 23 November 1999. Profile Productions, London

National Institute for Clinical Excellence. 2001. The Use of Electronic Fetal Monitoring: The Use and Interpretation of Cardiotocography in Intrapartum Fetal Surveillance. Inherited Clinical Guideline C. National Institute for Clinical Excellence, London

Newburn M, Singh D. 2003. Reconfiguring Maternity Services: Views of User Representatives. National Childbirth Trust, London

Newburn M, Singh D. Forthcoming. Creating a better birth environment – women's views about the design and facilities in maternity units: a national survey. In: Creating A Better Birth Environment – An Audit Toolkit. National Childbirth Trust, London

O'Cathain A, Walters SJ, Nicholl JP et al. 2002. Use of evidence-based leaflets to promote informed choice in maternity care: randomised controlled trial in everyday practice. BMJ, 324(7338): 643–646

Royal College of Obstetricians and Gynaecologists Clinical Effectiveness Support Unit. 2001. Induction of Labour: Evidence-Based Clinical Guideline Number 9. Royal College of Obstetricians and Gynaecologists, London

Royal College of Obstetricians and Gynaecologists, Royal College of Midwives and National Childbirth Trust. 2001. The Rising Caesarean Section Rate – Causes and Effects for Public Health. Conference report of a one-day national conference organised by Royal College of Obstetricians and Gynaecologists, Royal College of Midwives and National Childbirth Trust, London, 7 November 2000. National Childbirth Trust, London

Royal College of Obstetricians and Gynaecologists, Royal College of Midwives and National Childbirth Trust. 2002. The Rising Caesarean Section Rate – From Audit to Action, Report of a joint conference organised by the Royal College of Obstetricians and Gynaecologists, Royal College of Midwives and National Childbirth Trust, London, 31 January 2002. National Childbirth Trust, London

Saunders D, Boulton M, Chapple J et al. 2000. Evaluation of the Edgware Birth Centre. Barnet Health Authority, Edgware

Scottish Executive. 2001. A Framework for Maternity Services in Scotland. Scottish Executive, Edinburgh

Singh D, Newburn M. 2000. Access to Maternity Information and Support: The Experiences and Needs of Women Before and After Giving Birth. National Childbirth Trust, London

Stapleton H, Kirkham M, Thomas G. 2002. Qualitative study of evidence-based leaflets in maternity care. BMJ, 324(7338): 639–643

Thomas J, Paranjothy S, Royal College of Obstetricians and Gynaecologists Clinical Effectiveness Support Unit. 2001. National Sentinel Caesarean Section Audit Report. RCOG Press, London

Welsh Assembly Government. 2002. Realising the Potential. A Strategic Framework for Nursing, Midwifery and Health Visiting in Wales into the 21st Century. Briefing paper 4, Delivering the future in Wales. A framework for realising the potential of midwives in Wales. Welsh Assembly Government, Cardiff

The Practising Midwife 2003; 6(8): 20–25

Drawing the line: caesarean sections on demand

Natasha Carr

It is acknowledged that there are many compounding influences on caesarean section rates that go beyond the clinical practice of obstetrics and midwifery. Medical, legal, psychological, social and financial considerations have all made contributions (FIGO, 1999), as have organisational factors, provision of one-to-one support in labour, women's choices in childbirth (Sakala, 1993) and obstetricians' characteristics (Thomas & Paranjothy, 2001).

However, performing a caesarean section without clinical indication has traditionally been considered inappropriate and not part of the accepted standard of medical practice (Hall, 1987). Reasons why it has been considered inappropriate may include the lack of necessity, the lack of legal force, the cost or resource implications, not being in line with beneficence and non-maleficence and the impingement on individual autonomy – the autonomy of both women and health care professionals.

The legal argument presented in this article forms a small part of this much larger, complex ethical and legal debate on why we should not make provisions for women to have caesarean sections on demand.

The legal perspective

In the context of the NHS, maternity care is generally accessible and free to all women. This right of access to maternity care does not, however, mean that just any health care or specific care must be provided (National Health Service Act, 1977). Access to maternity care is more likely to mean the conferring of a right to obtain only specified services to which every woman entitled has a valid claim.

In the context of women demanding to have caesareans in the absence of clinical need, it can be argued that the NHS does not have to provide a 'caesarean-on-demand service' as part of these specified services.

What the law says

In legal terms, it has been established repeatedly that non-provision of services does not give rise to an action. We are working in a climate where, as professionals, we often fear the consequences if we do, or do not do, something. However, case law has established that the government does not have a duty to provide everything that is asked for (R v Secretary of State for Social Services, ex parte Hincks 1980, 93). Furthermore, the notable case of R v Cambridge Health Authority, ex parte B (A minor) 1995 has also considered the effective use of limited resources and the needs of others. In fact, in this case it was acknowledged that difficult judgements have to be made to the greater advantage of the maximum number of patients.

This has since withstood judicial review. A legal case specifically concerning the provision of a caesarean section on demand has not been tested in the courts; however, similar reasoning could be used. Women should not be able to exercise the choice to demand a caesarean section without clinical need, which could have negative consequences for many other pregnant women by diverting resources from where they are truly needed, such as for labouring women or for those with a genuine need for a caesarean section (Table 1.3.1). It may be argued that there would be no fairness in this and the courts are unlikely to back women who claim caesareans on demand.

Table 1.3.1 Traditional reasons for a caesarean section (Telfer, 1997)

Breech presentation
Malposition of the fetus
Emergency – for example, cord prolapse, antepartum haemorrhage
Fetal abnormality
Fetal distress
Cephalopelvic disproportion
Maternal conditions – for example, placenta praevia, eclampsia, delay in labour progress

A counter argument can be formed with regard to psychological distress and demanding a caesarean section. The intention is, however, not for a carte blanche approach to denying all women caesarean sections; indeed, recognition of psychological distress as a reason for caesarean section may be valid. One needs to take a holistic interpretation of clinical or health need as it is often not just physical need, as Telfer (1997) lists among reasons for a caesarean.

As long as a health authority 'asked the appropriate questions prior to its deciding not to fund a range of services or a particular treatment for a particular patient' (Kennedy & Grubb, 1998, p. 479), then its decision was justifiable. It is difficult to see, therefore, how an individual who was not provided with a caesarean on demand could take action against a trust.

Standards of care

It can be argued that the legal standard of care would not oblige a clinician to carry out a caesarean section on demand either. The standard of care is determined by the Bolam test, which originates from the case of Bolam v Friern Hospital Management Committee ([1957] 121):

When you get a situation which involves the use of some special skill or competence, then the test as to whether there has been negligence or not is … the standard of the ordinary skilled man exercising and professing to have that special skill.

If a practitioner fails to measure up to this principle test, the practitioner is negligent and is so adjudged. However, even if the standard of care has been breached (i.e. a negligent act), there can be no action in negligence unless there is some harm caused or loss experienced as a result of the negligent act.

Failing to provide health care in an appropriate manner can have disastrous consequences clinically, legally and ethically. It can be argued that harm can clearly be foreseen with certain types of care (see Table 1.3.2 for examples). Caesarean section in the absence of clinical need could indeed be regarded as inappropriate care. Subsequent judgements since Bolam have stated that the standard of care must have a logical basis that would involve the weighing of risks against benefits and then reaching a defensible conclusion (Bolitho v City and Hackney HA [1997] 4 All ER 771). If the body of professional opinion could not withstand logical analysis, one could hold it as not reasonable or responsible.

It was also further emphasised in this case that it was necessary to judge whether the clinical practice under consideration puts the patient at unnecessary risk. One could argue that unnecessary surgery does just that; it places both the mother and baby at risk. And to midwives who work 'with women' – being the guardians of normality – it certainly has no logical basis.

Table 1.3.2 Caesarean section risks: examples

Emergency obstetric hysterectomy (Gould, 1999)
Fetal laceration injury of caesarean delivery (Smith et al., 1997)
Long-term effects of caesarean section: ectopic pregnancies and placental problems (Hemminki & Merilainen, 1996)
Postoperative morbidity following caesarean section (Hillan, 1995)
Association between method of delivery and maternal rehospitalization (Lyndon-Rochell, 2000)

Guidelines may also be considered. The courts may refer to any guidelines from professional bodies in determining whether a practice is defensible or not. FIGO (1999, p. 321) has provided a position statement specifically regarding caesarean delivery for non-medical reasons. It explicitly states that:

Physicians have a professional duty to do nothing that may harm their patients. They also have an ethical duty to society to allocate health care resources wisely to procedures and treatments for which there is clear evidence of a net benefit to health. Physicians are not obligated to perform an intervention for which there is no medical advantage.

Professional expertise must include moral consideration of their actions and one awaits the NICE guidelines on caesarean section with anticipation.

Conclusion

It can be demonstrated and argued in law that there is no obligation on behalf of the government, the NHS or the clinician to provide specific services such as caesarean sections on demand for non-medical reasons. This may be a provocative position to take, but it appears to be the legal position. Arguments levelled at appealing that a legal right to care exists have no legal foundation and, in the past, the courts appeared reluctant to interfere with what seems to be ethical decision-making at the ground level. The courts will not force doctors, midwives or trusts to treat patients in a manner contrary to their clinical judgement or professional duty.

It truly is an ethical decision for the practitioner responsible for the allocation and use of resources to ask appropriate questions of an ethical nature. If we do, we will surely have to question whether women requesting caesarean sections without health or medical need ought to have their demands entertained. Certainly, taking a legal perspective, it is believed that this cannot be the case. The line must be drawn at demonstrating professional, ethical and legally sound practice – and not along the bikini line.

REFERENCES

7FIGO. 1999. FIGO Committee Report. FIGO committee for the ethical aspects of human reproduction and women's health. International Journal of Gynecology and Obstetrics, 64: 317–322

Gould D. 1999. Emergency obstetric hysterectomy – an increasing incidence. Journal of Obstetrics and Gynaecology, 19: 580–583

Hall M. 1987. When a woman asks for a caesarean section. British Medical Journal, 294: 201–202

Hemminki E, Merilainen J. 1996. Long-term effects of caesarean section: ectopic pregnancies and placental problems. American Journal of Obstetrics and Gynecology, 174: 1569–1574

Hillan E. 1995. Postoperative morbidity following caesarean section. Journal of Advanced Nursing, 22(6): 800–806

Kennedy I, Grubb A. 1998. Principles of Medical Law. Oxford University Press, Oxford

Lyndon-Rochell M. 2000. Association between method of delivery and maternal rehospitalization. Journal of the American Medical Association, 283: 2411–2416

Sakala C. 1993. Medically unnecessary caesarean births: introduction to a symposium. Soc Sci Med, 37: 1177–1198

Smith W, Hernandez C, Wax JR. 1997. Fetal laceration injury of cesarean delivery. Obstetrics and Gynecology, 90: 344–346

Telfer FM. 1997. Anaesthesia and operative procedures in obstetrics. In: Sweet BR (ed.), Mayes' Midwifery: A Textbook for Midwives. Bailliere Tindall, London

Thomas J, Paranjothy S. 2001. The National Sentinel Caesarean Section Audit Report. Royal College of Obstetricians and Gynaecologists Press, London

List of cases

Bolam v Friern Hospital Management Committee [1957] 1 WLR 582

Bolitho v City and Hackney HA [1997] 4 All ER 771

R v Secretary of State for Social Services, ex parte Hincks [1980] 1 BMLR 93

R v Cambridge Health Authority, ex parte B (A minor) [1995] 6 MedLR 250

List of statutes

National Health Service Act 1977. HMSO, London

The Practising Midwife 2003; 6(9): 20–22

Searching for autonomy

Katherine Pollard

Objective: to gain an understanding of what midwives understand by the term 'autonomy', and to discover whether they consider themselves and their colleagues to be autonomous in practice.

Participants: a snowball sample of 27 midwives working in five National Health Service (NHS) trusts within the southwest of England, based both in hospitals and in the community.

Method: within a qualitative research design, semi-structured interviews with participants were tape-recorded and transcribed verbatim and analysed using thematic content analysis.

Findings: most participants did not fully understand the implications of professional autonomy, particularly in terms of interprofessional collaboration and control of their own practice. There were mixed views among respondents about whether they practised autonomously. Although good relationships with medical personnel were found to facilitate midwifery autonomy, the ongoing dominance of the medical profession was still perceived as a major barrier to autonomy. Many participants did not feel that their midwifery education had equipped them for professional autonomy, although midwives educated by the direct-entry route were perceived to be more capable of exercising autonomy in practice than were nurse-trained midwives. Some participants expressed doubts about the possibility of genuine midwifery autonomy within the present system, while others felt that many midwives do not support their own or other midwives' professional autonomy.

Implications for practice: midwives need to initiate major change at a collective level, or to consider the creation of obstetric nursing posts, both to afford women the choice of genuinely autonomous midwifery care and to alleviate the stresses of practising within a system that requires the accountability and responsibility of midwifery autonomy, yet neither recognises nor supports it.

Introduction

Autonomy is a concept central to the definition of a midwife (WHO, 1992). In the UK, midwives' legal responsibility for their practice rests on the assumption that they are autonomous practitioners (Dimond, 1994). Wagner (1997) asserts that autonomous midwifery is 'central to women's freedom to control their own health care' (p. 16). It is associated with favourable clinical outcomes and enhanced satisfaction for women (Hundley et al., 1994; Shields et al., 1998). Midwifery autonomy therefore affects the physical and emotional health of women and their families. It is difficult to define autonomy absolutely in the complex context in which midwives operate.

However, autonomy involves at least the exercise of choice, and the power to make and act upon decisions (Henry & Fryer, 1995). An autonomous profession must be self-governing and self-regulating (Fleming, 1998). Unfortunately, midwifery in the UK is not an autonomous profession; it has historically been, and still is, controlled by nursing and medical organisations, frameworks and priorities (Fleming, 1998; Jowitt, 2000). Midwifery education in the UK comprises an 18-month course for nurse candidates, or a three-year course for direct-entry candidates (introduced in the early 1990s). A few midwives practice independently, in both domiciliary and hospital settings. The vast majority are employed by National Health Service (NHS) Trusts, their salary and status linked to nurses' clinical grading. Rank-and-file midwives are usually graded E or F, senior midwives G (including many community midwives) and midwifery managers H. NHS Trusts administer maternity units (mostly situated within larger hospitals). Most maternity units are directed by obstetricians, although a few midwife-led units cater for women with uncomplicated pregnancies. NHS midwives practise in maternity units, or in the community linked to a particular unit, or increasingly, work in both settings. Recent changes in care provision have introduced localised Primary Care Trusts (PCTs), which purchase services for their clients from the NHS Trusts. PCT management boards comprise general practitioners (GPs), other health professionals and lay representatives from the local community. Where there are a number of NHS Trusts in an area, PCTs can influence care provision, following the laws of supply and demand. Not all PCT boards have distinct midwifery representation; however, where they do, a midwifery perspective can theoretically influence care within local maternity units (Ollerhead, 1999). All NHS Trusts have a legal obligation to provide evidence-based care to service users (Parnham, 1999). These and other developments within the NHS have created potential opportunities for midwives to raise their professional profile and to become more autonomous (O'Loughlin, 2001; Sinclair, 2001). There has been no research focusing on midwifery autonomy in the UK; findings have come from studies exploring the midwife's role, and relationships with other health professionals and service users. These studies show that many midwives believe autonomy is not possible when practising with other professionals (McCrea & Crute, 1991; Sikorski et al., 1995; Pope et al., 1997; Meerabeau et al., 1999). Perceived barriers to midwifery autonomy include lack of recognition for the midwife's professional role and the dominance of the medical profession (Garcia & Garforth, 1991; McCrea & Crute, 1991; Meah et al., 1996; Hosein, 1998; Levy, 1999; Meerabeau et al., 1999). In this paper, the author describes a study exploring midwives' understanding of the term 'autonomy', and their perceptions of themselves and their colleagues as autonomous practitioners.

A concept analysis of autonomy

A concept analysis of autonomy was undertaken to clarify issues for exploration. Morse et al. (1996) define a concept as 'an abstract representation of a phenomenon' (p. 389), facilitating a cognitive grasp of complex behaviours and providing the means to refer to them, and assert that research design can be influenced by the level of maturity of the concept under study. Four criteria

for evaluation of concept maturity are postulated: clear definition, the identification of attributes or characteristics, the description and demonstration of relevant preconditions and outcomes, and the clear delineation of conceptual boundaries. Rodgers' (1989) evolutionary model of concept analysis was adopted for this study, because its flexible, non-isolationist view of concepts seemed appropriate for the complex context in which midwives operate. Following this model, a search on 'autonomy' was made on the CINAHL database from 1997 to 1999. An enormous range of material was found, so the search was narrowed by adding the keywords 'practice' and 'professional'; as there was still far too much material for analysis, these keywords were associated firstly with midwifery and then with mental health nursing, since this field appears to demand a particularly sophisticated understanding of autonomy from its practitioners. From the resulting literature, two random samples of 15 articles each were selected after stratification for time, from midwifery (Brauer-Rieke et al., 1997; Davis-Floyd, 1997; Fitzgerald & Wood, 1997; Fitzsimons, 1997; Garland & Jones, 1997; Germano & Bernstein, 1997; McKay, 1997; Barwise, 1998; Fleming, 1998; Hamilton, 1998; Rowan, 1998; Vann, 1998; Griffith et al., 1999; Rosser, 1999; Silverton, 1999) and from mental health nursing (Gibson, 1997; Godin & Scanlon, 1997; Howard & Greiner, 1997; Porter et al., 1997; Carnall, 1998; Dawkins, 1998; Gibb, 1998; Latvala et al., 1998; Olsson & Hallberg, 1998; Pang, 1998; Torn & McNichol, 1998; Wells et al., 1998; Hayter, 1999; Hobbs et al., 1999; Marland, 1999). Regular references to autonomy were also found in various fields of psychology. A convenience sample of 15 articles was drawn from psychology publications between 1980 and 2000 (Yalom, 1980; Smith, 1983; Wachtel, 1987; Warr, 1987; Schein, 1988; Argyle, 1989; Mullins, 1989; Atkinson et al., 1990; Rowan, 1993, 1997; Fontana, 1995; Fraser, 1995; Hixenbaugh & Warren, 1998; Rose, 1999; Stewart & Tilney, 2000). Etymologically, 'autonomy' comes from the Greek *autos* (self) and *nomos* (law) (Thompson, 1995), and is commonly defined as 'self-government' and 'self-regulation'. 'Independence' and 'freedom' are alternative definitions, although they can be viewed as related but distinct concepts, not sharing all the characteristics of 'autonomy'. In the literature, autonomy is considered to be a personal quality which enables individuals to express its associated characteristics; these are summarised in Box 1.4.1. Antecedents and consequences are those events or phenomena which commonly precede and follow its occurrence (Rodgers, 1989). The antecedents and consequences of autonomy found in the literature are summarised in Box 1.4.2. A key element of the evolutionary model of concept analysis is the identification of a model case demonstrating all the concept's attributes (Rodgers, 1989). Temple (1999) describes a case in which a newly qualified midwife agreed to attend independently a primiparous client labouring at home. The required antecedents were present: options existed and needed assessment (whether or not to assume professional responsibility for the client), and a decision was required. The midwife exercised her autonomy by choosing to attend the birth, having the professional capacity to do so. She took responsibility for her decision; her client and other professionals involved recognised her right to make this decision. She reported increased self-esteem and confidence after the exercise of her professional autonomy. References of a concept demonstrate the range of situations in which it can occur (Rodgers, 1989). The references of autonomy are very broad, including any situation in which individuals have the capacity to make and act on choices about themselves. Related concepts include 'freedom' and 'independence', but the former does not necessarily imply either responsibility or the capacity to make decisions, while characteristics of the latter may not include external validation. Since 'autonomy' can be distinguished from these related concepts, it has clearly delineated conceptual boundaries. The analysis demonstrated that 'autonomy' fulfils the criteria of a 'mature' concept (Morse et al., 1996). Conducting research about perceptions of autonomy was therefore meaningful, as there was sufficient clarity and consensus about its usage to allow realistic judgements to be made about its application in real-life settings.

Box 1.4.1 Associated characteristics of autonomy

Determining the sphere of activity under one's control

Having the right and the capacity to make and act upon choices and decisions in this sphere

Having this right acknowledged by others affected by or involved in these decisions

Taking responsibility for decisions made

Box 1.4.2 Antecedents and consequences of autonomy

Antecedents necessary for the exercise of autonomy:

A situation exists in which a course of action is required, and in which options are available

There is a need for the situation to be assessed

There is a need for a decision to be made and acted upon

Consequences of the exercise of autonomy:

Responsibility is taken for the decision made

The right to have made the decision is accepted as valid by others involved in the situation (even if disagreeing with the decision itself)

Personal esteem and confidence increase

Methods

The impetus for this study arose from the author's own experiences and observations in her professional practice. Her midwifery colleagues appeared to interpret the nature of professional autonomy inconsistently and, in some cases, to put themselves at professional risk by doing so. She consequently embarked on this study in order to add to the knowledge base concerning a concept that is highly significant for the profession. The study design incorporated a process typical of qualitative research, aiming both to 'see through the eyes' of the participants and to go below the surface (Bryman, 2001), to discover how midwives linked their practice and their understanding of autonomy. The author felt that conducting the concept analysis and consulting the available literature prior to fieldwork would help offset the disadvantages of her 'insider' perspective, by giving her a broader frame of reference with which to approach the topic. The data collection tool selected was in-depth semi-structured interviews, as this method would allow both a focus on the issues raised in the literature and the flexibility for participants' responses to reflect their lived reality (Rees, 1997; Bryman, 2001).

A conceptual framework

A conceptual framework for midwifery autonomy (see Figure 1.4.1) was developed from the results of the concept analysis and relevant research findings (McCrea & Crute, 1991; Hundley et al., 1994; Sikorski et al., 1995; Meah et al., 1996; Shields et al., 1998; Levy, 1999; Meerabeau et al., 1999). This provided a basis for developing an interview guide (see Appendix), the evolution of which continued throughout the period of data collection (Holloway & Wheeler, 1996).

Ethics

When this study commenced (1999), there was no obligation to gain formal ethical approval for research only involving NHS staff; the onus was on the researcher to ensure a sound ethical approach. This was achieved by adopting the principles advocated by Holloway and Wheeler (1996) and Rees (1997):

- the need to inform participants fully about the purpose and process of the study;
- the need to ensure that participation would not be detrimental to informants;
- the need to treat informants fairly.

Managers of five maternity units in the southwest of England were asked for permission to approach staff. Initial recruitment was made through the researcher's

Figure 1.4.1 A conceptual framework for midwifery autonomy

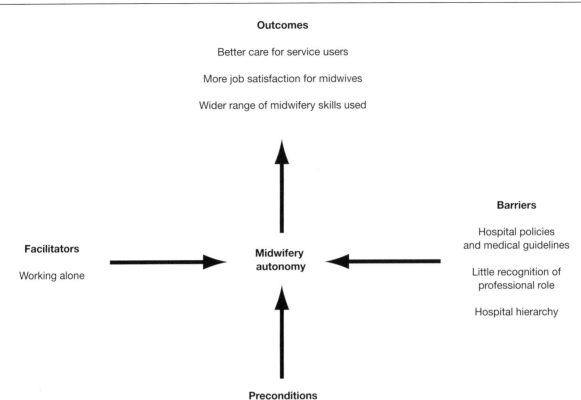

existing contacts, with care taken not to exert any undue pressure on individuals; this was followed by a snowball approach – that is, all initial and subsequent informants were asked to suggest other midwives who might participate in the study (Rees, 1997). If a midwife agreed in principle to participation, she was sent a letter outlining the research and explaining the interview process, including the fact that interviews would be taped. The letter stated that the researcher was a practising midwife, that participation was voluntary and that withdrawal was possible at any time. Anonymity was assured. The potential informant was then contacted by telephone and if she consented to participate, arrangements were made for interview. As each interview started, the researcher checked again that the informant gave consent to being tape recorded. Participants received verbatim interview transcripts for verification and further comment. Unit managers and

participants received a copy of the findings and recommendations made. Midwives were not interviewed in groups, to avoid placing pressure on them to disclose information in a situation which could potentially jeopardise their position in the workplace. Participation was considered to benefit informants, as it highlighted an area of professional importance both for practitioners and clients.

Sample

Opinions vary about appropriate sample size in qualitative research (Holloway & Wheeler, 1996). The researcher wished to explore any influences that differences in working conditions, training route, length of qualification and grade might have on perceptions of practice, and recruited midwives accordingly. Only one midwife approached declined to participate, on the

Table 1.4.1 The sample by grade, unit and type of base

Grade	Major unit		Low-risk unit		Midwife-led unit	
	Hospital	Community	Hospital	Community	Hospital	Community
E	5	0	0	0	0	0
F	7	1	0	1	0	0
G	1	4	1	0	0	6
H	1	0	0	0	0	0
Total	14	5	1	1	0	6

Table 1.4.2 The sample by grade, education route and length of qualification

Grade	Direct entry	Nurse trained	Years qualified				
			<3	3–5	6–10	11–15	>15
E	3	2	3	1	0	0	1
F	4	5	0	5	3	0	1
G	1	11	0	1	2	4	5
H	0	1	0	0	0	0	1
Total	8	19	3	7	5	4	8

grounds that she was planning to leave the profession and so felt that she could not contribute constructively to the study.

Recruitment ceased when no new data were being generated (Bryman, 2001), after 27 midwives from five NHS Trusts had been interviewed (see Tables 1.4.1 and 1.4.2). As 12 community midwives were interviewed, the sample had a relatively high proportion of G-grade midwives. Many of these had been in practice for more than 10 years, so only one of them had trained by the direct-entry route.

Data collection and analysis

Interviews were conducted between April 2000 and January 2001. Respondents were offered a choice of interview venue; most chose their own homes. Where the interview was conducted in the workplace, it was usually in a room designed for midwife–client interaction, familiar to the respondent. The author subscribes to the feminist standpoint on interviewing, and consequently incorporated self-disclosure and a two-way flow of information into interviews where appropriate (Bryman, 2001). The guide formed the basis for the interview, but the author also followed participants into other areas of discussion. Question order was not set, but varied with the flow of each interview. Data analysis commenced before the completion of data collection, and informed the continuing development of the interview guide. Analysis followed the schema outlined by Burnard (1991). The transcripts were read closely and coded for

categories; an examination and grouping of these categories produced a number of themes. The researcher subsequently returned to the transcripts, searching for further/alternative categories and/or themes. This process was repeated until no new themes or categories emerged. A selection of transcripts and their corresponding categories and themes was checked by two independent readers with research expertise, one of whom also had midwifery qualifications and experience. These readers also commented on the evolution of the interview guide.

Findings

The main findings from the study are presented here. They include midwives' understanding of their autonomous role, factors perceived to facilitate and bar midwifery autonomy, perceptions of professional position and the effectiveness of professional education. The Trusts have been numbered from 1 to 5: three ran major obstetric units; the other two units, one obstetrician-led and one midwife-led, were for low-risk women with uncomplicated pregnancies.

Understanding of autonomous role

Respondents commonly defined 'autonomy' as including the ability to make decisions, and the need to take responsibility for actions and decisions. Some informants also stated that autonomy involved recognising the scope of their practice. Only four hospital-based midwives and six community midwives felt they could always practise autonomously. Two community midwives and seven hospital-based midwives felt they could not practise autonomously at all. The remaining eight midwives reported being able to practise autonomously sometimes. These differences seemed to arise from informants' personal views of their working conditions combined with their basic understanding of autonomy. Some respondents only defined autonomy in terms of their employment conditions. A G-grade midwife from the obstetrician led low-risk unit (Trust 3) said:

... you are accountable ... to the Trust that employs you. Um, it's essential that you follow Trust guidelines ...

Most respondents' perceptions of their degree of autonomy accorded with their description of their practice – for example, clinical decision-making. However, there were discrepancies: for example, an E-grade midwife in a major obstetric unit (Trust 1) said that she was autonomous in practice, but stated that she always followed policies, whatever her opinion of them. Informants working in the same areas expressed opposing opinions; another E-grade practising in Trust 1 felt that her environment prevented her from working autonomously. This phenomenon was not limited to midwives practising in major units; one G-grade community midwife based in the midwife-led unit (Trust 4), unlike the rest of her colleagues, felt that she was denied autonomy by the local GPs. Only two informants actively viewed autonomy as a state involving collaboration with other professionals; over half the sample stated specifically that autonomy is only possible where midwives are working alone, a finding which accords with those from other studies (McCrea & Crute, 1991; Sikorski et al., 1995; Pope et al., 1997; Meerabeau et al., 1999). The researcher had the following exchange with an F-grade midwife from Trust 1:

Can you tell me what you understand by autonomy in that context? (Researcher)

... that women only ever need to see a midwife ... (F-grade midwife)

Other comments demonstrated confusion about how autonomy applies to midwifery practice. Some respondents thought that midwives could choose whether to assume autonomy; some also thought that senior midwives were responsible for the practice of junior midwives.

Facilitators of autonomy

Many informants felt that medical staff appreciated the midwife's role. One G-grade community midwife from a major unit (Trust 2) commented:

I have established an excellent working relationship with my GPs, and ... my GPs will ring me, not to tell me what they're doing, but to ask me if it's OK ...

Such an attitude from medical practitioners was considered a major factor facilitating midwifery autonomy. However, many respondents indicated that this was mainly a matter of luck, depending on the stance of individual doctors. Only one respondent intimated that the quality of her interprofessional relationships depended on her own efforts and ability. A significant marker of autonomy appeared to be the capacity to operate outside the constraints of the traditional hierarchical system of the NHS. Some community

midwives offered their ability to refer women directly to obstetricians as proof of their autonomy. Similarly, an absence of hierarchy between midwives was seen to facilitate autonomy. This was most notable in Trust 4:

I think it's an advantage having everybody on the same grade ... we're working autonomously together, which is much nicer than working autonomously alone (laughs).

Barriers to autonomy

The above findings notwithstanding, one of the greatest barriers to midwifery autonomy was thought to be the medical profession's power. This was sometimes expressed quite vehemently, as in the case of a G-grade community midwife from Trust 2:

... we have quite a struggle with GPs at the moment, we seem to be the lowest of the low, as far as GPs are concerned.

The negative attitude of other midwives was also identified as a barrier to autonomy. According to an E-grade midwife (Trust 1):

I think the senior midwives don't respect autonomy, not necessarily mine, but any midwives'.

Nineteen midwives in the sample made this type of comment about midwifery colleagues. They came from all five Trusts, were both community and hospital based, graded from E to H, and had been qualified from six months to 19 years. A factor seen to contribute to these problems was the lack of distinction between midwifery and nursing. An F-grade community midwife in Trust 3 commented:

... we are still wearing nurses' uniforms, so the medical staff see us as nurses who will do as they're told ...

Even within the profession, this distinction could be unclear, with data suggesting a gap between the theoretical understanding of the midwife's obligations and the reality of her being seen as a 'specialised nurse'. An F-grade in Trust 2 remarked:

... as long as they sign that piece of CTG [cardiotocograph], that's, you know, that's 'well, I'm OK then, the doctor's signed it' ...

Some respondents thought that this situation had arisen partly because midwives fall under the authority of a senior nurse who may be unaware of the midwife's distinct role and responsibilities. The following exchange occurred between the researcher and an H-grade midwifery manager:

Does the Director of Nursing appreciate midwives' professional accountability and autonomy? (Researcher)

Um – if she does, she's hiding it well ... it's sort of still that very nursing orientated culture ... they are looking at midwifery through nursing eyes ... (Midwife)

A further consequence of the lack of clear boundaries between nursing and midwifery was seen to be the general public's continuing ignorance about the extent of midwives' professional responsibilities and obligations

(McCrea & Crute, 1991; Sikorski et al., 1995). A community midwife in Trust 4 stated:

I think some of them probably don't realise we are (autonomous), there's still an element of 'you're nurses'.

Many respondents felt that the obligation to follow hospital policies and guidelines prevented them from being autonomous practitioners. An E-grade in Trust 5, the third major unit, said:

… there is a hospital-based policy … which sometimes is more rigid than I think is appropriate for me as an autonomous practitioner. I'm robbed of autonomy in that respect.

In the major units, policy-making was medically controlled, as previous studies have found (Garcia & Garforth, 1991; Meah et al., 1996). In the low-risk units, policies went to the medical staff for 'comments'. There was little agreement about the amount or quality of midwifery input into policy-making. Respondents who thought they practised autonomously, at least some of the time, felt they played a major part in drawing up guidelines, or said they did not follow policy when they considered it clinically inappropriate. There was a feeling that in some situations autonomy was only achievable through stealth. A hospital-based F-grade in Trust 2 said:

… I find that I'm being very quiet about it (going against policy) … I have to be a bit crafty; and I know a lot of midwives that'll do that …

Perception of professional position

The combined effects of difficult relationships with both medical and midwifery colleagues and the restrictive nature of hospital policies and guidelines, together with the obligation to be advocates for the women in their care, appeared quite overwhelming for some midwives. An E-grade midwife in Trust 1 spoke for many respondents:

… in these big units, with obstetricians who have more power than us, and other doctors, I just don't think that midwives can be autonomous.

Another E-grade, from Trust 2, raised the question of whether midwives are holding on to an ideal of midwifery whose time is past:

… (maybe) we're clinging on to something that women don't want any more … I think our ideas of our training, of autonomy, and independent practitioners, don't fit, and either we have to completely change society's view, or their expectations of midwifery, or we have to just accept the fact that it's gone.

It appears that midwives may not recognise the full implications of their professional role, and some respondents questioned whether all midwives want to be autonomous. Comments included the following, made by community midwives in Trusts 3 and 4, respectively:

… I don't think amongst midwives there is a feeling that

we are autonomous practitioners, generally I don't think there is …

… I think there are midwives who are happy not to have autonomy …

Education

There was a general perception that direct-entry midwives found it easier to be autonomous. However, whatever their education route, over half of the respondents felt they had not been equipped for professional autonomy. Disturbingly, these included midwives who had qualified relatively recently; of 10 midwives who had qualified within the previous five years, only three felt that they had been prepared for professional autonomy. The following comment was made by a direct-entry midwife who had been qualified for six months:

… do you feel that your training equipped you to be an autonomous practitioner? (Researcher)

No, not at all (laughs); I feel like it equipped me to be the opposite. (Midwife)

An F-grade who had been qualified for three years questioned her midwifery teachers' understanding of the concept, suggesting that they had not transcended the limitations placed upon them in their own education:

Do you feel that your training equipped you to be autonomous? (Researcher)

– it tried to, desperately, you know. But I think that the midwifery tutors, you see, were so much part of the same system, it's very difficult, because I think they were having a battle as well, because I don't think they believed what they were saying … (Midwife)

If there is any accuracy in this suggestion, there are serious implications for the ability of the profession to prepare its members for their autonomous role.

Discussion

If the findings from this study are examined in relation to the conceptual framework for midwifery autonomy (Figure 1.4.1), it appears that preconditions for midwives to practise autonomously are still not in place, and barriers to autonomy continue to operate. Disturbingly, senior NHS personnel, medical staff and even some midwives may still not appreciate that midwives have to assume autonomy. Although there have been concerted efforts to raise the profile of midwifery over the last decade, this seems to have failed in the broader context (Lewis, 2000). Perhaps the inability of midwives to understand and consolidate their professional autonomy, particularly in terms of interprofessional collaboration and control of their own practice, has contributed to this failure. This limited understanding may partly result from the lack of distinction between midwifery and nursing, both inside and outside the profession, demonstrated by the data here. Community midwives who practised before the NHS was established considered that their public visibility contributed significantly to their professional status (Hunter, 1999). By contrast, the widespread move into hospital practice seems to have rendered midwifery almost invisible to the public, by placing it firmly into the NHS hierarchy. This invisibility is reinforced by the continued regulation of midwives by nurses in the UK, as in the recently established Nursing and Midwifery Council (Jowitt, 2000). There is also no guarantee that employers are aware of the midwife's distinct role and responsibilities (Anderson, 1994). It appears that midwifery practice is still largely determined by medical principles. The National Institute for Clinical Excellence (NICE) provides guidelines to clinicians so that all service users can receive evidence-based care (Dimond, 2001); however, these guidelines depend on who is evaluating the available research. Evidence suggests that medical knowledge is always considered superior to midwifery knowledge (McCrea & Crute, 1991; Meah et al., 1996). Members of the NICE committees are drawn mainly from the medical profession and NHS management (NICE, 2000; Thornton, 2001); it appears that NICE guidelines affecting midwifery practice have been developed based on obstetric and paediatric principles, rather than on midwifery principles (Jowitt, 2001). So a number of entrenched factors appear to mitigate strongly against midwifery autonomy, while midwives are still obliged to assume the legal responsibilities of autonomous practice (Dimond, 1994). This inherently incongruous situation has been described as unethical, and can result in the loss of registration and employment for the individual midwife (Clarke, 1996; Rosser, 1999). Although not explored in this study, lack of autonomy in practice is associated with high stress levels and the ongoing haemorrhage of midwives from the profession (Barber, 1998; Stafford, 2001). Although some respondents felt that autonomy within the current system may be unachievable, this pessimistic view may have been a cultural phenomenon, rather than an accurate reflection of reality. Current conditions in the NHS, including the creation of consultant midwife posts, could help to establish midwifery autonomy (Ollerhead, 1999; O'Loughlin, 2001; Sinclair, 2001); however, this would require a major initiative, both at individual and collective levels. Education about the extent and detail of midwives' professional obligations would be required for midwives, NHS management and the medical profession; some doctors still interpret a midwife's mandatory referral for abnormality as an unwillingness to take responsibility for clinical decisions (Meerabeau et al., 1999). Prequalifying education would also need examining. There is an assumption that midwives are equipped for autonomous practice (Robotham, 2000); this is contradicted by the data. Midwifery educators may need to explore their own understanding of autonomy. Midwives would need to promote research based on midwifery principles to influence policy-making, a crucial area for professional control. Most significantly, the regulatory framework for midwifery practice would require change. This would probably depend on a campaign for a new Midwives' Act; it would be gratifying to see the Royal College of Midwives take the lead in this matter. As legal power regarding choice of care rests with service users in the UK (Harcombe, 1999), midwives would do well to strengthen their ties with consumer organisations, if they are serious about being autonomous professionals. This appears to be the central issue: do midwives want to be autonomous practitioners? The data here suggest that this is debatable: there is certainly very little support within the profession for independent midwives, who may be the only genuinely autonomous midwives in the UK (Milan, 1996). Perhaps, as one of the respondents suggested, the ideal of the autonomous midwife is no longer appropriate for our society at large. There may be an argument for the introduction of the obstetric nurse into the UK health care system, so that candidates can choose the profession they want to enter. To many this might seem a road leading to the end of midwifery in the UK, but as it is, data from this and other recent studies suggest that midwifery as an autonomous profession barely exists (Meah et al., 1996; Hosein, 1998; Levy, 1999; Meerabeau et al., 1999). Providing the alternative of obstetric nursing might allow the emergence of a smaller, but well identified and delineated, midwifery profession, which would be able to offer women genuinely autonomous care. It could mean that midwives would no longer struggle for recognition in an environment where the emphasis on medically controlled birth constantly conflicts with the ethos of expertise supporting natural physiological processes, and perhaps it would promote wider understanding about what midwives actually do, and about what care choices exist for pregnant women in the UK. In reality, neither the above option nor a drive towards true autonomy appears likely, given the size and nature of the problem, the poor intraprofessional attitudes mentioned by respondents in this study and midwives' noted cultural difficulties with change (Kirkham, 1999). Midwives will probably continue to interpret their obligation to practise autonomously according to local conditions and personal understanding and inclination. Unfortunately, this means that most women will continue to be denied the choice of autonomous midwifery care; and on a daily basis, midwives will continue to risk either their professional registration or their employment prospects, or both (Anderson, 1994; Rosser, 1999).

Conclusion

Most midwives in this study did not understand the implications of their autonomous role fully. There were mixed views among respondents about whether they practise autonomously, based on their attitude to their working environment and their basic understanding of the concept. The decisive factor seemed to be the degree to which midwives felt their practice was independent of both medical control and the NHS hierarchy. Respondents' perceptions of their own autonomy (or lack of it) generally agreed with the details of their practice, although occasional discrepancies did occur. There still appears to be little recognition for midwifery as an autonomous profession in its own right. However, midwives could exploit current conditions within the NHS to improve the situation. Education appears to be a key issue, both within the profession itself, and among NHS management and relevant professional groups. More midwifery control of policies governing practice is required. Regulation of the profession needs to be addressed as a matter of urgency. Midwives do not appear to support their own autonomy. There may be a place for the obstetric nurse in the UK health care system, which could allow the emergence of a truly autonomous midwifery profession. However, it is more likely that the status quo will persist. This means that many women will continue to be denied the choice of autonomous midwifery care, and every midwife will continue to risk the consequences of practising in a system that requires the accountability and responsibility of midwifery autonomy, yet neither recognises nor supports it.

Acknowledgements

I thank Colin Rees for his constructive comments and suggestions during the conduct of this research.

REFERENCES

Anderson T. 1994. Trust betrayed: the disciplining of the East Herts midwives. MIDIRS Midwifery Digest, 4(2): 132–134

Argyle M. 1989. The Social Psychology of Work, 2nd edn. Penguin Books, London

Atkinson RL, Atkinson RC, Smith EE et al. 1990. Introduction to Psychology, 10th edn. Harcourt Brace Jovanovich, Orlando

Barber T. 1998. Stress and the management of change. RCM Midwives Journal, 1(1): 26–27

Barwise C. 1998. Episiotomy and decision making. British Journal of Midwifery, 6: 787–790

Brauer-Rieke G, Connolly-DeTura P, Wilson L. 1997. Question of the quarter. In what ways is autonomy important to your practice? Midwifery Today and Childbirth Education, 42: 12

Bryman A. 2001. Social Research Methods. Oxford University Press, Oxford

Burnard P. 1991. A method of analysing interview transcripts in qualitative research. Nurse Education Today, 11: 461–466

Carnall L. 1998. Developing student autonomy in education: the independent option. British Journal of Occupational Therapy, 61: 551–555

Clarke R. 1996. Midwifery autonomy and the code of professional conduct: an unethical combination. In: Frith L (ed.), Ethics and Midwifery: Issues in Contemporary Practice. Butterworth-Heinemann, Oxford

Davis-Floyd R. 1997. Autonomy in midwifery: definition, education, regulation. Midwifery Today, 42: 21–22

Dawkins VH. 1998. Restraints with the elderly and mental illness: ethical issues and moral reasoning. Journal of Psychosocial Nursing and Mental Health Services, 36: 22–27, 36–37

Dimond B. 1994. The Legal Aspects of Midwifery. Books for Midwives Press, Hale

Dimond B. 2001. Legal issues: end of year review and some predictions for 2001. British Journal of Midwifery, 9(1): 49–52

Fitzgerald SM, Wood SH. 1997. Advance practice nursing: back to the future. Journal of Obstetric Gynecologic and Neonatal Nursing, 26: 101–107

Fitzsimons B. 1997. Professional issues. First class delivery: a review of the Audit Commission report, first in a series of articles based on the Audit Commission's national review of maternity services. British Journal of Midwifery, 5: 388–392

Fleming VEM. 1998. Autonomous or automatons? An exploration through history of the concept of autonomy in midwifery in Scotland and New Zealand. Nursing Ethics: An International Journal for Health Care Professionals, 5(1): 43–51

Fontana D. 1995. Psychology for Teachers, 3rd edn. MacMillan, Basingstoke

Fraser W. 1995. Learning from Experience: Empowerment or Incorporation? The National Institute of Adult Continuing Education (England and Wales), Leicester

Garcia J, Garforth S. 1991. Midwifery policies and policymaking. In: Robinson S, Thomson AM (eds), Midwives, Research and Childbirth, Vol. 2. Chapman & Hall, London

Garland D, Jones K. 1997. Waterbirth: updating the evidence. British Journal of Midwifery, 5: 368–373

Germano E, Bernstein J. 1997. Home birth and short-stay delivery: lessons in health care financing for providers of health care for women. Journal of Nurse Midwifery, 42: 451–455, 489–498

Gibb H. 1998. Reform in public health: where does it take nursing? Nursing Inquiry, 5: 258–267

Gibson C. 1997. Ethical dilemmas faced by mental health nurses. Nursing Standard, 11: 38–40

Godin P, Scanlon C. 1997. Supervision and control: a community psychiatric nursing perspective. Journal of Mental Health, 6: 75–84

Griffith R, Tengnah C, Grey R. 1999. Professional issues. Consent and women in labour: a review of the issues. British Journal of Midwifery, 7: 92–94

Hamilton M. 1998. Professional issues. Patterns of postnatal visiting: the views of women and midwives. British Journal of Midwifery, 6: 15–18

Harcombe J. 1999. Power and political power positions in maternity care. British Journal of Midwifery, 7(2): 78–82

Hayter M. 1999. Burnout and AIDS care-related factors in HIV community clinical nurse specialists in the North of England. Journal of Advanced Nursing, 29: 984–993

Henry C, Fryer N. 1995. Organisational ethics: the ethics of care. In: Henry C (ed.), Professional Ethics and Organisational Change in Education and Health. Edward Arnold, London

Hixenbaugh P, Warren L. 1998. Diabetes. In: Pitts M, Phillips K (eds), The Psychology of Health, 2nd edn. Routledge, London

Hobbs H, Wilson JH, Archie S. 1999. The Alumni program: redefining continuity of care in psychiatry. Journal of Psychosocial Nursing and Mental Health Services, 37: 23–29, 41–42

Holloway I, Wheeler S. 1996. Qualitative Research for Nurses. Blackwell Science, Oxford

Hosein MC. 1998. Home birth: is it a real option? British Journal of Midwifery, 6(6): 370–373

Howard PB, Greiner D. 1997. Constraints to advanced psychiatric-mental health nursing practice. Archives of Psychiatric Nursing, 11: 198–209

Hundley VA, Cruickshank FM, Lang GD et al. 1994. Midwife managed delivery unit: a randomised controlled comparison with consultant led care. British Medical Journal, 309: 1400–1404

Hunter B. 1999. Oral history and research part 2: current practice. British Journal of Midwifery, 7(8): 481–484

Jowitt M. 2000. Modernising regulation – the new Nursing and Midwifery Council consultation document. Midwifery Matters, 86: 3

Jowitt M. 2001. Not very NICE: induction of labour draft guidelines – a commentary. Midwifery Matters, 89: 23–25

Kirkham M. 1999. The culture of midwifery in the National Health Service in England. Journal of Advanced Nursing, 30(3): 732–739

Latvala E, Janhonen S, Moring J. 1998. Ethical dilemmas in a psychiatric nursing study. Nursing Ethics: An International Journal for Health Care Professionals, 5: 27–35

Levy V. 1999. Protective steering: a grounded theory study of the processes by which midwives facilitate informed choices during pregnancy. Journal of Advanced Nursing, 29(1): 104–112

Lewis P. 2000. Daring to be different: future resolution. British Journal of Midwifery, 8(1): 4–6

Marland GR. 1999. Atypical neuroleptics: autonomy and compliance? Journal of Advanced Nursing, 29: 615–622

McCrea H, Crute V. 1991. Midwife/client relationships: midwives' perspectives. Midwifery, 7(3): 183–192

McKay S. 1997. The route to true autonomous practice for midwives. Nursing Times, 93: 61–62

Meah S, Luker KA, Cullum NA. 1996. An exploration of midwives' attitudes to research and perceived barriers to research utilisation. Midwifery, 12(2): 73–84

Meerabeau L, Pope R, Graham L. 1999. Changing childbirth: who should be the lead professional? Journal of Interprofessional Care, 13: 381–394

Milan M. 1996. Independent midwifery: why the UK needs independent midwives. Modern Midwife, 6(8): 14–15

Morse J, Mitcham C, Hupcey JE et al. 1996. Criteria for concept evaluation. Journal of Advanced Nursing, 24(2): 385–390

Mullins J. 1989. Management and Organisational Behaviour, 2nd edn. Pitman, London

NICE. 2000. National Institute for Clinical Excellence, http://www.nice.org.uk, accessed on 12 June 2002

Ollerhead K. 1999. Primary care trusts: new opportunities for midwives in the new NHS? Practising Midwife, 2(11): 13

O'Loughlin C. 2001. Will the consultant midwife change the balance of power? British Journal of Midwifery, 9(3): 151–154

Olsson A, Hallberg IR. 1998. Caring for demented people in their homes or in sheltered accommodations as reflected on by home-care staff during clinical supervision sessions. Journal of Advanced Nursing, 27: 241–252

Pang MS. 1998. Information disclosure: the moral experience of nurses in China. Nursing Ethics: An International Journal for Health Care Professionals, 5: 347–361

Parnham J. 1999. Clinical governance and evidence-based health care: is there a governance–evidence gap? MIDIRS Midwifery Digest, 9(2): 144–146

Pope R, Cooney M, Graham L et al. 1997. Aspects of care provided by midwives – part one: an overview. British Journal of Midwifery, 5(12): 766–770

Porter CP, Pender NJ, Hayman LL et al. 1997. Educating APNs for implementing the guidelines for adolescents in Bright Futures: guidelines of health supervision of infants, children and adolescents. Nursing Outlook, 45: 252–257

Rees C. 1997. An Introduction to Research for Midwives. Books for Midwives Press, Hale

Robotham M. 2000. Special delivery. Nursing Times, 96(18): 49–51

Rodgers BL. 1989. Concepts, analysis and the development of nursing knowledge: the evolutionary cycle. Journal of Advanced Nursing, 14(4): 330–335

Rose N. 1999. Governing the Soul: The Shaping of the Private Self, 2nd edn. Free Association Books, London

Rosser J. 1999. Struck off – the midwife who obeyed doctor's orders. Practising Midwife, 2(4): 4–5

Rowan C. 1998. Court-ordered caesareans – choice or control? Nursing Ethics: An International Journal for Health Care Professionals, 5: 542–544

Rowan J. 1993. The Transpersonal: Psychotherapy and Counselling. Routledge, London

Rowan J. 1997. Healing the Male Psyche. Routledge, London

Schein E. 1988. Organisational Psychology, 3rd edn. Prentice-Hall, New Jersey

Shields N, Turnbull D, Reid M et al. 1998. Satisfaction with midwifery – managed care in different time periods: a randomised controlled trial of 1299 women. Midwifery, 14(2): 85–93

Sikorski J, Clement S, Wilson J et al. 1995. A survey of health professionals' views on possible changes in the provision and organisation of antenatal care. Midwifery, 11(2): 61–68

Silverton L. 1999. Caesarean section: the effects of women's choice. RCM Midwives Journal, 2: 172

Sinclair M. 2001. Birth technology: cameos from the labour ward. RCM Midwives Journal, 4(3): 85–87

Smith RM. 1983. Learning How to Learn: Applied Theory for Adults. Open University Press, Milton Keynes

Stafford S. 2001. Lack of autonomy: a reason for midwives leaving the profession? Practising Midwife, 4(7): 46–47

Stewart I, Tilney T. 2000. Transactional analysis. In: Palmer S (ed.), Counselling and Psychotherapy: The Essential Guide. Sage, London

Temple K. 1999. A tale of two midwives: Kate's story. Midwifery Matters, 80: 7–8

Thompson D. 1995. The Concise Oxford Dictionary of Current English, 9th edn. Clarendon Press, Oxford

Thornton J. 2001. Not so NICE clinical guidelines. British Journal of Midwifery, 9(8): 470, 472

Torn A, McNichol E. 1998. A qualitative study utilizing a focus group to explore the role and concept of the nurse practitioner. Journal of Advanced Nursing, 27: 1202–1211

Vann MK. 1998. Collaborative practice issues. Hospital admission privileges: professional autonomy for midwives: an essential component of collaborative practice. Journal of Nurse Midwifery, 43: 41–45

Wachtel PL. 1987. Action and Insight. Guilford Press, New York

Wagner M. 1997. Autonomy: the central issue of midwifery. Midwifery Today, 42: 16–18

Warr PB. 1987. Job characteristics and mental health. In: Warr P (ed.), Psychology at Work, 3rd edn. Penguin Books, London

Wells N, Johnson R, Salyer S. 1998. Interdisciplinary collaboration. Clinical Nurse Specialist, 12: 161–168

WHO. 1992. Definition of a Midwife. WHO, Copenhagen

Yalom ID. 1980. Existential Psychotherapy. Basic Books, New York

Appendix: interview guide

1. Please tell me how long you've been qualified, what grade you are, and what your main area of midwifery practice currently is. Are you nurse-trained or direct-entry?
2. What sort of a unit do you work in/are you associated with?
3. The WHO defines midwives as autonomous practitioners; the Midwives' Rules stress their accountability in law. What do you understand by autonomy in this context?
4. Do you think you are an autonomous practitioner where you're practising at the moment? Why/Why not? (*Yes to 4 – explore issues around decision making*)
5. If you're looking after somebody in labour, and you have decisions to make, what do you base those decisions on?
6. What part do the policies play in the decisions that you make?
7. Who makes the policies in your unit?
8. Do you ever go against hospital policy?
   a. (Yes) Do you feel supported by your colleagues when you do this?
   b. (No) Do you always agree with the policies?
9. Do your midwifery colleagues recognise and respect your autonomy?
10. Please tell me about your professional relationship with midwives of other grades.
    a. (*Snr*) Do you ever question junior midwives' clinical decisions?
    b. (*Jnr*) Are your clinical decisions ever questioned by senior midwives?
11. Do other health professionals recognise and respect your autonomy?
12. Last year there was a case of a senior midwife who was struck off because she followed a registrar's inappropriate instructions for the care of a woman in labour. She was struck off because she didn't use her own clinical judgement, she just assumed that the registrar was responsible. Please tell me what you think about this case.
13. What effect, if any, do you think midwifery autonomy has on the care that women who use the maternity services receive?
14. Have you ever had to use your autonomy to defend a woman's right not to follow midwifery or medical advice?
15. What was your colleagues' reaction to this situation?
16. Do you think that general-trained and direct-entry trained midwives differ in the degree to which they're prepared to exercise their autonomy? If so, how?
17. Do you feel that your training equipped you to be an autonomous practitioner?
18. Do you feel that you use the full range of skills that you acquired during your training?
19. Have you done any post-registration study, other than mandatory updates?
20. (*Only if they answered No to question 2*) Can you tell me, in the time that you've been practising, have you ever been in a situation where you have felt that you were practising autonomously?
    a. Yes – explore issues around decision making in that situation
    b. No – go on to question 21
21. Do you think that women realise that you are an autonomous practitioner?
22. Do you think it matters whether they realise this or not? Why?
23. Are there any other issues that you think are relevant to your professional autonomy?

Midwifery 2003; 19(2): 113–124

The risky business of normal birth

Jenny Fraser

I witnessed an interesting scenario on the delivery suite recently. Jo and her partner Sam had first visited the suite at about 06.00 hours. Jo was a primigravida at term, with a healthy and straightforward pregnancy, and had referred herself because she thought she was in labour. She was assessed on admission and found to be in early labour. An admission CTG showed a healthy reactive trace.

After discussion with the midwife, Jo decided to stay in the unit and transfer to the antenatal ward rather than go home, as she lived an hour's drive away and there was a great deal of holiday traffic on the roads. She was anxious not to find herself in a difficult situation.

Jo's labour picked up speed on the antenatal ward. She chose to keep upright and generally mobilised, with occasional rests on the bed when she felt like it. Another CTG was undertaken on the ward and, again, the trace was healthy and reactive.

At 16.00 hours, Jo asked to return to the delivery suite as she felt that labour was beginning to advance speedily. Prior to transfer, a vaginal examination showed that Jo's cervix was thin, well applied and six centimetres dilated. The baby's head was at the ischial spines and membranes were intact.

Jo was duly returned to the delivery suite soon afterwards. I overheard the handover from the midwife on the antenatal ward to Sophie, a delivery suite midwife. While this conversation was taking place at the midwives' station, the call bell rang from Jo's room and I went to see what was needed. The bed had been pumped up high to enable Jo to remain upright and to lean forward across a beanbag, which was on top of the bed. She had removed some of her clothes and was dressed in a shirt and knickers. Her hips swayed with the contractions as she hung on to her beanbag, which appeared to be at a perfect height for her.

Jo had been given the Entonox by the midwife handing over care; Jo was in control of this and was using it expertly. Meanwhile, Sam was encouraging Jo with appropriate words and actions; they looked very much like they were in harmony. Sam looked up when I entered and asked if I could possibly get some cold water for them, as it was a hot day. Jo's eyes stayed closed throughout this encounter as she was concentrating on what she was doing.

I got the water and returned to the room. Jo was starting to make grunting sounds and she looked as if she was beginning to feel the urge to push. I left as Sophie entered the room and commented to her that Jo was showing external signs of being in the second stage.

Sophie rang the bell about an hour later and I again went into the room. Jo was lying on her back on the bed, with the CTG running continuously, which had obviously been on for some time. The trace was healthy and reactive. Jo was pushing hard, encouraged appropriately by Sam and Sophie, and the baby was delivering spontaneously. Jo pushed her feet hard every time she was pushing with the contractions, so much so that the bottom half of the mattress had almost slipped off the edge of the bed, leaving a gap in the middle of the bed, which Jo kept sliding into. She looked uncomfortable each time this happened and needed help to extricate herself out of this position after every contraction. Very soon after my arrival in the room, a healthy, noisy baby emerged.

Midwives' fears

Out of curiosity, I later asked Sophie why she had felt the need to put the CTG monitor on Jo. Sophie's answer was surprising and worrying. She commented that, even though she was aware of evidence that did not support a routine admission CTG, she felt that she was under pressure to undertake one. I pointed out that Jo had been admitted earlier in the day and had had two CTGs since admission, both of which showed no sign of fetal compromise.

Sophie continued that she was aware of this and wanted to just intermittently auscultate, but felt it was an expectation that any woman arriving at or transferring to the delivery suite ought to have a trace. Sophie mentioned defensive practice, litigation and risk management as forming part of her concerns and felt she would be less likely to be swept up into a situation where she would have to explain her actions if she did undertake a CTG. She felt it was possible – should something go wrong and she had not obtained a CTG trace – that explanations would be demanded.

I felt very concerned after this conversation, as I am well aware that Sophie is a caring, safe and considerate midwife. She would have been more than capable of just being with Jo, listening intermittently and unobtrusively to the fetal heart, placing herself behind Jo and catching the baby when it emerged. Jo, by all accounts, had a good experience of birth. She had a 'normal' delivery, a lovely midwife to care for her, no medical input and a healthy baby.

During my conversation with Sophie I reminded her that my role incorporated risk management and I felt concerned that 'risk management' was one of the reasons she had given for her actions. She replied that it was not me personally, as she was well aware of my 'hands-off' approach to normal childbirth. So what is this faceless risk management that causes midwives like Sophie to feel that they must place a CTG on a woman with no untoward history in the final throes of labour?

What is risk management?

Risk management, as the name suggests, is about reducing risk in order to achieve a healthy outcome for mother and baby, and hopefully a positive experience for the woman. Risk management can weed out those individuals who you would not wish to care for your sister or your best friend. However, it is imperative for risk management to uphold and create an atmosphere where normal midwifery practice is encouraged. This can be achieved by legitimising such practice that was actually warranted within the scenario of Jo's birth.

Sophie should know that it was perfectly acceptable to have given care in the way that she wanted and not feel forced by some unknown domain to practise 'defensively'. In actual fact, not to have placed a CTG on Jo at that time would have been easily defended, and risk management must ensure that it enables such practice. How else will we reverse the trend toward more managed births? Is it the risk management culture that seeks to apportion blame when things go wrong that is the problem? If so, then midwifery practice will become as defensive as most obstetric practice and midwifery skills will be lost – an everyday cry from midwives.

The challenge for risk management is there. It is for those in everyday risk management to embrace good midwifery practice and give confidence to midwives like Sophie to practise in the way that they know in their hearts is appropriate. Otherwise, we will continue to lose such midwives.

Risk management is frequently tied up with claims and complaints in the perception of health professionals. It is therefore worth stressing that it is not about avoiding litigation but about enhancing clinical safety and improving standards of care (Edozien, 2003). Risk management can also be about enhancing the clinical experience as well as safety.

Maintaining normal birth

Scenario training 'skills and drills' workshops have become a regular feature in maternity units, but these tend to be centred on acute clinical situations such as a PPH (post partum haemorrhage), vaginal breech birth or prolapsed cord. Such scenarios dealing with these acute situations, whereby maternal and fetal mortality and morbidity are reduced, are to be applauded. Any midwife being presented with such a situation should feel more confident and competent in handling such a crisis. This is risk management leading to risk reduction.

However, it is just as important for midwives to have the skills to deal with normality, and some units have started workshops on how to keep birth within this arena. Such workshops can sit within the 'skills and drills' programme and this may ultimately increase the rate of normal birth, while decreasing the number of caesarean sections. Any results from such units already holding these workshops will be greeted with eager anticipation.

The RCM's Virtual Institute for Birth has a key objective of seeing pregnancy and birth as a normal physiological process, with commitment to a positive reduction in unnecessary medicalisation of pregnancy and birth. It is also committed to the promotion of midwifery skills rooted in normality across the UK (Day-Stirk & Palmer, 2003).

The Institute will engage in sophisticated media dissemination of evidence around normality in pregnancy and birth. The evidence will be rigorous and evidence based, and hopefully will give the desired confidence that midwives appear to be lacking at present.

Conclusion

In most circumstances, any birth other than a normal one has higher risk implications and so risk management should take a lead in reducing risk and its inherent costs, both in monetary and human terms.

Risk management and the normality of birth can coexist. Risk management can be a lever to uphold good midwifery skills, whether in a complicated, high-risk birth or a straightforward, uncomplicated one, in order to embrace woman-centred, safe and proper midwifery care. However, those charged with the day-to-day responsibility for risk management must make sure that they have no fears about the normality of birth themselves and must strive for a just and honest risk management culture, where discussion on clinical issues takes place so midwives learn positively from each other, and the confidence to practise fittingly becomes the norm.

REFERENCES

Day-Stirk F, Palmer L. 2003. The RCM Virtual Institute for Birth: promoting normality. RCM Midwives Journal, 6(2): 64–65 (the RCM Virtual Institute for Birth can be accessed at http://www.rcm.org.uk/data/info_centre/data/virtual_institute.htm)

Edozien L. 2003. An opportunity for safer childbirth. Clinical Risk, 9(3): 85

The Practising Midwife 2003; 6(9): 23–24

Where might we go from here?

At the beginning of this section, I invited you to list what you thought would be the five most important issues affecting women and midwives today, as if you were on a game show and trying to guess the most common responses to this question. As I'm not a game show host, I haven't got a poll to hand to tell you what the answers really are, but I would imagine that a good few of them were discussed in the articles in this section.

Concepts such as normality, control, risk and autonomy have been discussed in the midwifery literature for a number of years. Our theoretical understanding of these issues is becoming far deeper as more midwives carry out research and analysis of these questions and a number of woman-centred, midwifery-led projects are demonstrating what can be achieved, yet, as Jenny Fraser's story in this section illustrates, the practical reality often differs from the theory because of the culture in which we work. Given that we are a part of – and therefore co-create – this culture, we have the potential to influence it in any manner of ways.

So, as a follow-on to the 'game show' list of what the issues or priorities might be for women and midwives, I invite you to consider whether any of the things that you have listed are problematic in the area in which you work and, if so, whether there is something you could do within your sphere of influence to help create change…

Focus on...
Diversity (1)

Building bridges: involving Pakistani women

Yana Richens

The main focus of this article is on how maternity services are delivered to women of Pakistani origin whose first language is not English. As a practising midwife I would like you to reflect on several areas as you read this paper. I would like you to think about what strategies you employ in order to involve Pakistani women in decisions about their maternity care, and how you communicate with them about their treatment and care choices, as well as considering the kinds of information you provide for these women. I would also like you to consider whether you make assumptions based on stereotypical ideas about what we think these women want.

What's the problem?

It is widely acknowledged that since some people hold stereotypical ideas about different ethnic minority groups this influences the way these groups are treated when they require health services (Bowler, 1993; Hunt & Richens, 1999). Research exploring Pakistani women's experiences of maternity services has highlighted a range of problems, especially in relation to choice, communication and information (Richens, 2003).

Singh and Newburn (2000) recommend that special emphasis should be placed on contacting ethnic minority and socially disadvantaged groups in order to ensure that their needs are incorporated into the planning and funding of services.

Patient and public involvement and participation is a major focus of Government attempts to modernise the NHS over the last decade (Department of Health, 1993, 1997a, b, 1998, 1999a, b, 2001). The NHS Plan for England (Department of Health, 2000) devotes an entire chapter to this. In addition, Coulter (2002, p. 108) has argued 'that learning to see things through a patient's eyes should be a central part of professional training and continuing development'. This is a major challenge for health care

professionals, and doubly so when they are charged with caring for people whose first language is not English.

Our failure to actively involve Pakistani women in the planning of care and services, as well as our failure to ask them about their experiences, has been identified as arising from both insufficient funding and a lack of patient satisfaction questionnaires being made available in a variety of different languages. In addition, it may also be true that some people remain firmly entrenched in a stereotypical belief that even if these patient satisfaction measures were available, Pakistani women would still not be able to understand them because they are illiterate.

A review of the literature indicates that Pakistani women's experiences may be subject to a range of factors that impact on access, information and the quality of care that they receive. Studies have identified specific problems encountered by ethnic minority women when accessing maternity services. However, while the literature identifies priorities and factors that may contribute to how Pakistani women experience maternity services, it also highlights the need for additional research exploring women's actual experiences (Bowes & Meehan Domokos, 1996).

There is also a growing literature highlighting how women from ethnic minority groups are not satisfied with their care (Homans, 1980; Currer, 1986; Dobson, 1988; Parsons & Day, 1992; Cochrane, 1996; Katbamna, 2000; Hirst & Hewison, 2001).

The wider context

Beating institutional racism

In addition to the policy initiatives identified above, the Government has also recognised the fundamental issues around inequalities, and the belief that 'institutional racism' is a feature of government organisations (MacPherson, 1999).

Institutionalised racism has been defined by MacPherson (1999, pp. 6, 17, 22) as follows:

[Institutionalised racism] … can arise because of lack of understanding, ignorance or mistaken beliefs. It can arise from well intentioned but patronising words or actions. It can arise from unfamiliarity with behaviour or cultural traditions of people or families from ethnic minority communities. It can arise from racist stereotyping.

In a recent report entitled Tackling Health Inequalities (Department of Health, 2001), the Government decrees that a reduction in inequalities and institutional racism is a national priority. The report also highlights the role of midwives in reducing health inequalities. In order for this to happen, however, midwives need to know and understand the problems that are experienced by Pakistani women when they become users of maternity services.

Whether or not midwives feel comfortable about the notion of institutional racism is a bit of a moot point, since there is evidence to suggest that racism continues to be a factor in the way Pakistani women experience maternity services (McKenzie, 2003). McKenzie (2003, p. 59) proposes that:

Developing a deeper understanding of possible links between racism and health is a prerequisite for initiatives to decrease impact at a community and individual level.

To do this, midwives need to be aware of current policy, and they must be supported in ensuring that the needs of all their clients are met (Henderson, 2002).

What can midwives do?

1. Improve communication

Previous research exploring the experiences of ethnic minority women does provide some insight into the problems associated with communication (Currer, 1986; Bowler, 1993; McLeish, 2002). These authors suggest that language, culture and the ethnic origin of both the woman and her carers affect communication. A recent report from the Ombudsman (2002) identified failures in communication as being at the heart of complaints. Since communication is identified as a serious problem even where people speak the same language, it is reasonable to suggest that it is exacerbated in situations where professionals and patients do not share a common language.

Bradby (2001, p. 131) has suggested that communication is, however, more than simply talking to each other. It is also about '… facial expressions, body language, gestures and assumptions shared between communicants about the context and purpose of the exchange'.

2. Banish negative attitudes

Research has also shown that women from an ethnic minority background experience different treatment options, choice in pain relief and position in labour. These factors have been partly attributed to the negative attitudes of staff (Theodore-Gandi & Shaikh, 1988; Bowler, 1993; McLeish, 2002).

However, the difference in treatment options is not restricted to maternity care and women; it extends across general practice both in the UK (Sheikh et al., 2001) and the USA (Schneider et al., 2002). Furthermore, referral to secondary care is less frequent for ethnic minority people in the general population (Gilliam et al., 1989).

Some researchers (Hirst & Hewison, 2001; Garcia et al., 1998), however, have shown that the negative attitudes and behaviour of staff are not just restricted to ethnic minority women. Hirst and Hewison (2001) found that negative staff attitudes not only affected Pakistani women but also white women. However, women in the latter group were more likely to report these incidents. One possible explanation for this may be that white women are more aware of how hospital staff should behave and the appropriate standards of a hospital environment, as well as being more likely and able to articulate their views.

3. Be kind!

Some research has shown that what the majority of women value is a midwife who is kind and respectful, regardless of colour, class or ethnic origin (Langer et al., 1993). This finding was reinforced in a study undertaken in Australia (Small et al., 1999), which explored the views of Vietnamese, Turkish and Filipino women. Women who experienced the greatest difficulty in communication with their caregivers reported negative experiences. They reported that staff were unsympathetic towards them, and it was not uncommon for them to be scolded or shouted at. The authors suggested that women were not so much concerned about the fact that their caregivers knew little about their cultural practices; they were more concerned that the care was unkind, rushed and unsupportive. Similar findings are reported by Garcia et al. (1998, p. 63), who suggest that:

Unfortunately, women's comments often refer to the absence of kindness – of being ignored, told off or criticised. Good care is also care that feels safe and competent, and that includes good communication.

4. Stop stereotyping

Stereotyping has been defined as making inaccurate judgements or assumptions about an individual in a whole group based on the supposed characteristics of that group (Allport, 1954), and unfortunately it is still the case that many stereotypes of Asian women persist and can lead to inequalities of maternity care (Bowler, 1993; Hunt & Richens, 1999).

One example is described by Torkington (1987), whereby a Muslim woman was stereotyped by staff as coming from a large, supportive, Asian family who brought her food. In fact, she had not eaten for two days.

As described above, what women want, regardless of their ethnicity, is good, competent care. Hundt (2002) argues that 'without communications skills ... a clinician is just a technician ...'.

5. Provide information

In order to deliver good, competent care to women whose first language is not English, it is necessary to provide good information. Pakistani women need access to information even before they conceive, and this should continue throughout antenatal, birth and postnatal care.

Research has shown that effective communication and information go hand in hand. In a study exploring the experiences of Pakistani women, one reported the consequences of her failure to understand the importance of the midwives' instructions (Richens, 2003). The woman did not speak English. She was in her late twenties, had four children and was pregnant with her fifth child. She attended an antenatal appointment at her GP's surgery at 36 weeks. Examination showed that she had experienced reduced fetal movements and the midwife told her that she should go to the hospital. However, the woman did not go until two weeks later when she was in spontaneous labour. As a result, the baby was born severely asphyxiated with the umbilical cord tightly around the neck. The child is now severely disabled. When asked why she did not go straight to the hospital, the woman reported that she felt scared, she did not have anyone to look after her children and that she had not realised the importance of going straight away.

It is possible, from this example, to consider two things: first, the role and actions of the midwife in the antenatal situation and, second, the actions of the woman. What is needed is a way of checking this process. Where a client does not speak the same language as the midwife, then the midwife needs to ensure that a correct interpretation of the specific language occurs. This must take into account conceptual equivalence, cultural interpretation and understanding.

Midwives need to act as advocates in representing the needs of all women clients. In order to undertake this advocacy role in relation to women whose first language is not English, midwives need to be supported to do this through the provision of interpreters and translators. They need to know how to access such services, which are available 24 hours a day.

Conclusion

The findings from a study by the Audit Commission (1997) suggest that women want the same from maternity services regardless of their ethnicity: choice, communication and information. It is the responsibility of health care organisations to provide midwives with the resources, skills and training required, and it is the responsibility of midwives to ensure that women have choice, that they engage in effective communication, and that they provide good, accurate sources of information in the relevant language. Fulfilling these needs forms an essential part of the midwives' role and duty to all women. To achieve this in practice, an understanding of the problems, together with a co-ordinated strategic approach and vision (Hart & Lockey, 2002), is required by managers.

Acknowledgements

Thanks to Lynne Currie for reading the draft of this article. I am also grateful to the Department of Health for the Mary Seacole Award, which made the study possible.

REFERENCES

Allport GW. 1954. The Nature of Prejudice. Addison-Wesley, Wokingham

Audit Commission. 1997. First Class Delivery: Improving Maternity Service in England and Wales. Audit Commission, Abingdon

Bowes AM, Meehan Domokos T. 1996. Pakistani women and maternity care: raising muted voices. Sociology of Health and Illness, 18(1): 45–65

Bowler I. 1993. 'They're not the same as us': midwives' stereotypes of South Asian women. Sociology of Health and Illness, 15(2): 157–178

Bradby H. 2001. Communication, interpretation and translation. In: Culley L, Dyson S (eds), Ethnicity and Nursing Practice. Palgrave Macmillan, Basingstoke

Cochrane R. 1996. Women's experience of antenatal care in Tower Hamlets. In: McKie L (ed.), Researching Women's Health Methods and Processes. Quay Books, Wiltshire

Coulter A. 2002. The Autonomous Patient: Ending Paternalism in Medical Care. The Nuffield Trust.

Currer C. 1986. Health concepts and illness behaviour: the case of some Pathan mothers in Britain. PhD Thesis, University of Warwick

Department of Health. 1993. Changing Childbirth: Report of the Expert Maternity. HMSO, London

Department of Health. 1997a. The New NHS: Modern and Dependable. The Stationery Office, London

Department of Health. 1997b. A First Class Service. The Stationery Office, London

Department of Health. 1998. The New NHS: Modern and Dependable. A National Framework for Assessing Performance (Consultation Document, NHS Executive). The Stationery Office, London

Department of Health. 1999a. Saving Lives: Our Healthier Nation. The Stationery Office, London

Department of Health. 1999b. Making a Difference: Strengthening the Nursing, Midwifery and Health Visiting Contribution to Health and Healthcare. The Stationery Office, London

Department of Health. 2000. The NHS Plan. The Stationery Office, London

Department of Health. 2001. Tackling Health Inequalities. Consultation on a Plan for Delivery. The Stationery Office, London

Dobson S. 1988. Ethnic identity: a basis for care. Midwife, Health Visitor and Community Nurse, 24(5): 172.

Garcia J, Redshaw M, Fitzsimons B, Keene J. 1998. First Class Delivery: A National Survey of Women's Views of Maternity Care. Audit Commission, Belmont Press.

Gilliam SJ, Jarman B, White P, Law R. 1989. Ethnic differences in consultation rates in urban general practice. British Medical Journal, 299: 953–957

Hart A, Lockey R. 2002. Inequalities in health care provision: the relationship between contemporary policy and contemporary practice in maternity services in England. Journal of Advanced Nursing, 37(5): 485–493

Henderson C. 2002. Terms and conditions: midwives hold the key. British Journal of Midwifery, 10(6): 344

Hirst J, Hewison J. 2001. Pakistani and indigenous white women's views and the Donebedian Maxwell grid: a consumer-focused template for assessing the quality of maternity care. International Journal of Health Care Quality Assurance, 14(7): 308–316

Homans HY. 1980. Pregnant in Britain: a sociological approach to Asian and British women's experience. PhD thesis, University of Warwick

Hundt G. 2002. Local voices on global health issues. Inaugural lecture, Warwick University, 10 September

Hunt SC, Richens Y. 1999. Unwitting racism and midwifery care. British Journal of Midwifery, 7(9): 358

Katbamna S. 2000. Race and Childbirth. Open University Press, Buckingham

Langer A, Victora C, Victora M et al. 1993. The Latin American trial of psychosocial support during pregnancy: a social intervention evaluated through an experimental design. Social Science and Medicine, 36(4): 495–507

MacPherson W (Chair). 1999. The Stephen Lawrence Inquiry, Vols 1 and 2. HMSO, London

McKenzie K. 2003. Racism and health (editorial). British Medical Journal, 326: 65–66

McLeish J. 2002. Mothers in Exile – Maternity Experiences of Asylum Seekers in England. The Maternity Alliance

Ombudsman. 2002. The Parliamentary Ombudsman: Annual Report. The Stationery Office, London

Parsons L, Day S. 1992. Improving obstetric outcomes in ethnic minorities: an evaluation of health advocacy in Hackney. Journal of Public Health Medicine, 14(2): 183–191

Richens Y. 2003. An exploration of women of Pakistani origins experience of UK maternity services. Mary Seacole Report 2001 (unpublished)

Schneider EC, Zaslavsky AM, Epstein AM. 2002. Racial disparities in the quality of care for enrolees in Medicare Managed Care. JAMA, 287(10, March): 13

Sheikh S, Williamson K, Kearley K et al. 2001. Danger of stereotyping in suspected osteomalacia. British Medical Journal, 323: 149–151

Singh D, Newburn M. 2000. Access to Maternity Information and Support – The Experiences and Needs of Women Before and After Giving Birth. NCT, London

Small R, Liamputtong RP, Yelland J, Lumley J. 1999. Mother in a new country. The role of culture and communication in Vietnamese, Turkish and Filipino women's experiences of giving birth in Australia. Women and Health, 28(3)

Theodore-Gandi B, Shaikh K. 1988. Maternity Services Consumers' Survey Report. Bradford Health Authority

Torkington NKP. 1987. Racism and health. Women's Health Information Centre Newsletter, 7, Spring

The Practising Midwife 2003; 6(8): 14–17

What's it like to work in Siberia?

Rachel Simpkins

About Siberia

Siberia is a vast region covering the Asian part of Russia. It shares borders with China, Mongolia and Kazakhstan, and is larger than Canada (the second largest country in the world after Russia). Siberia boasts the world's deepest lake (Lake Baikal) and is the source of most of Russia's oil and natural gas.

Siberia has a notorious past. From the 17th century, criminals and political offenders were exiled there. When the region was part of the Union of Soviet Socialist Republics (USSR), millions were sent to the work camps and prisons known as the 'Gulag' during the 1930s and 1940s.

Introduction

Having been a qualified midwife for less than 12 months, I felt I needed more experience before fulfilling my ambition to work in Africa. When a friend approached me to travel with her to Siberia to deliver a baby, I jumped at the chance and felt this might be an ideal 'taster'. Dreams of African heat soon turned to Siberian snow!

Jessica and Jonathan are a young Canadian/English couple working for a Florida-based church-planting mission in Ulan Ude, Siberia. Their four-year-old daughter was born in a Canadian hospital, and their two-year-old son arrived quickly in England with Jonathan's mother conducting an unplanned homebirth! Having seen the local hospital, they decided on a second, planned homebirth. Ulan Ude doesn't have the luxury of community or even independent midwives, and so they decided to import an English midwife.

Five weeks before our planned departure my friend fell ill and was advised not to fly. Anxious not to let Jessica and Jonathan down, but not confident enough to travel alone, I frantically searched for someone to accompany me. Unable to find a midwife, I looked further afield – and my friend Kate, an archaeologist, conveniently had some time off between excavations.

Plans went ahead, and D-day quickly approached. Jonathan regularly emailed to say that Jessica was feeling so heavy that she thought she might give birth at any moment. We wondered whether we would be there before the delivery since Jessica would already be 38 + 6 weeks pregnant by the time we arrived.

We set off early on a wet Friday in April. The plane was late arriving in Moscow, where we joined an hour-long queue through passport control. This left us with just 30 minutes before our connecting flight departed from another terminal. On the advice of a friendly fellow traveller, we found our luggage in lost property despite being told it would be transferred for us. With no time to spare, we caught a taxi to the other terminal three miles away only to be charged $65 (about £50) for it – welcome to Russia! Fortunately, we caught our plane despite arriving at the airport just as it was due to leave. From then on the journey went smoothly. After a six-hour flight we were met by two girls in Irkutsk who accompanied us on a spectacular eight-hour ride on the Trans-Siberian Railway to Ulan Ude.

We arrived at Jessica and Jonathan's home on Saturday evening to a warm welcome and a much needed meal. Jonathan was especially relieved to see us as Jessica had been having Braxton Hicks contractions all day. After a chat over dinner, I was able to discuss a birth plan with Jessica, palpate her abdomen and look at the antenatal notes Jonathan had been keeping. Kate and I then went to the nearby apartment that we were to share with four Russian girls for the next two weeks. We literally fell into bed at 11 p.m. We were woken by the phone at 3.15 a.m. – Jessica was in early labour. We arrived to find her having weak contractions every five minutes. She pottered around the apartment while I prepared the delivery equipment I had brought with me.

At about 5 a.m., Jessica had a small show and her labour quickly established. She now needed to breathe through each contraction. Early decelerations were heard with the sonicaid, although they recovered quickly. Jessica's membranes ruptured spontaneously, and three minutes later the baby arrived at 5.34 a.m. He cried immediately and, at Jessica's request, was dried before being placed skin-to-skin. After the delivery of the placenta, Jessica relaxed in a bath before breastfeeding baby Nathan. We left the happy family together as the two children awoke to find their new brother had arrived overnight. Kate and I couldn't believe that we'd travelled halfway around the world to deliver this baby, and he arrived just nine hours after we did!

The Siberian system

A few days later, I went with Jonathan to the gynaecological hospital to get the documentation necessary to register the birth. It was documented that Nathan was actually born there, since homebirths were unheard of. Jonathan arranged a tour of the maternity unit, where 1600 births a year took place – half the number of a decade ago due to a declining birthrate.

The unit was split into two identical levels – a 'physiological' ward for 'normal' births and an 'acute' ward for more problematic cases. These were set along a long, bare corridor with a small nurse's desk in the middle. At one end was the 'labour room', consisting of four uncomfortable-looking beds with no curtains to separate them, and a CTG monitor. Women in the second stage of labour were transferred to the 'delivery room' next door. This was larger and with space for two women to give birth together – again with no curtains. There were two three-quarter-length beds, both with stirrups, which were routinely used. While midwives cared for labouring women, a doctor oversaw the birth. Cultural norms dictated that partners were not present during childbirth. The two delivery rooms were used on alternate days, and during our tour the midwife actually showed us a room with a birthing woman in it! After delivery, mother and baby were transferred to one of the bare four-bedded postnatal rooms.

Because the hospital was a specialist referral unit, it had a high caesarean section rate (20%). Facilities to perform ventouse deliveries were available, but caesareans were preferred. The four-bedded intensive ward area was full during our visit, with a ventilated woman receiving suction in full view of the other patients.

The special-care baby unit took a maximum of eight babies, although those of less than 30 weeks' gestation were transferred to another hospital. The incubators and other equipment looked modern compared with the general state of the hospital.

The other babies were kept with their mothers, and were swaddled extremely tightly. This is traditional in Russia, and has been shown to calm and comfort babies. All babies received hepatitis C and TB vaccinations within the first three days of life. The breastfeeding rate within the hospital was high. Most women were discharged on day 5 (day 8 if post-caesarean), with a paediatrician visiting them at home two days later. I left the tour feeling very relieved that Nathan's birth went smoothly, and a hospital admission was not needed.

Getting to know the locals

Due to Nathan's well-timed arrival I was able to provide two weeks postnatal care as well as have time to explore. Ulan Ude (home to the world's largest Lenin's head!) has a population of 300,000, many of whom are Buryat – who originate from Mongolia. The city had a typically Eastern European flavour – bland, with lots of run-down apartment blocks. The weather was a lot warmer than we had expected (15–20°C), and so the piles of jumpers we had brought with us lay redundant.

The roads around the city were often covered with potholes. Taxis would hurtle down a street at 80 m.p.h. and then swerve suddenly to miss a pothole. The lack of seatbelts did nothing to quell our nerves! Trams travelled at a more relaxed pace, but were a haven for pickpockets. I got off the tram one day to find my bag open and a six-inch knife slit down one side. Fortunately, nothing was taken.

The countryside outside the city made a refreshing change. It was mostly hills and mountains covered with pine forest. Native animals include the Siberian tiger and the bear. Although we didn't encounter these, we did see a wild wolf! We spent a day by Lake Baikal – the world's deepest lake (one mile deep). In winter it freezes to a depth of 20 metres, allowing a road to be built on it. Although it was beginning to thaw, we were able to walk on part of the ice.

During our stay we spent two nights in a village that had electricity but no running water. We were therefore able to experience an outhouse. This 'toilet' was basically a small wooden shed with a hole in the floor. It snowed during our stay, so we both prayed that we wouldn't need to pay a visit during the night.

Our host taught in the village school, and I was asked to teach first aid to a Year 8 and Year 10 class with the aid of a translator. The children treated us like celebrities, even asking for our autographs. We chatted to the English teacher, who, despite having never spoken to an English person before, was completely fluent.

It was apparent that many people, especially in the village, were living in poverty. Everything they had was put to use and they couldn't afford to waste anything –

especially food. One lunchtime we had Russian pancakes. The leftovers reappeared at teatime and again the following day for breakfast. And, despite being so poor, villagers were also extremely generous. When they realised it was my birthday, they gave me an ornamental cup, bowl and spoon, which were actually household decorations.

Everyone we met was extremely friendly. Jonathan and Jessica opened their home to us, despite having just had a new baby. We both had an amazing and often humbling trip and would love to return – perhaps when baby number four is on the way!

The Practising Midwife 2003; 6(7): 32–34

What's it like to work in Ontario?

Elizabeth Fulton-Breathat

Across Canada, regulated midwifery is a fairly recent phenomenon. Although health care is funded for the entire nation, each of the 10 provinces and three territories has different regulations governing the practitioners who provide care in that jurisdiction. The Province of Ontario, located roughly in the middle of Canada, is the second largest and most heavily populated of all the provinces. In January 1994 it became the first to recognise and fund midwifery as a regulated health profession.

The resurrection of midwifery in Ontario was a consumer-driven movement. Women in the province wanted an alternative to the medical birth model, and they sought out midwives who had received their training through apprenticeships or in other countries. The midwives who practised were considered to be *alegal* – unfunded, unregulated and without status. Midwives had no hospital privileges or direct access to laboratory testing or diagnostic imaging.

Over a number of years the Ontario government responded to pressure from both consumers and midwives, and worked to include midwifery in the Regulated Health Professions Act. A consortium of three universities (Laurentian, McMaster and Ryerson) was chosen to offer the four-year Midwifery Education Programme. The College of Midwives of Ontario was created to govern midwifery practice across the province.

Input from midwives, consumers and other health care professionals shaped the midwifery model of care in Ontario (see Box 2.3.1). Today, midwifery is a self-regulated profession independent of both medicine and nursing.

Compensation for midwifery practice is part of the provincial health budget, and remuneration falls somewhere between that of physicians and nurses. Full-time salaries currently range from C$55,000 to 77,000 (£22,500–31,600), and malpractice insurance is subsidised. Practice groups are financially independent and receive C$575 per client for overhead expenses.

Box 2.3.1 Midwifery model of care in Ontario

Continuity of care Midwives provide care from conception to approximately six weeks following birth. The care is provided by a small group of no more than four midwives known to the woman.

Informed choice While the midwife is recognised as having a unique body of knowledge, all decisions such as tests, procedures and choice of birthplace are jointly made by the woman and the midwife.

Appropriate use of technology Midwives are expected to provide evidence-based care. Decisions regarding which forms of technology are used can be one of the woman's informed decisions.

Choice of birthplace Midwives are expected to offer both home and hospital birth care (although some women may be screened out for health reasons). Practising midwives must attend a minimum of five home and five hospital births each year to maintain their registration.

Time with women Midwifery appointments normally last from 30 to 45 minutes to ensure that the woman has the opportunity to know her care providers, and for health assessments and informed choice discussions to take place.

Two midwives at each birth While the second midwife is not usually present until the birth, this is a unique safety mechanism in Ontario's model of care.

A full-time midwife provides clients with antenatal/postnatal care, and attends approximately 40 births per year as the primary midwife. An equal number of births are attended as the second or back-up midwife. The provision of 24-hour on-call availability is easily the most challenging aspect of the model of care. Off-call time and holidays are determined within practice groups.

Midwives can choose which communities and settings they work in and who they work with. In rural communities, where birth numbers and overhead expenses may be lower, midwives may choose to work in smaller groups. The cost of leasing space in a large city can sometimes be the determining factor for the size of urban practices. Midwives now have access to laboratory testing, diagnostic imaging and hospital privileges.

In 1994, when midwifery was first regulated, only 60 midwives were registered to practise in Ontario. There are now more than 250 midwives working in the province. In addition to the BHScM graduates from the Midwifery Education Programme, the College of Midwives of Ontario assesses and registers midwives from other countries through the International Midwifery Pre-registration Program (IMPP). Reciprocity is available for midwives registered in the Canadian provinces that have regulated midwifery. These include British Columbia, Alberta, Saskatchewan, Manitoba and Quebec.

In the eight years since midwifery became regulated in Ontario, midwives have become an accepted part of the health care team. Demand for midwifery services continues to exceed the availability of registered midwives. As the profession expands within the province and across the country, midwives have the potential to significantly influence maternity services and the manner in which care is delivered.

USEFUL LINKS

The Association of Ontario Midwives
http://www.aom.on.ca
The Government of Ontario
http://www.gov.on.ca/health/english/pub/women/midwife.html
The College of Midwives of Ontario
http://www.cmo.on.ca/

McMaster University
http://www.fhs.mcmaster.ca/midwifery/
Laurentian University
http://www.laurentian.ca/midwifery
Ryerson University
http://www.ryerson.ca/programs/midwifery.html

The Practising Midwife 2003; 6(4): 27–28

Excerpts from a CNM's journal: Kosovo, winter 2000

Barbara Hammes

Diary excerpts chronicle the experiences of a nurse-midwife on assignment in Kosovo with Doctors of the World, USA, during the winter of 2000.

17 January 2000

Two days ago I celebrated my 50th birthday. Today, flying over familiar Midwest farms on a journey to a new country, I feel a mixture of exhilaration, pride, doubt, and fear. My husband and youngest son have assured me they will 'take care of the home front', and the three older children, away at universities, all promise to email. My teaching colleagues at the University of Wisconsin have granted me a semester's leave of absence. They all know how long I have wanted to be part of an international health project, and they encouraged me to accept an invitation by Doctors of the World (DOW), USA. I will be one of two nurse-midwives assigned to a midwifery-training project in Kosovo.

25 January 2000

It is 10:00 a.m. and I feel very much like a midwife, exhausted from being up all night. Yesterday the administrator of the Prishtinë University Obstetrical-Gynecological Hospital invited me to work alongside his midwives and doctors, and to take advantage of this opportunity I stayed on through the night. Fortunately, two medical students knew some English and could supplement my Albanian-English dictionary. Otherwise, we communicated by demonstration and universally recognized medical terms.

The hospital is built in the old-fashioned Communist style, with long glass and steel-walled patient wings that offer no privacy. During this freezing winter, doctors and midwives wear coats over their scrubs, and cats run from one radiator to the next in an attempt to keep warm inside the cold corridors. Patient gowns are scarce, and women in labor wear heavy, hand-knitted sweaters and layers of their own clothing. The city power plants are in need of repair, and power sources are highly variable, coming now from Macedonia and Greece. Electricity is often on for six hours, then off for six. The hospital has been without running water for up to six days at a time this winter. Latex gloves are washed, dried on towels on the floor near the electric space heaters, and reused. Despite the widespread use of antibiotics, high infection rates are an inevitable consequence.

When I arrived on the labor and delivery unit, a baby had just been born. A thin cloth was placed over its blue, limp body, and it was carried at arm's length down the long, unheated corridor to the nursery. Such practices frustrate the neonatalogists, who understand the importance of the 'warm chain' concept in caring for newborns. The chief neonatalogist described to me how, last week, a baby had a temperature of 34°C when it reached the nursery. There seem to be no protocols in this OB unit, and no planning ahead. There are fleece blankets and stethoscopes in a cupboard at the end of the hall, but not in the delivery room.

At midnight, the chief obstetrical resident hurriedly invited me to accompany him to the emergency unit, where a young woman lay bleeding from a ruptured ectopic pregnancy just diagnosed by ultrasound. Her family was instructed to return to their village to round up blood donors, and she was carried on a stretcher up four flights of stairs to the operating suite. The obstetricians and anesthesiologists scrubbed with water from a reused, 2-l Coke bottle and struggled with the cold temperature, malfunctioning equipment, and inadequate supplies and anesthetic agents. Amazingly, the young woman survived, and I witnessed the remarkable surgical skills and courage of my new colleagues.

After assisting with nine vaginal deliveries and observing one cesarean section, I was invited to demonstrate my own midwifery skills with a woman who had just reached the unit when she began to give birth. I was grateful that the DOW maternal-infant health (MIH) director, an Albanian obstetrician, appeared at the door. He saw the fear in my eyes, and understanding, stopped the fundal pressure that was being routinely and aggressively administered to expedite delivery. When the infant (who appeared to be approximately 32 weeks gestation) was born, I held it close to me, and we rushed down the hall to a semiwarm overhead radiant heater. Although there was an ambu bag with a term newborn-sized mask present, someone had to run down another hallway to locate a stethoscope to auscultate a pulse. After performing the required episiotomy and repair, and resuscitating the newborn, I was offered a job. Nice to know!

Midwives here have a high school education, whereas physicians have six years of medical education between high school and residency. The Midwifery Director has politely refused past offers of midwifery training updates, explaining that her midwives need only to 'follow the physicians' directions'. Midwives routinely cut episiotomies, but only physicians repair them, using external closing. This is very uncomfortable for the women, and nearly impossible to keep clean because there is only sporadic running water in the cities, and none in rural homes. When I shared photographs of births I had attended in the United States, the midwives and physicians explained that with over 1000 births a month, they do not have time to cater to the needs of childbearing families like we do in the United States. Yet I noticed no shortage of staff; each delivery had two midwives, an obstetrical resident, an obstetrician, and four medical students.

Women are forbidden to walk, eat, or drink during active labor, and most of the women I observed last night were given IM or IV-push oxytocin during transition and second stage. To hasten cervical dilatation during transition, an IV 'antispasmodic' (which seems to be a derivative of scopolamine) is also used. Although each woman receives a monitor strip upon entering the labor unit, I rarely observed FHR auscultation in the active labor and delivery suites. Before leaving the hospital this morning, I was reassured to see 'my' newborn, resting comfortably in the warmer in the premature unit. I am beginning to understand a common belief in Kosovo: 'What doesn't kill you makes you stronger!'

Our DOW MIH director readily accepted an invitation from the chief neonatologist to develop a modified neonatal resuscitation 'train the trainer' course. Within the next two weeks, I will team up with the DOW American obstetrician consultant and two United Kingdom pediatricians from the non-governmental organizations (NGOs) to write up, translate, and conduct the training. Fortunately, together we have the necessary resources, including the important coffee and cakes! Perhaps one of the best things we can demonstrate is teamwork among midwives, obstetricians, and newborn staff; all agree this is a problem worldwide.

27 January 2000

It's hard to believe that we have been here one week already. Today our DOW MIH medical director asked me to drive from our headquarters in Prishtinë to Klinë, to assess the feasibility of establishing a Klinë Health House birthing center. I was able to hitch a ride over the ice- and snow-covered roads with two consultants from another NGO. After morning coffee with the Klinë Health House director, a local English/Albanian-speaking ambulance driver took me to see the building that was to become the new birthing center. At present it houses 80 Albanians whose rural homes were burned during the war. There, they can stay warm for the winter as their homes are being rebuilt.

During my tour of the site, the caretaker invited me to have tea in his family's room that he shares with his wife and three daughters. We spent an hour together sitting on the floor cushions, as I listened to the stories of what people endured during the past three years and how they hid in the woods from the Serbian soldiers. Once, when a new mother had her throat slit, the ambulance driver tried to keep her one-week-old baby alive by encouraging the newborn to nurse from the dead mother's breasts. The baby expired after two days. Here we were, telling and listening to stories of war and incomprehensible horrors while sharing English and Albanian words, tea, cookies, and photos of our children.

17 February 2000

Every Wednesday and Thursday I travel to the mountainous city of Suharekë, where there is a Health House birthing center with nine midwives, two apprentices, and an obstetrician. Before the war, they delivered approximately 200 babies per month. Now, during the cold winter and with only sporadic electricity and running water, approximately 50 women give birth here each month. Other women remain at home or believe it is safer to travel over treacherous roads to the medical center hospitals in neighboring Përzeren or in the capital of Prishtinë.

Because of the damage caused by bombing, heavy tank transport, and winter freezing, the roads are almost impassable. It takes two hours to travel less than 50 miles from Suharekë to Prishtinë. To make matters worse, it is often necessary to pass oversized, slow-moving tanks and supply trucks that belong to the Kosovo Forces of the United Nations. Even so, with the breathtaking scenery and my skillful driver, these trips have become a welcome interlude of 'R and R'. It is comforting to see the rural farms, border fences of woven spindly tree trunks, hillside vineyards, and scrub oaks dotting the mountainous ravines, but I remain gripped with sadness and horror when I see the scattered mass graveyards alongside the roads. A colorful plastic-flowered shield covers each victim's raised mound, and a single red Albanian flag, printed with double black eagles, flies high above the graveyard.

Just as difficult to adjust to are the colorful yellow and red plastic warning tapes that read 'DANGER! MINES!' and are posted along the country roads. We have learned from others' mistakes not to venture off the hard road surfaces. How strange it is to see the posters hanging in the hospital maternity wards, warning mothers to keep their children from wandering into the farm pastures and wooded areas. Winter snow will prevent the mine specialists from the UN Mission in Kosovo from clearing these landmines until spring. Because of poor roads and landmines, getting to a birthing center or hospital in Kosovo can be dangerous. It is understandable why few women are willing to travel for prenatal care.

Since the war, the health system is in the process of being completely reorganized. Albanian health professionals, now in the majority, are updating their skills to take over the leadership of the main health centers. The Serbian health professionals, now the minority power, are trying to establish parallel systems of health care in their villages. It will take years to establish needed home and institutional services for both populations.

Today, the DOW obstetrical consultant, Dr Anne, accompanied me to demonstrate the physician-midwife team approach and to talk with the Suharekë obstetrician and encourage him to promote our training program. Our class was suddenly interrupted by a woman who was bleeding heavily after a fall climbed the stairs to the birthing center. She was supposedly in her fifth month of pregnancy and rapidly delivered a baby who appeared to be about 28 weeks' gestation. The nurses quickly wrapped it in a small towel and placed it on the side counter and turned their attention back to the mother, who was now stable with little bleeding.

The infant was wiggling and obviously struggling for life. Resuscitation was out of the question because there is no way to sustain life for such a small baby in this harsh environment. I instinctively picked up the baby and held it close. Through our interpreter, Dr Anne and I tried to explain our belief that the mother should be given an opportunity to see and hold her baby. The

midwives stated sensitively that this would only make her cry. We tried to explain why we thought it was healthy to cry for a lost baby. When the midwives understood that it might help her, they asked the young mother, who indicated she wanted her baby. I brought the still-warm body over and unwrapped the perfectly beautiful, now expired baby boy. The mother sat up on the delivery table, leaned over, and kissed her infant on his forehead. Time seemed to stand still as we all cried together in that freezing room. When we resumed our class, the head midwife described how she too had lost a newborn son 15 years ago at the Prishtinë University Hospital. She had never discussed it with anyone before. Together, we nine women shared the hurt that is still in her heart today.

25 February 2000

A wonderful week! On Wednesday when I went to the Suharekë birth center I was surprised to encounter the head midwife because she was to have attended a WHO conference in a nearby city. She said she didn't want to miss me, and I wondered if perhaps she didn't trust me to teach her midwives while she was gone. But as I quickly found out, she couldn't wait to discuss a birth she had attended the day before. After working with a primip who pushed for three hours with the vertex still high, the midwife became desperate enough to try out the techniques we had demonstrated in class to resolve prolonged second-stage labor. She had the woman stand upright and push leaning over the bed, using the force of gravity and allowing the baby to rotate from occiput posterior to occiput anterior. Within 15 minutes the baby was born, much to the joy of the midwives and of course the mother!

Earlier in the week, another midwife tried some position changes that also worked. Today the midwives proudly displayed on the delivery room walls the handouts of labor support techniques that I brought last week. They are enthused and want Dr Anne to return again to meet with their obstetrician. We agreed they should be charting fetal heart tones, vaginal exams, and labor progress. At present, the care they provide is conveyed to the doctor, who charts it whenever he comes in, which may be the next day.

At Suharekë, unlike at Pristinë Hospital, the midwives rarely use oxytocics or antispasmodics to hasten labor. The birthing center's supplies this winter are so scarce that when a woman arrives in labor, her family is sent to a nearby pharmacy to buy oxytocin, IV solution, and a needle and tubing in case an emergency develops. Families pay the equivalent of $8.00 for all of this, which is a great financial burden. It is ironic to find that the birthing center has a vast supply of IV magnesium sulfate, which was donated by a well-meaning NGO unaware that all complicated cases are transferred 30 miles away to Përzeren. However, breech births, even with first babies, are not transferred unless labor is protracted. I am learning from the midwives' skills and calmness, as they attend these breech births.

Arriving back at DOW headquarters, we learned that another case of infanticide occurred last night in the Prishtinë Hospital, when a mother killed her newborn son. She had been raped during the war and knew no other way. She left the hospital and has not been found. There is so much sadness and anger, and worse, numbness, in response to the widespread violence perpetrated against women during the war. Many mothers leave their infants in the hospitals. Tragically, until there is an official government, mechanisms for adoption are impossible. No social services exist here yet, although they are desperately needed.

29 March 2000

Because I wanted to know more about the midwives' lives and work, last month I accepted the Suharekë midwives' invitation to spend 36 hours with them. It was clear that the senior midwives wanted to demonstrate their expertise. Because the most senior midwife only worked nights, she was never present for our classes, and I had not yet met her. I knew that unless I could admire their skills, I would be unable to convince them to reconsider their firm belief in episiotomies for all primiparous and para-2 women. Although there was only one birth during my visit, I was richly rewarded. During our time together we shared much about ourselves as women and midwives.

Across the open hall from the delivery room there is a cramped lounge that serves as the midwives' classroom by day and sleeping room by night. Above the sink hangs a nonworking electric water heater donated by an NGO but never installed. For classes we must bring our own diesel fuel to operate the generator that powers either the space heater or the overhead projector. Through the cold night, without running water or electricity, we shared photos and stories of our families and hobbies. Along with great charade skills, the Albanian-English dictionary was in constant use! We worked by candles and my battery-operated reading light. The midwives taught me how to tat, and they shared traditional foods brought from home.

Finally, at about 1.30 a.m., after swapping endless birthing stories and tips, we settled down to sleep. I will never forget the sights, sounds, or smells of that night. Imagine, two 50-year-old overweight midwives, an eager young apprentice, and a cleaning lady sharing two single cots. I must say it was a perfect way to keep each other

warm! With no functioning washing machines in the hospital, blankets are reused and shared by midwives and laboring women. The odor is strong! Outside our large window, a wooden shutter clanged back and forth all night in the howling wind, and yet we were gratefully able to sleep.

The next morning, I walked the senior midwife to her bus stop and purchased juice and sweet rolls for the new shift. I felt comfortable with and respectful of my new colleagues. As I looked at their photographs and heard the stories of their burned-out homes, I felt their tragedy and understood their courage. With no official government, they are paid almost nothing for their skills and dedication, yet they continue to serve. Since that time, I have continued to come twice a week for classes, and the Suharekë midwives have attended an increasing number of births from the surrounding communities.

Today when I arrived there was much excitement. I was honored to receive a sweater, hand knit by a senior midwife. It was the traditional one worn by local women of postmenopausal stature. I will wear it proudly and warmly! A reporter came from the local radio and newspaper to interview the midwives and me. Imagine my surprise when the midwives opened the delivery record book and proudly pointed out that only two episiotomies had been cut the past month – out of 92 births! It was evident from the resulting article and radio program that these midwives are held in high esteem.

14 April 2000

The experience of teaching our curriculum to Serbian midwives in the clinic at Donja Gusterica was unexpected and unforgettable. One reason I signed up with DOW was because of its expressed neutrality; I wanted to be able to work with both the Albanian and Serbian midwives in Kosovo. For my first session with the Serbian midwives, I arrived to teach a postpartum course, complete with an overhead projector and Serbian-translated transparencies and handouts. But the electricity and generator were not functioning that day, and the small room in the temporary clinic shelter was damp, cold, and foul-smelling. Because the sun was shining, we all agreed to move our chairs outside. The front yard made a wonderful classroom for our growing group, and townsfolk passing by, and a few large pigs, chickens, and dogs soon joined the eight midwives. Fortunately, it was possible to teach with tanks driving by and soldiers calling out to the young midwives!

After returning twice the following week to practice neonatal resuscitation and discuss evidence-based obstetrical practices, the midwives asked for a session on internal repair of episiotomies and tears. Eager to help them practice this new suturing technique, I cut up the ends of an unused foam mattress that I found behind a storage cabinet in the DOW headquarters. Despite struggling to perfect the skill with inadequate suture materials and worn needle holders, the midwives were enthusiastic and appreciative.

Today was my final day with the DOW project in Kosovo. I am humbled as I pack up and prepare to return to the United States. I have learned so much about courage, stamina, making do, generosity, and the universal bond among women. After 25 years of practice in the States, this experience has taught me what midwifery means on a universal level. As a result, I enthusiastically encourage any American midwife to consider taking an international assignment. You will find the experience enriching and rewarding beyond measure!

Journal of Midwifery and Women's Health 2001; 46(2): 82–85

Midwifery in northern Belize

Diane B Boyer, Carrie Klima, Judith Jennrich, Jeanne E Raisler

During several volunteer experiences in the Corozal District in northern Belize, the authors worked with and interviewed traditional midwives, midwife educators, administrators, and professional midwives, who practice in public health clinics, rural health outposts, and a government hospital. One interview with a traditional midwife from a rural Mayan village garnered interesting information about her 63-year practice, which is compared with the practice of professional midwives. Issues important to midwifery and health care in Belize are discussed. The interviews and the authors' own experiences reveal changing birthing practices, as well as the continued importance of midwives in the care of childbearing women in northern Belize.

Introduction

Anselma Yam, a diminutive 81-year-old woman from the rural Mayan village of Patchakan in northern Belize, was 18 when her grandmother began teaching her the art of midwifery. During her 63 years of practice attending home births, she has delivered one footling breech and three sets of twins without complications and has never had a perinatal death. Her way of traditional birthing represents a declining aspect of midwifery practice in Belize. Although unsure of the reason, and not convinced that it is better for mothers and babies, Anselma believes that in their fear of birth, women are encouraged by their families and clinic workers to go to the hospital. She said that she loves midwifery and is very sad that no woman from the village has come forward to learn from her. She believes it takes 'much courage' to be a midwife and that there are few women in the village with this trait. When asked what she liked most about midwifery, she replied, *'Todo me gusta'* (I like it all). During a combined total of more than 52 weeks of volunteer practice and teaching in

the Corozal District of northern Belize from 1992 to 1999, the authors observed and interviewed Anselma, four other traditional birth attendants (TBAs), six professional midwives, midwife educators, and administrators. Informed consent was obtained before all interviews.

Belize and its people

Belize is a small country in Central America, just south of the Yucatan peninsula of Mexico, with Guatemala on the west and the Caribbean Sea on the east. Before its independence from Great Britain in 1981, Belize was known as British Honduras. Only 174 miles long and 68 miles wide, Belize had a population of 222,000 in 1996, estimated to rise to 245,000 by 2000 (Cubola Productions, 1991; Pan American Health Organization, 1995, 1998; National Committee for Families and Children and UNICEF Belize, 1997). Approximately one-quarter of the population is concentrated in Belize City. The country is divided into six administrative districts, the northernmost of which is Corozal District.

The economy is largely based on agriculture and fishing, with sugar cane, bananas, citrus, and rice as major crops (Cubola Productions, 1991). Tourism provides an increasingly important source of income. The main attractions are the islands, or cayes, off the coast, which are near the longest coral reef in the Western Hemisphere, and a lure for snorkelers and divers. Mayan ruins dot the countryside, which ranges from low, often swampy areas near the coast to rainforest in the south, and mountainous areas in the south and west. The climate is semitropical, and temperatures are often above 90°F with 90% humidity.

Belize is geographically in Central America but is similar to Caribbean countries in its culture, politics, and economy (Pan American Health Organization, 1998). Although the population is small, the people of Belize represent a fascinating mix of origins and cultures, with

Creoles, Mestizos, Mayans, Garifuna, Asians, and Europeans as the main groups. In the 1990s, Belize experienced an influx of immigrants from other Central American countries. English is the official language, but Spanish, Creole, and Garifuna are also spoken. According to the Pan American Health Organization (PAHO, 1998), the basic literacy rate in 1996 was 75%, and 33% of Belizeans were considered poor (unable to meet expenses on basic food and nonfood items).

Health status and services in Belize

Recent economic trends in Belize have led to decreased government spending on health services, resulting in cuts in services in rural communities and health posts. Although the government has provided health services at little charge over the years, efforts are now being made to recover costs. The National Health Plan 1996–2000 provides for universal access to comprehensive health services through primary health care, by using a decentralized approach and privatization of some health services. However, these reforms have not been fully achieved (Pan American Health Organization, 1998). In the National Health Plan, officials cite 'increased health costs and decreasing financial resources available at national and international levels as barriers which would have to be overcome to achieve the goals of the plan' (Belize Ministry of Health and Sports, 1996).

There are seven public hospitals in Belize, one in each district and the Karl Heusner Memorial Hospital, which is the national referral hospital, in Belize City (Belize Ministry of Health and Sports, 1996). In addition, there are two small private hospitals. There is a neonatal intensive care unit at Karl Heusner, but no adult or pediatric intensive care units in Belize. People with sufficient funds often seek care in Mexico or the United States. There are 40 public health centers and 35 rural health posts, providing maternal and child health services, public health nursing, treatment for minor ailments, health education, and some specialized services (Pan American Health Organization, 1998). In 1995, there were six physicians, 14 nurses, and 10 professional midwives per 10,000 population (Pan American Health Organization, 1993; Belize Ministry of Health and Sports, 1996; Central Statistical Office, 1996).

Data from the PAHO indicate that, in 1996, life expectancy at birth was 71.8 years for females and 69.9 for males. The average number of children per woman was 4.6. During the 1993–1996 period, heart disease was the leading cause of death for both males and females. Respiratory diseases were the main reason for hospitalization among males. Complications of pregnancy were the leading cause of hospitalization for females; 37% of these admissions were related to abortions, which are illegal in Belize. More than half (51.7%) of pregnant women have iron deficiency anemia. The main causes of infant mortality, which decreased from 31.5/1000 live births in 1993 to 26/1000 in 1996, were perinatal asphyxia, low birth weight, and infections, primarily respiratory. Leading causes of maternal mortality, which was 16.1/100,000 live births in 1993 and 13.9/100,000 in 1996, were hemorrhage, pulmonary embolism, eclampsia, and abortion. For comparison, the infant mortality rates were 34/1000 in Mexico, 52/1000 in Nicaragua, and 14/1000 in Costa Rica during this time period. Maternal mortality was 49/100,000 in Mexico, 60/100,000 in Nicaragua, and 19/100,000 in Costa Rica (Pan American Health Organization, 1998).

Belize has launched a 'baby-friendly hospital' initiative, with one of its goals the promotion of breastfeeding. However, fewer than half (46%) of babies are exclusively breastfed to four months (Pan American Health Organization, 1998). Corozal District Hospital is working toward 'baby-friendly hospital' status, and in 1998, the authors taught part of a workshop on breastfeeding held for TBAs, community health workers, nurses, midwives, and physicians in the district.

The Corozal District and its midwives

Corozal is the northernmost district in Belize, with a population of about 30,000. With a location close to Mexico, many people in the district speak Spanish. There are many Mayans in the area, but use of the Mayan language seems to be waning, although occasional Mayan words are incorporated into Spanish or English. Sugar cane is the primary agricultural crop.

The main health care facilities in Corozal District are the government-run 32-bed Corozal Hospital and Corozal Clinic, and the Presbyterian Clinic in Patchakan village, 12 miles from Corozal Town. The authors had the opportunity to work in all three facilities. The Corozal Hospital offers inpatient and outpatient services, whereas the Corozal Clinic provides maternal and child health services, sexually transmitted disease (STD) clinics, and some illness care. The clinic has an active community outreach program, and the immunization rate in the area is 80% (G. Heredia, personal communication), higher than many cities in the United States. Family planning services are offered in conjunction with the Belize Family Life Association, a nongovernmental organization associated with International Planned Parenthood. The Presbyterian Clinic in Patchakan is a private facility that offers primary care services with volunteer health care providers enlisted for blocks of service time. There are also approximately 10 private physicians who see outpatients in their offices and may admit patients to the hospital, where care is assumed by government doctors.

In addition, selected villagers have been trained as community health workers and traditional birth attendants.

Infectious diseases, including parasitic infections, are a major cause of morbidity and mortality in Corozal District, and chronic diseases, especially diabetes and heart disease, are common. Machete wounds related to sugar cane farming and fights are frequent, as are abscesses, resulting from numerous insect bites and poor sanitary conditions.

In 1998 there were 875 registered births for the 28,464 population in Corozal District, a birth rate of 30.7/1000 (M. Chavaria, personal communication). The overall birth rate in Belize was 30.9/1000 in 1998 (Pan American Health Organization, 1998). In 1996, Corozal District had the lowest infant mortality rate in Belize, at 13.8/1000 (Pan American Health Organization, 1995). Respiratory infections were the main cause of infant deaths (G. Heredia, personal communication).

Traditional birth attendants in the Corozal District

The area that is now Corozal District was inhabited by Mayans before the European invasion, and traditional midwives have no doubt been attending births in the area as long as there have been human populations. More recently, TBAs with government-supported training provide delivery services at home primarily in rural areas, with at least one home visit prenatally to observe conditions and advise the family. TBAs are taught to advise primigravidas and grand multiparas to go to the hospital for delivery. Women are also encouraged to go to the Corozal Clinic for prenatal and postpartum care, where many of the TBAs also participate in providing care (G. Heredia, personal communication).

According to Guillermina Heredia, Director of Maternal-Child Health in Corozal District, formal TBA training in the district began in the 1980s. Traditional midwives practising without formal training, as well as new candidates selected by vote in their villages, are recruited into the training program. Although TBAs trained in earlier years may not be able to read and write, new candidates must be literate. Other selection criteria are personality, kindness, and the people's confidence in them. It is illegal in Belize to practice as a TBA without formal training (G. Heredia, personal communication). However, according to the Belize Inspector of Midwives, if a nontrained TBA is reported to be practising, the approach is not punitive, but an attempt is made to enroll the TBA in a training program.

The purpose of the TBA training program is to 'provide TBAs with the knowledge and skills needed to safely manage the pregnant woman, who is living in rural areas, during pregnancy, labor, delivery, and the immediate care of the newborn infant' (Ministry of Health, 1986). Emphasis is on recognition and timely referral of deviations from normal. TBAs are also expected to give advice on child rearing and child spacing and to serve as role models in the community (Ministry of Health, 1986).

The TBA training program consists of one month of classes, one month of providing prenatal care in the Corozal Clinic, observation of 20 births, and then attendance at 20 in-hospital births. After the classroom and clinical aspects of the program are completed, a nurse evaluates the TBA while she works for one month in the community. If the evaluation is satisfactory, she can then work independently. Three or four TBAs are trained at a time for villages that need them. A TBA training manual is the principal tool for training (Ministry of Health, 1986). Nurse Heredia observed that the training has become much easier with the recent literacy requirements.

Refresher courses are held every three months for those who have completed the TBA program. The authors participated in one of these courses and found the 20 TBA participants to be a highly knowledgeable group. The course contained content about family planning as well as obstetrics. Issues raised by the TBAs included problems with clients not paying and perceived lack of proper attention to referrals they made to the hospital. The charge for the entire pregnancy is commonly $50 BZ ($25 US), including the delivery and daily home visits for 8–10 days postpartum to care for the mother and baby and to do laundry.

Interview with Anselma Yam

During their work at the Presbyterian clinic in Patchakan, a rural Mayan village of about 950 people, the authors became acquainted with Anselma Yam, the local traditional midwife. Interviews with Anselma were conducted in the kitchen of her home, a typical rural Belizean thatched-roof, earth-floored house. Woodsmoke from the cooking fire scented the air, and chickens, cats, dogs, and grandchildren wandered through during the visits.

Anselma has always lived in Patchakan, which is about 12 miles inland from Corozal Town. At the age of 18, she began to learn about midwifery from her grandmother, who, as the only midwife in the community, was the main source of health information for the village. When Anslema began her training 63 years ago, midwifery in rural villages in Belize was learned exclusively by apprenticeship. In addition to her grandmother, Anselma learned from a midwife in a neighboring village. Many years later, when formal TBA training began in Belize, Anselma took the course, even though by that time she had attended hundreds of births. She believes that the primary benefits were learning about cleanliness and infection control, as well as gaining access to the birth kits supplied to TBAs after their training. Anselma proudly showed her birth kit, which contained an apron, gloves, string, scissors, cord clamps, bulb syringe, alcohol, a pan for boiling instruments, and honey to feed the baby if the mother does not have milk. TBAs are required to record the births in a delivery log, and Anselma's log recorded 48 births between 1990 and 1994. Because Anselma cannot read or write, the community health nurse or Anselma's granddaughter writes the information in the log.

During pregnancy, most women obtain prenatal care from professional midwives at the government clinic. The TBAs, including Anselma, regularly rotate to the clinic to assist with prenatal care. Anselma visits each woman in her home three times before the birth of the baby to observe the cleanliness of the house and the preparations for the baby, iron sheets and diapers to disinfect them, perform an abdominal examination to determine the position of the baby, and listen to the fetal heart rate with a Pinard fetoscope.

The advice TBAs give to women during pregnancy about nutrition seems to be grounded in the theories of hot/cold, common in Latin American cultures. During pregnancy, Anselma encourages women to avoid chilies, eggs, and very cold or hot foods. She recommends papaya, although the reasons for this were not clear. Other TBAs interviewed advised eating many fruits and vegetables, fish, liver, and carrot juice, and avoiding cola drinks and sweets. Women are counseled to work for the first seven months of pregnancy and rest for the last two months. They are also advised to avoid sexual intercourse after seven months.

When labor begins, Anselma is usually summoned by a family member, sometimes in a large sugar cane truck, because very few Belizeans own their own vehicles. Most often she arrives early in the labor process and finds much to do in preparation for the birth. She always brings her birth kit and a picture of the Virgin Mary, because 'She is the Saint of Children and will watch over the baby during labor'.

It is unusual for the father of the baby to be present during the labor and birth. His role is more often to stand by to transport the mother to the hospital in case of emergency. In Belize, birth is considered the purview of women, and mothers and sisters are often present to provide support to the woman and her family during labor.

Women are encouraged to assume whatever positions they find comfortable in labor, and to take fluids and eat lightly. Anselma said that most women prefer to walk until the latter part of labor, but do not want to eat. She performs vaginal examinations infrequently, using a finger cot, and listens to the baby's heartbeat every hour. As the time of birth draws closer, the bed is readied with the previously prepared clean linens. Women usually give birth lying on their beds with their legs apart. Other TBAs interviewed also attend births with women in this position. Anselma frequently uses oil on the perineum and cannot remember encountering any serious lacerations. She proudly said that the biggest baby she had delivered was nine pounds. After the birth, she cuts the cord with sterile scissors, which she boiled upon her arrival and uses a sterile cord clamp provided by the government. She delivers the placenta and performs external uterine massage. TBAs are given ergotrate to use in case of postpartum hemorrhage, but Anselma rarely uses this. The baby is usually put to breast right after the birth.

Anselma described the types of problems experienced throughout her career and the traditional remedies for complications encountered during labor and birth. For long labors, she boils cloves for tea, which is given to the woman to drink to make contractions stronger and more frequent. She also uses *Oil of Essencia de Marvelosa* in water massaged on the abdomen to start labor or to relieve severe labor pains. This product comes from Guatemala and is the extract of a flower (E. Yam, personal communication). In cases of retained placenta, sitz baths are made with traditional herbs or garlic is roasted and given to the birthing woman to chew to facilitate placental expulsion. If serious problems develop, Anselma will send a woman to the hospital.

Anselma usually stays with the mother for about six hours after the birth and then returns daily for 10 days. During these visits, she washes the perineum with clean water, performs massage to hasten recovery, cleans the umbilical cord with alcohol, and assesses whether the baby is healthy and eating well and the new mother is without signs of infection. Because tetanus is endemic in Belize and a frequent cause of neonatal morbidity and mortality, Anselma assesses diligently for signs of infection of the umbilicus and warns against some dangerous traditional practices, such as placing feces or dirt on the umbilical cord. The usual charge for her services is $30 BZ ($15 US). 'Sometimes I have been given chickens, a pig, or a cow for my work', she said laughing.

Anselma said that she loves midwifery and is sad that few women are now learning to be TBAs. She is critical of midwives who do not keep confidences and gossip about the women and their homes. Anselma is not convinced that the trend for hospital births is better for mothers and babies. 'At the hospital they pay $70 BZ, and no one comes to their house before to help them prepare and no one visits them after.'

Professional midwives

The route into professional midwifery in Belize for Nurse S. (who wished to remain anonymous) was very different from Anselma's story. Midwifery is considered an advanced practice nursing role, and nursing and midwifery education have been free. After completing the three-year professional nursing program and 10 years of nursing experience, Nurse S. decided to become a midwife as a chance for professional advancement. She applied to the only program in the country, at the Belize School of Nursing in Belize City. This program admitted eight students in 1999 (P. Beet, personal communication). The applicant must be recommended by a nursing sister at the hospital where she has worked and by the district medical officer. The program is one year in length and contains 455 hours of theory and 1440 hours of clinical practice, including attending 25 births (P. Beet, personal communication). Upon passing a written, oral, and practical examination given by the Nurses and Midwives Council of Belize, midwifery graduates receive a midwifery license in addition to their nursing license.

Graduates must take a minimum of a two-year contract after graduation to pay back the government. There are few private employment opportunities, and almost all nurses and midwives in Belize work for the government and can be assigned to a post anywhere needed in the country. Nurse S. was fortunate to be assigned back to her home community. Salaries for midwives have improved recently, but they are still not well paid, considering the education required and the level of responsibility (F. Ogaldez, personal communication).

There are two other routes into midwifery practice in Belize. Practical nurses, after one year of training and two or three years of work experience, may apply to the one-year program for practical midwives. After passing their licensure examination, they work under the supervision of professional midwives in hospitals. Rural health nurses receive one year of education as practical nurses, one year of midwifery education, and additional training in community health. They work independently in public health in rural areas. As of May 2000, there were 60 professional midwives, 32 practical midwives, and 44 rural health nurses with midwifery training who were licensed in Belize (M. Castillo, registrar, personal communication). Continuing education for nurses and midwives is not mandated for continued licensure, although the Belize inspector of midwives anticipates that this will be a requirement in the future.

Professional midwives work in either the public health clinics or the hospital, but usually not both, so the only midwives in Belize doing comprehensive care are traditional midwives in the rural areas. Nurse S., who is providing intrapartum and postpartum care in a district hospital, thinks it would be beneficial if the midwives in the hospital and in public health cross-trained and kept current in both areas so there would be more flexibility in staffing. Although the professional midwives may attend a few home births during their training, they rarely do so after graduation.

Professional midwives staff the small labor and delivery unit at Corozal Hospital around the clock in eight-hour shifts, and they attend most of the births in the district, as is true throughout Belize. The delivery room contains two delivery tables separated by curtains. Mothers walk in early labor and can have fluids and some food if they want. Meperidine is sometimes used for pain, although most women receive no pain medication. Births occur with mothers in the lithotomy position, and episiotomies are frequently performed on primigravidas. The midwives cut and repair episiotomies but must have a physician order for inductions and other medications. If necessary, they may start an IV for dehydration and give pitocin for postpartum hemorrhage without a physician order. Mothers breastfeed right away, and there is very little bottlefeeding while in hospital. Family members are not present at delivery. Twenty-four-hour postpartum discharge is routine after an uncomplicated birth. Total cost for the delivery is $75 BZ ($37.50 US), but many people are unable to pay (F. Ogaldez, personal communication).

Physician collaboration for the midwives was variable during the authors' visits. For a time, a Cuban obstetrician was stationed in Corozal, but more often consultation was provided by a general practitioner, with a general surgeon doing cesarean sections. Lack of readily available obstetrician consultation and referral is a major practice issue mentioned by all professional midwives interviewed.

In the first eight months of 1999, there were 349 deliveries, with a 26% cesarean section rate. The most frequent indications for cesarean sections were cephalopelvic disproportion and prolonged labor. Spinal anesthesia was used, and the usual hospital stay was three to four days (F. Ogaldez, personal communication). Ultrasound and electronic fetal monitoring are not available in the Corozal Hospital or Clinic. In one instance when a breech presentation was diagnosed by the staff midwife and one of the authors, the physician disagreed, and the issue was settled by a physician-ordered X-ray (the baby was breech).

The professional midwives interviewed said that access to continuing education is a major issue for midwives, particularly in rural areas. They mentioned resuscitation of the newborn, management of pre-eclampsia, and breech delivery as examples of workshops most needed. Other practice issues and concerns mentioned by the professional midwives interviewed were the need for increased prenatal classes for mothers, the need to decrease the number of unplanned pregnancies, and the need for more incorporation of support persons in labor. Poor health of women before conception, especially anemia, late prenatal care, and a need for special programs for HIV-positive pregnant women are also of concern to these midwives. A major issue is a countrywide shortage of midwives. At Corozal Hospital in 1999 there were five midwives to staff three daily shifts seven days a week. One response by the government to the shortage has been to import nurses and midwives from Cuba, Nigeria, and Guyana to work on contract in Belize.

The Belizean midwives interviewed consider the fact that most of the births in the country are attended by midwives who usually are able to detect complications and to intervene in time to prevent bad outcomes as a major accomplishment of professional midwives. They also noted that midwives are placing increased emphasis on teaching the mother and on breastfeeding. They believe that midwives are respected in their communities, although respect from physicians is variable.

The professional organization for midwives in Belize is the Nurses' Association of Belize, which has district branches. This is a voluntary organization with nominal annual dues to which most midwives belong. The activities of the organization involve welfare, economics, education, and policy (P. Beet, personal communication). The Corozal branch of the Nurses' Association conducts fundraisers such as dances, variety shows, and a snack shop at the hospital to support continuing education for members. They select nurses to sponsor for international conferences by a random drawing and also give small short-term loans for members in need (F. Ogaldez, personal communication). None of the midwives interviewed voiced a need to have a separate professional organization.

Some midwives think that the professional organization should take a more active policy role nationally to make the views of midwives and nurses known to the Ministry of Health. These midwives perceive that they have little input into policy and administrative matters. One gave an example of how plans were made for renovation of the labor and delivery unit of a hospital without consulting the midwives who work there. However, on a recent visit to Belize, one of the authors noted that high-level nursing administrators are involved in frequent government meetings regarding the implementation of the National Health Plan. The published report of the Belize National Health Plan also lists a number of nurses and midwives, including some interviewed for this article, as participants in the planning process (Belize Ministry of Health and Sports, 1996).

The future of midwifery in Belize

A major change that one professional midwife has seen in more than 30 years of practice in Belize is that there are fewer prolonged labors because the decision to intervene is made much earlier. Other changes mentioned were discontinuation of enemas and perineal shaves in labor. There have been increased efforts to promote breastfeeding and, as the education of women has improved, use of family planning is increasing. Technology such as dopplers, fetal monitoring, and ultrasound may become more available.

Another trend is that the number of home births has decreased considerably. In 1995, 18% of registered births in the country took place at home compared to 38% in 1985, and home births will probably continue to decline as the numbers of TBAs decrease (Central Statistical Office, 1996). Although TBA training continues, with recruitment of a few new TBAs in small rural villages, it is obvious that traditional midwifery with home births is declining in Belize. Some women may prefer TBAs because they are familiar and conduct traditional practices such as massage, but unless younger TBAs can be recruited, they will not have a major role in childbearing in Belize in the future. However, one professional midwife believes that the current influx of midwives from other countries, with accompanying cultural and communication difficulties, may encourage some childbearing women to turn to their local TBAs for care.

Preparation of professional midwives is also changing. A new baccalaureate program in nursing matriculated its first class at the University of Belize in the fall of 2000. Midwifery education will remain postgraduate, although educators believe that the change in basic nursing preparation will lead to as yet unspecified changes in midwifery education as well (P. Beet, personal communication). Some midwives have expressed concern that the move to baccalaureate education will make nursing education less accessible. Nursing and midwifery education have been free at the Belize School of Nursing, but only limited funding is now available for students in the program at the University of Belize. Access to affordable continuing education will continue to be an issue.

Conclusion

Interviews with midwives, health care administrators, and educators as well as the observations of the authors support the prediction that professional midwives will continue to play an essential role for the foreseeable future in Belize, providing care for most childbearing women. At present, TBAs play a useful role, but this will decline unless new TBAs can be recruited. The economic and political forces that affect health care in Belize also affect the education and practice of midwives. The ultimate outcomes of the decentralization and privatization that are part of the National Health Plan and their effect on midwives remain to be seen. Midwives have made strides in improving care for women and newborns, but they continue to be challenged by health care forces that may not recognize their important role and the expertise they can provide toward women's health care. Some midwives at the local level believe that they need more input into health planning and policy. The division between midwives who work in the community and those who provide care in hospitals may limit their abilities to work together effectively. Some midwives support the idea of developing a new practice model that would allow them to work in both the community and the hospital. A unified model might facilitate cohesiveness that could lead to increased political effectiveness.

Future research on midwifery in Belize could investigate the trend toward fewer home births with TBAs, determining why women choose not to use them and whether there are ways to reverse the trend. TBAs have much to offer to women in rural villages who might have to travel long distances and be away from their families to have their babies in the district hospital. Determining reasons why local women choose not to become TBAs would also be useful. Other studies could investigate the traditional remedies used by TBAs. Professional midwives could study clinical questions such as effective ways to promote breastfeeding, inexpensive methods to reduce iron deficiency anemia, and ways to reduce transmission of STDs and HIV.

The recent efforts to provide universal health care have left Belizeans with more questions than answers. What health care services will be provided? Who will provide them? Where will they be given? Who will pay? These are questions that remain unanswered at this time. Belizean midwives, who are committed to improving health care for their communities, are concerned and waiting for answers. Anselma Yam looks back at the past and also toward the future. As the authors were leaving her home, she showed an old, framed photograph of her mother and grandmother and said, 'This is my history', then drew her nine-year-old granddaughter next to her. 'Maybe she will be a midwife when she grows up.' Whatever the future may bring, the authors feel privileged to have been able to work with the dedicated midwives of Belize and hope to continue this association (Pan American Health Organization, 1993).

Acknowledgements

The authors thank Sabina Dambrauskas, CNM, MSN and Maria Thibault, RN, FNP for their assistance with gathering the interview data for this article, and the Belizean midwives who were so generous in sharing their time and experiences with us.

REFERENCES

Belize Ministry of Health and Sports. 1996. The Quest for Equity: Belize National Health Plan, 1996–2000. Government of Belize, Belmopan, Belize

Central Statistical Office. 1996. Belize Abstract of Statistics. Ministry of Finance, Belmopan, Belize

Cubola Productions. 1991. Atlas of Belize. Cubola Productions, Benque Viejo del Carmen, Belize

Ministry of Health. 1986. Traditional Birth Attendants Manual. Government of Belize, Belmopan, Belize

National Committee for Families and Children and UNICEF Belize. 1997. The right to a future. The Government of Belize Central Statistical Office, Belmopan, Belize

Pan American Health Organization. 1993. Implementation of the Global Strategy for Health for All by the Year 2000, Vol. 3, Region of the Americas. World Health Organization, Washington

Pan American Health Organization. 1995. Health Statistics from the Americas. World Health Organization, Washington

Pan American Health Organization. 1998. Health in the Americas. World Health Organization, Washington

Journal of Midwifery and Women's Health 2001; 46(1): 33–39

Questions for debate

Do you think that all women should be entitled to ask to have a midwife who shares their cultural background and/or their spiritual or philosophical beliefs, or is it enough for midwives to have an understanding of different cultural, spiritual, philosophical and other differences?

In this ever-changing world, how can midwives develop an understanding of the diversity of cultures and belief systems held by the women they attend?

Exploring Pregnancy...

SECTION CONTENTS

Before you read the articles in this section, and especially the original article which Lorna Davies has written, you may like to write a few notes on each of the following questions:
- How do you feel about your own body?
- How do you feel about the bodies of pregnant women?
- If you have been pregnant yourself, how did you feel about your pregnant body?

No one is ever going to look at what you have written, so it is safe to be honest!

Risk and risk assessment in pregnancy – do we scare because we care?

Katja Stahl, Vanora Hundley

Objective: to assess whether being labelled 'high-risk' affects women's psychosocial state in pregnancy.

Design: prospective, cross-sectional, non-experimental, case–control study.

Setting: a large city in Germany.

Participants: women between 22 and 41 weeks gestation were identified at antenatal classes and invited to participate in the study. Of the 147 women who were given a questionnaire, 82% (122) responded but only 75% (111) were eligible for inclusion in the study. Of these 111 women, 57 were classified as 'labelled high-risk' and 54 as 'no-risk' according to the risks documented in their antenatal records.

Measurements: women's psychosocial state was assessed using a validated, anonymous, self-completed questionnaire, the *Abbreviated Scale for the Assessment of Psychosocial State in Pregnancy* (Goldenberg et al., 1997). Analysis of covariance (ANCOVA) was performed to test the effect of the risk label on psychosocial state. The effect of other variables, such as parity or education, was also tested.

Findings: the effect of the risk label on psychosocial state after adjusting for age was statistically significant ($R^2 = 0.07$, $F = 7.59$, df $= 1$, $p = 0.001$). No significant differences were found for the other independent variables. The data showed that a large number of women had one or more risk factors and that 71% were booked for obstetrician-led care. A high variability in obstetrician's documentation of women's risk factors was also found.

Conclusion: the data suggest that labelling women to be 'at risk' may negatively affect their psychosocial state. The findings highlight the need to re-evaluate the risk catalogue in the German antenatal record (*Mutterpass*) as well as the German maternity guidelines (*Mutterschaftsrichtlinien*). Although this study was conducted within the German system of antenatal care, the findings raise questions about the effects of risk labelling in maternity care wherever it is practised. Further research is needed to assess women's psychosocial state in a more representative sample, to explore women's experiences and satisfaction with the practice of risk assessment and to investigate the reasons for the high variability in documenting women's risk factors.

Introduction

In many countries the practice of trying to identify those women who are at high or low obstetric risk was initiated as a means of trying to reduce maternal and neonatal mortality. For example, in the UK, risk assessment seems to have begun in response to recommendations by the Cranbrook Committee in 1959 (Ministry of Health, 1959). The committee proposed criteria to help identify women who were 'suitable' for care in general practitioner units, with a view to reducing maternal mortality. In Germany, systematic risk assessment in pregnancy began with the incorporation of antenatal services into the standard health care plan of health insurance policies in 1966. This was a result of the then prevailing debate among politicians and the medical professions about the need for a stronger focus on prophylaxis and prevention in health care in general and the need to improve the antenatal care system in particular, as the perinatal mortality rates were still higher than those in other European countries (Schlieper, 1997; Schumann, 2000).

Contemporary antenatal care in Germany is predominantly obstetrician-led. The fact that midwives are also allowed to provide antenatal care for low-risk women is not very well known among pregnant women. The structure and content of the antenatal care programme is defined by maternity guidelines (*Mutterschaftsrichtlinien* – Bundesausschuss der Ärzte und Krankenkassen, 1998) and obstetricians are required to provide antenatal care accordingly; however, midwives are not. Prenatal care activities are documented in a hand-held antenatal record (the *Mutterpass*, literally 'mother passport'), which contains, among other things, a list of 52 risk factors that have to be assessed at 'booking' and during pregnancy (Box 3.1.1). The obstetrician completes this checklist, thereby identifying women who are 'high-risk' and putting a tick in a red box given for this purpose. Women who are not categorized as 'high-risk' are eligible to have antenatal care provided by a midwife.

The findings of a study by Haertsch et al. (1999) that compared seven guidelines for antenatal care from the USA, Canada, Australia and Germany illustrate the biomedical focus and technological dominance of all these guidelines. Only two of the seven guidelines were based on scientific evidence; the others, which included the recommendations of the German guidelines, were 'based primarily on expert opinion' (Haertsch et al., 1999, p. 30).

While the aim of risk assessment has been to improve mortality and sometimes morbidity outcomes, their effectiveness in achieving this aim is still very much debated (Alexander & Keirse, 1989; Tew, 1998; Enkin et al., 2000). Points of critique include the low sensitivity, specificity and predictive values of the tools used to assess risk, and the problems associated with the definition of risk factors. The issue of risk assessment is made more complex by the fact that professional groups and women often interpret the term 'risk' in very different ways. Health care practitioners, on the one hand, tend to rely heavily on epidemiological assumptions in discussing risk. Their understanding of risk reflects their specialised knowledge and training, as well as their personalised values and experiences (Handwerker, 1994; Lupton, 1999). Women's understanding of risk, on the other hand, tends to be far more contextual, individualised and embedded in their social environment and everyday lives (Handwerker, 1994; Lupton, 1999; Saxell, 2000), and women's self-rating of pregnancy risk may very well differ from the practitioner's assessment (Heaman et al., 1992).

Little attention has been paid to the effect of risk assessment in terms of maternal mental health and few studies have examined the effect of the label 'high-risk' on women's psychosocial state. A small qualitative Canadian study reported by Saxell (2000), which intended to probe the meaning that women and midwives placed on risk and on the label 'high-risk', found that half of the women in the study associated the label 'high-risk' with the possibility of complications occurring or of the baby not being healthy. Some women felt angry or resentful that a label was being placed on them that could drastically alter their care and some felt a loss of control and a sense of powerlessness by being labelled 'high-risk'. However, it was pointed out that the women in this study represented an exceptional minority whose views might not be shared by most women (Saxell, 2000). Handwerker (1994) examined interactions between pregnant women and health care professionals in a qualitative study and suggested that labelling poor pregnant women 'high-risk' implicitly and explicitly makes them accountable if they are unable to change their behaviour as prescribed by health professionals, leading to feelings of guilt and increased stress, which in turn may lower the uptake of antenatal care. Other studies point out that 'high-risk' women have less positive expectations for their childbirth experience and this leads to increased anxiety (Heaman et al., 1992), more stress and more negative emotions (Hatmaker & Kemp, 1998). In addition, these women perceived their overall risk and risk for specific outcomes as significantly higher than low-risk women (Gupton et al., 2001). However, the inclusion criteria for the 'high-risk' groups in these studies have either required hospitalisation for more than 48 hours (Heaman et al., 1992; Gupton et al., 2001) or enrolment in a home-uterine-activity-monitoring programme due to being at risk for preterm birth (Hatmaker & Kemp, 1998), and therefore it is not possible to distinguish between the effect of the actual condition of the women and the effect that the label 'high-risk' may have had. One Finnish study (Melender, 2002) suggested that alarming information received from health care providers contributed to fears associated with pregnancy and childbirth, but the study did not refer explicitly to the label 'high-risk'.

The scarcity of literature on the effects of being labelled 'high-risk', together with the fact that the German antenatal care system seems to lead to a considerably high number of pregnant women being labelled 'high-risk', raises the question of whether the label 'high-risk' affects the psychosocial state of pregnant women.

Method

Research question and operational definitions

This study was designed to examine whether the label 'high-risk' given to women who would be considered to be at low obstetric risk outside Germany affects the psychosocial state of these pregnant women. Psychosocial status was taken to mean a combination of

Box 3.1.1 Risk catalogue as displayed in the *Mutterpass*

Medical and family history/booking	Genuine 'high-risk'*	Labelled 'high-risk'†	Not mentioned‡
Family history (e.g. diabetes, hypertension, anomalies, genetic disorders, psychiatric disorders)			X
Allergy, e.g. against drugs			X
Previous blood transfusion			X
Psychological stress (family, job)			X
Social disadvantage (integration problems, economic problems)			X
Small of stature			X
Skeletal deformities			X
Previous pregnancy less than a year ago			X
Other (to be specified)			X
Obesity		X	
Age < 18 years		X	
Age > 35 years		X	
Multiparity (> 4)		X	
Infertility treatment		X	
More than two miscarriages/terminations		X	
Complications during previous delivery		X	
Previous postpartum complications		X	
Previous caesarean section		X	
Medical history (e.g. heart, lung, liver, renal, neurological or psychiatric disorder) (to be specified)	(X)§	(X)§	
Coagulation disorder	X		
Rhesus incompatibility in previous pregnancies	X		
Diabetes mellitus	X		
Previous pre-term birth (before completed 37 weeks)	X		
Previous small for gestational age	X		
Previous perinatal death or anomaly	X		
Other uterus surgery	X		
Conditions occurring during pregnancy			
General medical conditions needing treatment (to be specified)*			X
Regular medication			X
Psychological stress			X
Socio-economic problems			X
Risks from other blood tests			X
Hypotension			X
Other (to be specified)			X
Uncertain duration of pregnancy		X	
Anaemia		X	
Abnormal lie		X	
Drug or alcohol abuse	X		
Haemorrhage before 28 weeks	X		
Haemorrhage after 28 weeks	X		
Placenta praevia	X		
Multiple pregnancy	X		
Hydramnios	X		
Oligohydramnios	X		
Insufficient placenta	X		
Insufficient cervix	X		
Pre-term contractions/labour	X		
Urinary tract infection	X		
Indirect Coombs test positive	X		
Hypertension (BP > 140/90)	X		
Proteinuria > 1000 mg/l	X		
Moderate to massive oedema	X		
Gestational diabetes	X		

*Risk factors that would assign the woman to obstetrician-led care in Germany as well as in Scotland and the Netherlands.

†Risk factors that would assign the woman to obstetrician-led care in Germany but would leave the woman eligible for midwifery-led care in Scotland and the Netherlands (Area Maternity Service Committee for Grampian, 1998; Ziekenfondsraad, 1998).

‡Risk factors that are listed in the *Mutterpass* but are not mentioned in the *Mutterschaftsrichtlinien*; women with these risk factors are considered to be 'no risk' in this study (Box 3.1.2).

§May lead to categorisation either as 'genuine high-risk' or 'labelled high-risk' depending on specification.

the affective states and cognitive factors of anxiety, depression, self-esteem mastery and perceived stress as measured by the Goldenberg et al. (1997) scale. The label 'high-risk' was taken to be the label that was assigned to pregnant women when they showed a characteristic or condition that was perceived to be associated with an increased risk of an adverse pregnancy outcome.

Design

This was a prospective, cross-sectional, non-experimental, case–control study. This type of study design is typically used in retrospective ex post facto research, where the health outcome has already occurred and a person with a certain condition (a case) is compared with a similar person without that condition (a matched control) in terms of antecedents to the outcome (Carter, 1996; Polit et al., 2001). However, case–control studies can also be used prospectively to explore future outcomes in groups with certain conditions. Examples in maternity care have included Kilbride et al. (1999), Karsenti et al. (2001) and Sobande et al. (2002). Such studies are sometimes called cohort studies; however, this term is usually associated with longer-term follow-up (Costei et al., 2002) than was the case in this study. The women in this study had already been allocated their risk status, thus making them 'cases'; the outcome of interest was their psychosocial state at the time that they attended for antenatal education.

Tool

A structured, psychometric questionnaire, the *Abbreviated Scale for the Assessment of Psychosocial Status in Pregnancy* (Goldenberg et al., 1997), was used to measure the psychosocial status of pregnant women. The scale is a condensed version of five previously validated scales that each measure one aspect of psychosocial status. These include self-esteem (Rosenberg, 1965), trait anxiety (Spielberger et al., 1970), depression (Radloff, 1977), mastery (Pearlin et al., 1981) and stress (Schar et al., 1973). The abbreviated scale has a possible score range from 28 ('poor' psychosocial status) to 140 ('good' psychosocial status).

Participants were asked to specify their age, week of pregnancy, parity, marital status, education, form of professional training or education and antenatal care provider. A copy from the risk catalogue from the antenatal record was provided and women were asked to copy the ticks that the obstetrician had made in their *Mutterpass*. This was used to identify the risk status accorded to the woman by the obstetrician.

Defining risk category for the study

The 52 risk factors from the *Mutterpass* were compared with the maternity guidelines from the Netherlands (Ziekenfondsraad, 1998) and Grampian, Scotland (Area Maternity Services Committee for Grampian, 1998). It was clear that some factors would lead to obstetrician-led care in all three countries and therefore these factors were considered to indicate that the woman was at 'genuine high-risk' (Box 3.1.2). It was decided that women with these factors should be excluded from the study because differences in their psychosocial state might be due to the condition that made them 'high-risk' and not solely to the label 'high-risk' (the awareness that the pregnancy is not 'normal'). Other factors were more open to debate and it was decided to identify women as belonging to one of two groups.

Group 1 consisted of women who were 'labelled high-risk'. These were women who had risk factors ticked in their *Mutterpass* that would lead them to be labelled 'high-risk' in Germany, but in Scotland and the Netherlands they would still be eligible for midwifery-led care and would therefore be considered 'low-risk' in these countries.

Group 2 consisted of women who appeared to have 'no-risk'. This group included women without any documented risk factors and women who had risk factors that were listed in the *Mutterpass* but which were not listed in the guidelines (*Mutterschaftsrichtlinien*) that require the obstetrician to label the woman as 'high-risk' in their maternity records. The fact that only 36 of the 52 risk factors in the *Mutterpass* are also listed in the guidelines led to a situation where women from the 'no-risk' group could be said to have 'risk factors'. However, as these risk factors are considered to be very minor and would not lead them to be labelled 'high-risk' even in Germany (the effect of the label was the focus of the investigation of this study), these women were included in the 'no-risk' group.

Sample

The sample was a convenience sample of women attending antenatal classes in a large city of Germany. Recruitment took place from the last week of May to the third week of June 2002. Women between 22 and 41 weeks gestation were identified at antenatal classes and invited to participate in the study. The available number of antenatal classes in this time period (22) meant that 147 questionnaires could be distributed.

Midwives offering antenatal classes were approached, and the purpose, method and procedures of the study

Box 3.1.2 Study groups

Group 1: 'labelled high-risk'	Group 2: 'no risk'	'Genuine high-risk' (excluded)
Medical history (e.g. heart, lung, liver, renal, neurological or psychiatric disorder) (to be specified)*	Family history (e.g. diabetes, hypertension, anomalies, genetic disorders, psychiatric disorders)	Coagulation disorder
		Rhesus incompatibility in previous pregnancies
Obesity	Allergy, e.g. against drugs	
Age < 18 years	Previous blood transfusion	Diabetes mellitus
Age > 35 years	Psychological stress (family, job)	Previous pre-term birth (before completed 37 weeks)
Multiparity (> 4)	Social disadvantage (integration problems, economic problems)	Previous small for gestational age
Infertility treatment	Small of stature	Previous perinatal death or anomaly
More than two miscarriages/terminations	Skeletal deformities	Other uterine surgery
Complications during previous delivery	Previous pregnancy less than a year ago	Drug or alcohol misuse
Postpartum complications	General medical conditions needing treatment (to be specified)	Haemorrhage before 28 weeks
Caesarean section	Regular medication	Haemorrhage after 28 weeks
Uncertain duration of pregnancy	Psychological stress	Placenta praevia
Anaemia	Socio-economic problems	Multiple pregnancy
Abnormal lie	Risks from other blood tests	Hydramnios
	Hypotension	Oligohydramnios
		Placental insufficiency
		Cervical incompetence
		Pre-term contractions/labour
		Urinary tract infection
		Indirect Coombs test positive
		Hypertension (BP > 140/90)
		Proteinuria > 1000 mg/l
		Modcrate to massive oedema
		Gestational diabetes

There was the option for other factors to be added by the obstetrician; these factors may lead to categorisation as 'genuine high-risk' or 'labelled high-risk' (when red box ticked) depending on specification.

*May lead to categorisation as 'genuine high-risk' depending on specification.

explained to them. They discussed the issue with the women in their classes and when the women agreed, questionnaires were handed out to them in the following class either by the researcher or the midwife.

Research Ethics approval was sought from the appropriate local research ethics committee of the *Landesärztekammer* (Local Medical Association). However, ethical approval was not deemed to be necessary, as according to German guidelines ethical approval is only needed for research led by doctors. The research was peer-reviewed and approved in line with the Research Governance Strategy of the educational institution where KS was registered as a student.

Of the 147 women who were given a questionnaire, 82% (122) responded. Women's responses regarding their risk assessment were used to identify women to be excluded from the study and the two groups of women to be compared. Two women sent the questionnaire back without completing it and therefore had to be excluded at this stage.

Nine women were considered to be 'genuinely high-risk' and were excluded from the study. The remaining 111 women who were eligible for inclusion were classified according to the two groups described above (Box 3.1.2).

Sample size

A sample size calculation based on the data from the Goldenberg et al. (1997) study indicated that a sample size of 35 women per group was needed to detect a 10% difference in the total score for psychosocial state between the groups (80% statistical power, 5% significance level). This calculation was based on previous findings from the full scale (Goldenberg et al., 1997) rather than the shortened scale (Goldenberg et al., 1997) used in this study, as data from the shortened scale were not available. Therefore, a decision was made to do a retrospective sample size calculation prior to commencing inferential data analysis. The retrospectively calculated sample size, based on data from this study, showed that 15 women per group were needed to detect a difference of this size, therefore the number of women per group was sufficient for significance tests to be undertaken.

Data collection

Questionnaires were distributed in antenatal classes either by the researcher (100) or by the midwives (47) when they felt it was not feasible for the researcher (KS) to come to class. The purpose of the study and the questionnaire was explained personally by the researcher and midwives were also asked to do this in the researcher's absence. A covering letter including this information was also handed to the women. Women took the questionnaire home and were asked to send it back to the researcher in the prepaid envelope provided. The questionnaire guaranteed the participants complete anonymity. The questionnaires had no identifying numbers and no other identifying information was asked, therefore the questionnaires could not be linked to the participants. The return of the questionnaire was taken as consent to take part in the study.

Analysis

Descriptive statistics were produced for all variables. To check for differences between the groups with regard to the demographic variables, continuous variables with a normal distribution were tested using Student's t-test. Normal distribution was tested for using the Kolmogorov–Smirnov test for normality. Categorical variables were analysed using the χ^2-test. The Yates continuity correction is given for 2×2 tables and Pearson's χ^2 for 2×3 tables. Fisher's Exact test was used when more than 20% of the cells had a count of less than five. Findings were considered to be statistically significant at the 5% level.

A total score to assess overall psychosocial status was calculated and divided into quartiles to illustrate the distribution of women's scores. Following Copper et al. (1996), a score in the lowest quartile was defined as 'poor psychosocial status'; however, the authors did not give labels for the remaining score quartiles. Therefore, in this study the second lowest quartile was defined as 'poor to moderate psychosocial state', the third quartile as 'moderate to good psychosocial state' and the highest quartile as 'good psychosocial state'.

To investigate the effect of the risk label on overall psychosocial state, the difference in means of the total score between the two groups was tested with analysis of covariance using the GLM univariate model. Using this general linear model procedure, the effects of individual factors as well as interactions between factors could be investigated (Norusis, 1999). Using the total score quartiles to test for the difference in proportions between the groups would have meant losing some information through the grouping of the continuous variable. In addition, results would have been influenced by the setting of the cut-off points introducing a possible source of bias. An analysis of covariance was also performed to test the main and interaction effects of parity, pregnancy week, form of care, marital status, school degree and further education on the scores for psychosocial state.

The variables were entered individually into the model to test for the main effect on psychosocial state. Next, to test for interaction effects the variables were entered simultaneously into the model.

Findings

Of the 111 women included in the study, 57 had risk factors that led to them being categorised as 'labelled high-risk' and 54 women were categorized as 'no-risk'. The characteristics of the sample are shown in Table 3.1.1. The 'labelled high-risk' group was significantly older than the 'no-risk' group ($t = 7.11$, $p = 0.001$, 95% CI for difference in means 3.2–5.6). No significant differences between the groups were found in terms of marital status, school degree and further education. The women in the sample were well educated; the majority (69%) were expecting their first baby. The women were rather advanced in their pregnancies, the mean week of pregnancy being 34.1 (SD 3.7).

The number of risk factors per woman varied between 0 and 5, and 78% of women reported that they had at least one risk factor (Table 3.1.2). The most common risk factor in the 'labelled high-risk' group was 'aged over 35', with 27 (48%) women having this, followed by 'infertility treatment', ticked in 12 (21%) risk catalogues. The most common risk factors in the 'no-risk' group were 'allergy', with 22 (41%) of the women being positive for this risk factor, and 'family history' (9; 17%).

The red box was ticked in only seven of the 57 cases that should have been categorised as 'high-risk' according to the guidelines. In one case the red box was ticked when only 'allergy' was present. Further inconsistencies included failure to fully complete the risk catalogue, mistakes in completing it, such as not ticking aged over 35 or multiparity when it actually would have been appropriate, and no specification of risk factors given when required in order to be of informative value.

Only one woman had a low psychosocial status score of 83 (Figure 3.1.1); all other women had scores in the third and fourth quartiles representing 'moderate to good' and 'good' psychosocial states. More than half of the women scored in the highest quartile. Over two-thirds of the women from the 'no-risk' group had scores in the fourth quartile compared to a little more than half of the women from the 'labelled high-risk' group.

The analysis of covariance showed a significant difference in mean scores ($R^2 = 0.07$, $F = 7.592$, 1 df, $p = 0.007$) between the groups after adjusting for age (Table 3.1.3), with the scores being significantly lower in the 'labelled high-risk' group. The main effect of the risk

Table 3.1.1 Demographic characteristics of the sample

	Total ($n = 111$) Mean (SD)	Group 1 'labelled high-risk' ($n = 57$) Mean (SD)	Group 2 'no risk' ($n = 54$) Mean (SD)	p (95% CI)
Age (years)	32.4 (3.9)	34.5 (4)	30.1 (2.8)	0.001 (3.2–5.6)
Pregnancy week	34.1 (3.7)	34.1 (4)	34.1 (3.9)	0.94 (–1.5 to 1.3)
	n (%)	n (%)	n (%)	1.00*p
Marital status				
Single	6 (5)	3 (5)	3 (6)	
Partner	105 (95)	54 (95)	51 (94)	
School degree[†]				0.12 ($\chi^2 = 2.4$, df = 1)
Abitur (13 years)	83 (75)	47 (83)	36 (68)	
Other (9–10 years)	27 (24)	10 (18)	17 (32)	
Further education				0.58[‡] ($\chi^2 = 1.1$, df = 2)
University	50 (45)	28 (49)	22 (41)	
Vocational training	42 (38)	19 (33)	23 (43)	
Both	13 (12)	7 (12)	6 (11)	
None	6 (5)	3 (5)	3 (6)	
Parity				0.096 ($\chi^2 = 2.8$, df = 1)
Primipara	77 (69)	35 (61)	42 (78)	
Multipara	34 (31)	22 (39)	12 (22)	
Form of antenatal care				0.42 ($\chi^2 = 0.7$, df = 1)[§]
Obstetrician only	79 (71)	43 (75)	36 (67)	
Obstetrician/midwife	29 (26)	13 (23)	16 (30)	
Midwife only	3 (3)	1 (2)	2 (4)	

* Fisher's Exact test.

[†] One missing value.

[‡] As proportions were similar in each group and the count per group was small, the category 'none' was excluded in the analysis in order to avoid having a cell count of less than five in more than one group for the χ^2-test.

[§] Obstetrician/midwife and midwife only were grouped and compared with obstetrician only in order to avoid having a cell count of less than five in more than one group for the χ^2-test.

label on women's psychosocial state remained significant when risk group was entered together with one or two of the other independent variables in the model. The sample size did not allow for more than three independent variables to be tested simultaneously.

No significant difference in mean scores was found when parity, pregnancy week, form of care, marital status, school degree and further education were entered individually as the independent variable in the model, suggesting that these variables had no influence on women's psychosocial status. In addition, no interaction effects were found (Table 3.1.3).

Discussion

In line with findings from previous studies (Collatz, 1983; Wulff, 1992; Behrens & Goeschen, 1995; Urbschat, 2001), over three-quarters (78%) of women in this study had at least one risk factor. However, it could be argued that this indicates a considerable difference in practice from some other developed countries, namely the UK (Anonymous Personal Communication, 2003), although this needs further exploration. The high percentage of women regarded as being 'at risk' in this study raises the question of whether this process is still consistent with

Table 3.1.2 Number and kind of risk factors (count (%))

	Total sample	'Labelled high-risk' group	'No risk' group
Number of risk factors			
0	24 (21.6)	0 (0.0)	24 (44.4)
1	50 (45.0)	24 (42.1)	26 (48.1)
2	20 (18.0)	18 (31.6)	2 (3.7)
3	14 (12.6)	12 (21.1)	2 (3.7)
4	2 (1.8)	2 (3.5)	0 (0.0)
5	1 (0.9)	1 (1.8)	0 (0.0)
Risk factors that led to inclusion in the 'labelled high-risk' group			
Age > 35 years	27 (47.7)	27 (47.7)	
Infertility treatment	12 (21.1)	12 (21.1)	
Medical history (to be specified)*	10 (17.5)	10 (17.5)	
Caesarean section	6 (10.5)	6 (10.5)	
Anaemia	6 (10.5)	6 (10.5)	
More than two miscarriages/terminations	4 (7.0)	4 (7.0)	
Complications during previous delivery	3 (5.3)	3 (5.3)	
Obesity	2 (3.5)	2 (3.5)	
Multiparity (> 4)	1 (1.8)	1 (1.8)	
Abnormal lie	1 (1.8)	1 (1.8)	
*Risk factors that led to inclusion in the 'no risk' group**			
Allergy, e.g. against drugs	42 (37.8)	20 (35.1)	22 (40.7)
Family history	21 (18.9)	12 (21.1)	9 (16.7)
Psychological stress	3 (2.7)	1 (1.8)	2 (3.7)
Other	7 (6.3)	6 (10.5)	1 (1.9)
Skeletal deformities	3 (2.7)	2 (3.5)	1 (1.9)
Risks from other blood tests	1 (0.9)	1 (1.8)	0 (0)

*Women with risk factors from the 'labelled high-risk' group could also show risk factors from the 'no risk' group but were included into the 'labelled high-risk' group.

the original intention of the concept of risk assessment in pregnancy – namely, to decrease perinatal and maternal mortality by identifying those women who are at risk of an adverse outcome and referring them to the appropriate treatment.

The most common risk factors in this study, 'aged over 35', 'allergy' and 'family history', mirrored Graham's (1998) findings, indicating the continued reliance of risk assessment systems on socio-demographic or physical characteristics and demonstrating that this can result in a large proportion of pregnant women being at risk. However, this kind of risk factor is neither closely linked to nor predictive of the adverse pregnancy outcomes of interest; thus, it contributes to a poor sensitivity, specificity and positive predictive value of the risk assessment tool. Despite the introduction of ever more screening tools and methods,

Figure 3.1.1 Proportion of women per total score quartiles

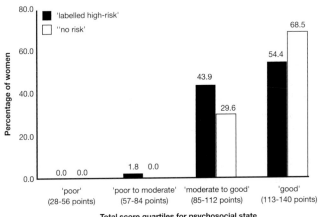

Table 3.1.3 Effect of different independent variables on total score

Independent variable	Observed means of total score (SD)*	Predicted means of total score (95% CI)†	R^2	F	df	p
Risk group			0.07	7.592	1	0.007
'Labelled high-risk'	112.2 (13.8)	110.9 (107.6–114.3)				
'No risk'	116.9 (8.6)	118.2 (114.8–121.7)				
Pregnancy week			0.001	1.535	1	0.218
22 to 28 weeks	114.6 (11.9)	11.1.6 (110.3–118.8)				
29 to 40 weeks	114.6 (11.8)	114.6 (111.9–117.3)				
Parity			0.02	1.590	1	0.210
Primipara	115.4 (11.9)	115.4 (112.7–118.1)				
Multipara	112.4 (11.7)	112.3 (108.3–116.4)				
Form of care			0.004	0.266	1	0.607
Obstetrician only	114.9 (12.0)	114.9 (112.6–117.6)				
Obst./midw.	113.3 (11.4)	113.3 (109.1–117.5)				
Midwife only						
Marital status			0.003	0.399	1	0.592
Single	112.2 (14.0)	112.0 (102.2–121.7)				
Partner	114.6 (11.7)	114.6 (112.3–116.9)				
School degree			0.00	0.002	1	0.969
9 or 10 years	114.2 (10.9)	114.3 (109.6–118.6)				
13 years	114.4 (12.1)	114.4 (111.8–117.0)				
Further education			0.02	0.801	3	0.496
University	114.7 (12.0)	114.9 (111.4–118.3)				
Vocational	114.7 (12.3)	114.6 (110.8–118.3)				
Both	115.9 (8.6)	116.0 (109.3–122.6)				
None	107.3 (12.8)	107.1 (97.4–117.0)				

*Means of total score and standard deviations that were actually observed in the sample.

†Means of total score based on the model adjusted for age; these are means that are predicted by the model and not actually observed means.

and a continuously increasing number of risk factors (leading to more women being categorised as 'high-risk'), there is no evidence that this is actually reducing maternal and perinatal morbidity and mortality in developed countries (Alexander & Keirse, 1989; Collatz, 1993; Tew, 1998).

In this study only nine women were excluded because they showed risk factors that would have led to obstetrician-led care according to the Dutch and Scottish guidelines. This means that 93% of the women who responded would have been eligible for midwifery-led care at booking in these countries; however, the majority (71%) had obstetrician-led care. It seems likely that women having obstetrician-led care had more antenatal visits and experienced more interventions and more prenatal diagnostic procedures (Collatz, 1993; Urbschat, 2001) than would be deemed beneficial for women who are actually not 'high-risk'. The low predictive value of the screening tests performed during antenatal care visits

is likely to produce a high number of false-positive results, leading to a considerable number of unnecessary medical interventions and possibly greater anxiety (Chalmers, 1982; Alexander & Keirse, 1989).

Rather than reducing morbidity, the findings of this study suggest that risk labelling may actually have a negative effect on women's psychosocial state. This supports the findings of Saxell's (2000) qualitative study that the label 'high-risk' led to feelings of loss of control and powerlessness. The finding that labelling pregnant women 'high-risk' has a negative effect on women's psychosocial state highlights the need to re-evaluate the risk assessment system used in Germany in terms of its ability to correctly identify those women for whom the label is justified. Those who are labelled 'high-risk' need to be provided with appropriate support and reassurance to alleviate the consequences it may have on their psychosocial state. However, it is questionable whether the current practice of obstetrician-led care, where the epidemiological model of risk dominates and the emphasis lies on medical aspects with usually little time being spent with the woman, can achieve this even with a revised risk assessment tool.

The issue of risk in pregnancy is very complex, and many social and cultural factors have an influence on whether a woman is 'at risk'. It is conceivable that midwives who usually spend more time with the women and do home-visits, thus often having a better insight into the women's individual situation, are in a better situation to assess the actual risk, refer the women if necessary, and to provide the support and reassurance that may be needed. Moreover, women appear to be more open during antenatal visits with midwives because they feel that they are taken seriously and supported (Abraham-van der Mark, 1996; Waldenström & Turnbull, 1998), which is an essential prerequisite for successful risk assessment as the women themselves are the source of the information that is needed (Alexander & Keirse, 1989). Research from other countries suggests that midwives can effectively deliver routine antenatal care to women with normal pregnancies and refer them to specialist care if the need arises (Tucker et al., 1996); however, evaluation of a midwifery-led antenatal care programme within the German health system would be required. Furthermore, referral to specialist care due to a genuine risk should not be a 'one-way street'. There should be an option that would allow referral back into midwifery care when the problem is solved. A study conducted in the UK has shown that this leads to fewer women having specialist care for the most part of their pregnancy (Midwifery Development Unit, 1995).

The fact that a high percentage of German women receive obstetrician-led care, which is not in line with the evidence that shows midwifery-led care to be beneficial for low-risk women compared to obstetrician-led care (Enkin et al., 2000), and the inconsistent use of the risk assessment tool also highlight the need to re-evaluate the risk catalogue in the *Mutterpass* as well as the *Mutterschaftsrichtlinien*. Sound evidence-based maternity guidelines would be a first step in the direction of correctly identifying those women who are 'at risk'. Pregnant women need more than a mere medical assessment of their risk status; support and reassurance play an important part in the process of risk assessment whether women are at risk or not.

Limitations

There are a number of limitations to this study. First, the difference in total psychosocial score amounted to only 7.3 points and explained only 7% of the variability in psychosocial score, posing the question whether this difference is of clinical relevance. Although a validated scale was used, there was little guidance in the literature on the interpretation of the size of the difference (Copper et al., 1996; Goldenberg et al., 1997). A 10% difference (11 points) in total score might be thought clinically important. However, given the fact that the majority of the women scored in the top quartile and all the women, apart from one, scored in the two highest quartiles, it could be argued that one is unlikely to find large differences and that a difference of 6.5% (7.3 points) of the total scale is acceptable as a clinically relevant difference.

Psychosocial state was assessed at only one point in time and for most women this was relatively late in pregnancy. The literature suggests that the way women feel may change during pregnancy (Lubin et al., 1975; Lundgren & Wahlberg, 1999), with the first trimester being a particularly psychologically vulnerable period. It is conceivable that to be classified as being at risk may have had a greater impact at that time. The experience of the pregnancy progressing well despite being labelled 'high-risk' may have a stabilising effect on women's well-being and may result in less of an effect from the label later in pregnancy. Future research should consider the effect of gestation on psychosocial state.

In addition, it was difficult to say whether it was really the risk label itself that had an influence on how women felt because obstetricians ticked the red box in only seven cases, thus 'visibly' applying the label to only those women. Of those seven women, only one scored in the top quartile of the total score (she reported that she had been reassured by her obstetrician that her risk factor was no reason for being worried); the other six had scores in the third quartile, suggesting that the risk label affects psychosocial state in some way and reassurance may be helpful in alleviating the effect. However, the number of women is too small to draw conclusions about whether the lower scores were associated with the risk label. It may well be that the effect of the interventions that usually follow a risk factor, and the emphasis on the possible danger that goes along with them, cannot be separated from the effect that the risk label (the increased awareness of not having a 'normal' pregnancy) had, although this cannot be directly concluded from the data. The documentation of risk factors, even when consistently performed, provides little information about the content and quality of the antenatal care received. A qualitative study exploring women's experiences and satisfaction with the practice of risk assessment could be useful in terms of shedding light on the different aspects of this process that are important to women and on the effect it has on them.

Comparison of women's responses with actual maternity records would have validated the information provided by the women. However, there is evidence of good agreement between medical records and women's perceptions, whether elicited by interview (Joffe & Grisco, 1985) or by postal questionnaire (Martin, 1987), and therefore this is unlikely to have shed any further light on the inconsistencies. The inconsistencies in completing the risk catalogue sometimes made it difficult to decide which study group a woman belonged to. A study to explore the reasons for the high variability in using the risk assessment tool would be desirable. The findings may contribute to informing the revision of the risk assessment tool and the maternity guidelines.

There are limitations to using antenatal classes as a means of identifying women for research studies. The characteristics of the sample in this study were in keeping with the typical 'middle-class' profile of antenatal class attenders (Lumley & Brown, 1993; Nichols, 1995; Nolan, 1995) and therefore no conclusions can be drawn about the effect of the risk label on psychosocial status of pregnant women not fitting this profile. Also, the convenience sample means that generalising the findings to the wider population of pregnant women is not possible. Furthermore, although the sample size calculation indicated that the number of women per group was large enough to perform significance tests for psychosocial status, small numbers in the subgroups meant that some grouping within variables was necessary. Therefore, it is not possible to say anything about the subgroups that have been subsumed into other groups. Further research is needed to assess pregnant women's psychosocial state as a consequence of risk labelling in a more representative sample with a repeated measures design to inform the discussion about whether the effect of the risk label found in this study is of clinical relevance.

A causal relationship cannot be inferred due to the non-experimental design and although a case–control design was used and post hoc statistical control of extraneous variables was performed, bias cannot be completely ruled out.

Nine women who filled out the questionnaire were excluded from the study and their data were not used. Although problematic from an ethical point of view, the researcher did not see a way to avoid this problem. Checking the risk profile of women before asking them to participate would have focused the attention on this particular issue, which then may have altered the answers to the questionnaire.

Conclusion

The findings of this study suggest that labelling women to be 'at risk' may negatively affect their psychosocial state. However, the difference found between the study groups was small and its clinical relevance may be debatable. The fact that a high percentage of German women receive obstetrician-led care and the inconsistent application of the risk assessment tool used in German antenatal care highlight the need to re-evaluate the risk catalogue in the German antenatal record (*Mutterpass*) as well as the German maternity guidelines (*Mutterschaftsrichtlinien*). Although this study was conducted within the German system of antenatal care, the findings raise questions about the effects of risk labelling in maternity care wherever it is practised. Further research is needed to assess women's psychosocial state in a more representative sample, to explore women's experiences and satisfaction with the practice of risk assessment and to investigate the reasons for the high variability in documenting women's risk factors.

REFERENCES

Abraham-van der Mark E (ed.). 1996. Successful Home Birth and Midwifery: The Dutch Model. Het Spinhuis, Amsterdam
Alexander S, Keirse MJNC. 1989. Formal risk scoring during pregnancy. In: Chalmers I, Enkin M, Keirse MJNC (eds), Effective Care in Pregnancy and Childbirth, Vol. 1. Oxford University Press, Oxford
Area Maternity Services Committee for Grampian. 1998. Antenatal Care in Grampian. Area Maternity Services Committee, Aberdeen
Behrens O, Goeschen K. 1995. Sind die Mutterschaftsrichtlinien zu verbessern? [Can the maternity guidelines be improved?]. Geburtshilfe und Frauenheilkunde, 55: M129–M131 (in German)
Bundesausschuss der Ärzte und Krankenkassen. 1998. Richtlinien über die ärztliche Betreuung während der Schwangerschaft und nach der Entbindung (Mutterschaftsrichtlinien) [Guidelines for obstetricians for the provision of pre- and postnatal care (maternity guidelines)]. Stand, 24 April.
Carter D. 1996. Descriptive research. In: Cormack D (ed.), The Research Process in Nursing, 3rd edn. Blackwell Science, Oxford
Chalmers B. 1982. Psychological aspects of pregnancy: some thoughts for the eighties. Social Science and Medicine, 6: 323–331

Collatz J. 1983. Analysen zur Mutterschaftsvorsorge. Prozesse der Versorgung und ihre Beeinflussung durch psychosoziale und biomedizinische Faktoren [Analysis of antenatal care. Psychosocial and biomedical influences on care provision]. PhD thesis at the Department of Human Biology at the Medical University, Hanover (in German)
Collatz J. 1993. Entspricht die derzeitige Versorgung dem Betreuungs- und Beratungsbedarf schwangerer Frauen? [Does today's antenatal care programme meet the needs of pregnant women?]. Gesellschaft für Geburtsvorbereitung – Rundbrief 1(93): 33–49 (in German)
Copper RL, Goldenberg RL, Das A Elder N et al. 1996. National Institute of Child Health and Human Development Maternal-Fetal Medicine Units Network. The preterm prediction study: maternal stress is associated with spontaneous preterm birth at less than thirty-five weeks' gestation. American Journal of Obstetrics and Gynecology, 175: 1286–1292
Costei AM, Kozer E, Ho T et al. 2002. Perinatal outcome following third trimester exposure to paroxetine. Archives of Pediatrics and Adolescent Medicine, 156(11): 1129–1132

Enkin M, Keirse MJNC, Neilson J et al. 2000. A Guide to Effective Care in Pregnancy and Childbirth, 3rd edn. Oxford University Press, Oxford

Goldenberg RL, Hickey CA, Cliver SP et al. 1997. Abbreviated scale for the assessment of psychosocial status in pregnancy: development and evaluation. Acta Obstetrica et Gynecologica Scandinavica, Supplement, 165(76): 19–22

Graham W. 1998. Every pregnancy faces risks. Safe Motherhood Fact Sheet. Family Care International and the Safe Motherhood Inter-Agency Group, New York

Gupton A, Heaman M, Cheung LWK. 2001. Complicated and uncomplicated pregnancies: women's perception of risk. Journal of Obstetric, Gynecologic and Neonatal Nursing, 30(2): 192–201

Haertsch M, Campbell E, Sanson-Fisher R. 1999. What is recommended for healthy women during pregnancy? A comparison of seven prenatal clinical practice guideline documents. Birth, 26(1): 24–30

Handwerker L. 1994. Medical risk: implicating poor pregnant women. Social Science and Medicine, 38(5): 665–675

Hatmaker DD, Kemp VH. 1998. Perception of threat and subjective well-being in low-risk and high-risk pregnant women. Journal of Perinatal and Neonatal Nursing, 12(2): 1–10

Heaman M, Beaton J, Gupton A et al. 1992. A comparison of childbirth expectations in high-risk and low-risk pregnant women. Clinical Nursing Research, 1(3): 252–265

Joffe M, Grisco JA. 1985. Comparison of antenatal records with retrospective interviewing. Journal of Biosocial Science, 17: 113–119

Karsenti D, Bacq Y, Brechot JF et al. 2001. Serum amylase and lipase activities in normal pregnancy: a prospective case–control study. American Journal of Gastroenterology, 96(3): 697–699

Kilbride J, Baker TG, Parapia LA et al. 1999. Anaemia during pregnancy as a risk factor for iron-deficiency anaemia in infancy: a case–control study in Jordan. International Journal of Epidemiology, 28(3): 461–468

Lubin B, Gardener SH, Roth A. 1975. Mood and somatic symptoms during pregnancy. Psychosomatic Medicine, 37(2): 136–146

Lumley J, Brown S. 1993. Attenders and nonattenders at childbirth education classes in Australia: how do they and their births differ? Birth, 20(3): 123–130

Lundgren I, Wahlberg V. 1999. The experience of pregnancy: a hermeneutical/phenomenological study. Journal of Perinatal Education, 8(3): 12–20

Lupton D. 1999. Risk. Routledge, London

Martin C. 1987. Monitoring maternity services by postal questionnaire: congruity between mothers' reports and their obstetric records. Statistics in Medicine, 6: 613–627

Melender HL. 2002. Experiences of fears associated with pregnancy and childbirth: a study of 329 pregnant women. Birth, 29(2): 101–111

Midwifery Development Unit. 1995. The establishment of a Midwifery Development Unit based at Glasgow Royal Maternity Hospital. Midwifery Development Unit, Glasgow Royal Maternity Hospital, Rottenrow

Ministry of Health. 1959. Report of the Maternity Services Committee (Cranbrook Committee report). HMSO, London

Nichols M. 1995. Adjustment to new parenthood: attenders versus non-attenders at prenatal education classes. Birth, 2(1): 21–26

Nolan M. 1995. A comparison of attenders at antenatal classes in the voluntary and statutory sectors: education and organisational implications. Midwifery, 11: 138–145

Norusis MJ. 1999. SPSS for Windows 9.0. Reference Manuals. SPSS, Chicago

Pearlin LI, Liberman MA, Menaghan EG et al. 1981. The stress process. Journal of Health and Social Behaviour, 22: 337–356

Polit DF, Beck CT, Hungler BP. 2001. Essentials of Nursing Research, Methods, Appraisal and Utilization, 5th edn. Lippincott Williams & Wilkins, Philadelphia.

Radloff LS. 1977. The CES-D scale: a self-report depression scale for research on a general population. Applied Psychological Measurement, 1: 385–401

Rosenberg M. 1965. Society and Adolescent Self Image. Princeton University Press, Princeton, NJ

Saxell L. 2000. Risk: theoretical or actual. In: Page LA (ed.), The New Midwifery: Science and Sensitivity in Practice. Churchill Livingstone, Edinburgh

Schar M, Reeder LG, Kirken JM. 1973. Stress and cardiovascular health: an international cooperative study, II: the male population of a factory at Zurich. Social Science and Medicine, 7: 585–603

Schlieper B. 1997. Die Rolle der Hebamme in der Schwangerenvorsorge [The role of the midwife in the provision of antenatal care]. Dissertation for the German equivalent to a Masters Degree in Sociology at the University of Bielefeld (in German)

Schumann M. 2000. Die Bedeutung des Risikodenkens in Schwangerschaft und Geburt. Zur Karriere eines medizinischen Konzepts [The effects of risk-oriented thinking in childbirth. The career of medical concept]. Dissertation for the German equivalent to a Masters Degree in Social Sciences (in German)

Sobande AA, Archibong EI, Akinola SE. 2002. Pregnancy outcome in asthmatic patients from high altitudes. International Journal of Gynaecology and Obstetrics, 77(2): 117–121

Spielberger CD, Gorsuch RL, Loshene RE. 1970. Manual for the State-trait Anxiety Inventory. Consulting Psychology Press, Palo Alto, CA

Tew M. 1998. Safer Childbirth? A Critical History of Maternity Care, 4th edn. Free Association Books, London

Tucker JS, Hall MH, Reid ME et al. 1996. Should obstetricans see women with normal pregnancies? A multicentre randomised controlled trial of routine antenatal care by general practitioners and midwives compared with shared care led by obstetricians. British Medical Journal, 312: 554–559

Urbschat I. 2001. Die Medikalisierung schwangerer Frauen. Eine Auswertung der niedersächsischen Perinataldaten von 1992 bis 1996 [The medicalisation of pregnant women. An analysis of the perinatal register of Lower Saxony from 1992 to 1996]. Hebammenforum-online, Thema März 2001, www.hebammen-forum.de, accessed 9 July 2002

Waldenström U, Turnbull D. 1998. A systematic review comparing continuity of midwifery care with standard maternity services. British Journal of Obstetrics and Gynaecology, 105: 1160–1170

Wulff KH. 1992. Schwangerenvorsorge – Inanspruchnahme und Effektivität [Antenatal care – uptake and effectiveness]. Deutsches Ärzteblatt, 89(40): B2038–B2042

Ziekenfondsraad. 1998. Obstetric manual. Final report of the Obstetric Working Group of the National Health Insurance Board of the Netherlands (abridged version). Translation by Beddow CE, Herschderfer K. Original Dutch title: Verloskundig Vademecum. Amstelveen, the Netherlands

Midwifery 2003; 19(4): 298–309

Reduced frequency prenatal visits in midwifery practice: attitudes and use

Deborah S Walker, Stephanie Day, Corinne Diroff, Heather Lirette, Laura McCully,

Candace Mooney-Hescott, Victoria Vest

Recent research supports the use of reduced frequency prenatal visit schedules (RFVS) for women of low obstetric risk. However, for the RFVS to be widely adopted for use in practice, health care providers must implement and support its use. The purpose of this study was to explore midwives' attitudes toward and use of reduced frequency prenatal care visit schedules for the care of low-risk women. A descriptive, correlational study was conducted at the 1999 Annual Meeting of the American College of Nurse-Midwives with completed surveys received from 234 midwives. Seventy-two percent ($n = 170$) responded that they were familiar with the reduced frequency visit schedule. Of those, 71% agreed that they could give effective prenatal care by using reduced frequency scheduling, although few (17%) reported using it in practice. Significant differences were found between the midwives who were familiar versus those who were unfamiliar with the visit schedule in their perceptions for five central themes: (1) quality of care of the RFVS; (2) women's empowerment or self-care with the RFVS; (3) ability to manage practice; (4) patient satisfaction; and (5) barriers to the use of RFVS. Providers' responses to the use of RFVS have been mixed. Successful integration of this schedule into prenatal care services may require more than knowledge of its safety for low-risk women. Careful selection of women for whom the schedule is appropriate and a commitment from midwives to tailor prenatal care to the individual women's needs is indicated. Further research is also needed to evaluate the barriers that prevent midwives from using a reduced frequency visit schedule for the prenatal care of low-risk clients.

Introduction

Early and continuous prenatal care is recognized as one of the most effective means of reducing unfavorable pregnancy outcomes for women and infants, including reduced infant mortality and low-birth-weight rates. In the United States, health care providers have traditionally followed the American College of Obstetricians and Gynecologists (ACOG, 1997) recommended prenatal visit schedule. Although use of this 'traditional' schedule of care is widespread, its efficacy has not been supported through research.

In the past 20 years, there has been an increasing awareness and implementation of reduced frequency prenatal visit schedules. In 1982, England's Royal College of Obstetricians and Gynecologists established guidelines for low-risk pregnancies, reducing their standard 13 prenatal visits to eight for primiparas and five visits for multiparas (Sikorski et al., 1995a). Other European countries (e.g. France, Switzerland, and Luxembourg) have incorporated similar schedules involving fewer visits. In 1989, the United States Department of Health and Human Services' (USDHHS) Expert Panel on the Content of Prenatal Care (1989) recommended a reduced frequency prenatal visit schedule for low-risk, healthy women. As a result of these guidelines and policies, a growing body of literature examining the clinical effectiveness of reduced frequency prenatal visit schedules has evolved.

Several studies from Europe, Africa, and the United States have compared the traditional visit schedule to the reduced visit schedule. Although these studies varied in the number of reduced visits, research design, and participant demographics, they found no statistically significant differences in perinatal outcomes between women following a reduced frequency schedule of approximately eight visits and those attending prenatal care using the more traditional schedule of 14 visits

(Binstock & Wolde-Tsadik, 1995; Sikorski et al., 1995a; McDuffie et al., 1996; Munjanja et al., 1996; Berglun et al., 1997; Walker & Koniak-Griffin, 1997). Perinatal outcomes studied were preterm delivery, pre-eclampsia, cesarean delivery, and low birth weight. In addition, some studies were also able to demonstrate that the reduced schedule led to fewer ultrasounds and fewer antenatal inpatient hospital admissions, with no differences in perinatal outcomes (Munjanja et al., 1996; Berglun & Lindmark, 1997).

A thorough review of the literature, which was written as part of this research project, was published in the May/June 2001 issue of the *Journal of Midwifery and Women's Health (JMWH)* (Walker et al., 2001). Other reviews have been published on this subject as well (Villar & Khan-Neelofur, 2000; Guillermo et al., 2001). Since the earlier review (Walker et al., 2001), the World Health Organization (WHO) antenatal care trial (Villar et al., 2001), an impressive multicenter, randomized, controlled trial that included 27 clinics and more than 30,000 women participants from four different countries, was published. This trial provided further support for reduced frequency visit schedules (RFVS) by demonstrating no differences in maternal or perinatal outcomes between women in the traditional versus reduced frequency groups. In addition, focus groups exploring provider's perceptions of prenatal care were conducted in each country followed by a questionnaire to all the study providers ($n = 174$). Providers reportedly expressed satisfaction with the RFVS because of their belief that paperwork would be reduced and they would be allowed to spend more time with their patients (Villar et al., 2001). About two-thirds of providers in both models were satisfied with the number of visits offered. However, more of those using the new model said that the time they spent with women at each visit was right (Villar et al., 2001).

Assessing the attitudes of health care providers is key when planning changes in the delivery of care. Providers' beliefs must be carefully examined, and those beliefs must be addressed if the successful adoption of a new model of care is to occur. Sikorski et al. (1995b) examined the professional caregivers' responses and attitudes toward the implementation of a new reduced frequency prenatal visit schedule in Great Britain. Most (63.8%) practitioners surveyed supported a reduction in the number of prenatal visits, with midwives being the most intent on seeing changes made to the organization of prenatal care (Sikorski et al., 1995b).

Sanders et al. (1999) conducted focus groups with midwives ($n = 14$) who participated in a clinical trial (Jewell et al., 2000) evaluating a flexible (women decided the number and timing of their visits) versus traditional schedule of prenatal care in Great Britain. The midwives

interviewed felt the flexible schedule reinforced the normality of pregnancy. These midwives felt that a gap of eight weeks between visits was unacceptably long and that the maximum amount of time between visits should be six weeks. They also recognized that a flexible schedule would not always equate to a reduced number of visits. The midwives supported the move away from the traditional schedule in principle, but they had reservations related to their concerns that women's psychosocial needs would go unmet and were reluctant to integrate change into their practice (Sanders et al., 1999). Although this study's sample is small and comes from one geographic area, it provides some insight into midwives' attitudes toward using reduced frequency scheduling.

More than a decade has passed since the USDHHS proposed a reduced frequency prenatal visit schedule (Public Health Service Expert Panel on Prenatal Care, 1989). Several trials have documented that reduced frequency prenatal visit schedules are safe for women of low obstetric risk (Binstock & Wolde-Tsadik, 1995; Sikorski et al., 1995a; McDuffie et al., 1996; Munjanja et al., 1996; Berglun & Lindmark, 1997; Walker & Koniak-Griffin, 1997; Villar et al., 2001), but findings have been mixed as to whether providers are satisfied with the quality of care achieved with RFVS (Sikorski et al., 1995b; Sanders et al., 1999; Villar et al., 2001). Compelling reasons for providers to implement the RFVS in low-risk prenatal care may include, but are not limited to, the following: (1) an unwarranted burden may be experienced by pregnant women and the health care system when healthy women attend greater numbers of prenatal care visits than are necessary to achieve optimal perinatal outcomes; (2) frequent visits may promote the idea that pregnancy is an illness and requires high levels of scrutiny and intense surveillance; and (3) research has demonstrated that women who are seen more frequently may be subjected to higher rates of unnecessary interventions (Sikorski et al., 1995a; Munjanja et al., 1996; Berglun & Lindmark, 1997) leading to increased levels of anxiety, stress, and unnecessary worry. For the change to a RFVS to occur, however, prenatal care providers must be satisfied with the quality of the care provided and committed to the belief that it is the best means of providing care for pregnant women of low obstetric risk.

Midwives, as expert providers of prenatal care, reportedly agreed in principle with reduced scheduling (Sanders et al., 1999) and were the most intent on seeing changes made to the organization of prenatal care (Sikorski et al., 1995b). A survey of their attitudes and use of RFVS was conceived as an important undertaking in assessing the potential for implementing this change in health care delivery. The purpose of this study, therefore, was to evaluate midwives'* attitudes toward and use of

---

*CNMs/CMs and midwives used herein refer to midwives who are certified by the American College of Nurse-Midwives (ACNM) or the ACNM Certification Council Inc., and midwifery refers to the profession as practised in accordance with the standards promulgated by the ACNM.

reduced frequency prenatal visit schedules for pregnant women of low obstetric risk.

Methods

Sample

Midwives attending the 1999 American College of Nurse-Midwives' Annual Meeting were asked to participate in this study. The ACNM Annual Meeting is a national gathering of midwifery practitioners, students, and others interested in the profession, thus providing a broad representation of the midwifery profession in the United States. All midwife attendees who were able to speak or read English were eligible to participate in the study. Student midwives who had not yet practised outside of their educational programs were not eligible. Participation was anonymous and voluntary.

Procedure

Permission to conduct the study was obtained from the University of Michigan's Institutional Review Board and from the ACNM Division of Research before data collection began. Questionnaires were distributed at various times throughout the 1999 ACNM Annual Meeting, with a total of 243 questionnaires returned, resulting in 234 completed surveys and representing a response rate of 32.3% of conference attendees.

Instrument

Data were collected by using an instrument developed specifically for this study. The first section of the instrument included questions about the participants' demographic characteristics, knowledge, and use of the reduced frequency prenatal visit schedule. The remainder of the questionnaire consisted of 27 statements about participants' attitudes toward reduced frequency prenatal visit schedules, to which the participants were asked to respond by using a five-point Likert-type scale (1 = strongly disagree to 5 = strongly agree).

To assist participants in completing the questionnaire, definitions of key terms (Figure 3.2.1) and an introductory paragraph were included. The introductory paragraph explained the research project and provided instructions for its completion. Consent to participate was indicated by completion and return of the questionnaire.

To assess content validity, an expert panel consisting of four nursing faculty members who had master's degrees and one faculty member who had a doctoral degree reviewed and critiqued the questionnaire before data collection occurred. Revisions were made on the

Figure 3.2.1 Definition of terms used in the study questionnaire

ACOG prenatal visit schedule: (approx. 14 visits) every 4 weeks up to 28–32 weeks gestation, every 2 weeks to 36 weeks, then weekly until birth.

Reduced-frequency visit schedule: (approx. 8 visits) one visit in each of the following weeks gestation 6–8, 14–16, 24–28, 32, 36, 38, then weekly until birth.

Prenatal care visit: a regularly scheduled, in-person visit between the pregnant woman and the health care provider.

Health care provider: a nurse-midwife/midwife, nurse practitioner, physician assistant, or physician.

Low-risk: The absence of health or obstetric complications such as hypertension, multiple gestation or chronic illnesses which would increase the likelihood for further development of complications during the pregnancy, labor, birth and postpartum period.

basis of the critiques, and the revised surveys were used in a pilot test with a sample of practising midwives ($n = 6$). On the basis of comments obtained from the pilot test, no further revisions were necessary.

Psychometric evaluation

The 27 statements concerning attitudes toward the RFVS were grouped using an extraction method of principal component analysis. This analysis identifies groups of highly correlated questions and revealed six clusters or themes out of the related questions. Nine statements were not grouped with any factor, either because they did not fit into a category or because they were poorly worded. After completing further analyses, the sixth factor, which contained only three items, was discarded, because the questions could not be cognitively determined to form a concept. The five related themes that emerged were as follows: (1) midwives' perception of the quality of care of the RFVS; (2) women's empowerment or self-care with the RFVS; (3) midwives' ability to manage their practice; (4) patient satisfaction; and (5) barriers to the use of the RFVS. These groups of questions explained 52.35% of the variance. Cronbach's α coefficients for factors 1–4 demonstrated α scores ranging from 0.85 to 0.62, indicating acceptable reliability for a new instrument. Scheduling and reimbursement were the focus of the fifth factor. This factor had an α of 0.35, which was low despite the limitation of only two questions in this factor.

Data analysis

Two members of the research team independently entered the data into computer spreadsheets. Data were cross-referenced and checked independently to eliminate data entry errors and were analyzed using the Statistical Package for the Social Sciences (SPSS, 1997), with the assistance of a statistician from the University of Michigan's Center for Statistical Computing and Research.

Statistical tests appropriate to the level of the specific variable were chosen. For example, internal consistency and reliability of the questionnaire were assessed by using Cronbach's α. Pearson's correlation coefficients were used to explore the relationship between demographic characteristics and users versus nonusers of the RFVS. A Student t-test compared users versus nonusers of RFVS, and those familiar versus those unfamiliar with RFVS and the five factors. All analyses used an α of 0.05 and 95% confidence intervals.

Results

Demographic characteristics of the study participants and their practices are shown in Table 3.2.1. Midwife participants practised in 42 of the 50 United States, as well as the District of Columbia and Puerto Rico. Most respondents were CNMs, and more than half held master's degrees. Years of active practice ranged from zero to 35 (mean = 10.2, SD = 8.4). Very few midwives responded to the question on charges; those who did reported the average amount charged for the total prenatal care package as $2040.00 (SD = $754.22).

Participants reported their client base as largely white (51.0%), with the next largest groups being black (22.6%) and Hispanic (18%). Almost half of the participants' clients were reported to be Medicaid recipients (45.6%) – see Table 3.2.1. There were no statistically significant differences found between the demographic characteristics of the midwives who were familiar with the RFVS versus those who were unfamiliar with it, nor between those who used RFVS and those who did not use reduced frequency scheduling.

For those reporting use of reduced frequency scheduling ($n = 40$), we examined the relationship between satisfaction with RFVS and both personal and practice demographic characteristics. Statistically significant positive correlations were found between midwives with a higher proportion of Medicaid clients and greater satisfaction with the quality of care afforded by the RFVS ($r = 0.169$, $P = 0.013$), as well as midwives' perception that women who followed the schedule were more empowered with better self-care skills ($r = 0.140$, $P = 0.039$). Conversely, a statistically significant negative correlation was found between perception of the quality of care achieved with the RFVS in practices serving a higher percentage of black clients ($r = -0.41$, $P = 0.013$). No other correlations approached significance at the 0.05 level; however, the small sample size of this subgroup limited the power to detect differences in attitudes (see Table 3.2.2).

Table 3.2.1 Characteristics of the respondents ($n = 234$)

Variable	%
Credentials	
CNM	97.9
CM	0
CPM	0.4
Direct entry midwife	0.4
Other	0
Missing	1.3
Highest degree attained in Midwifery Education Program	
Certificate	25.5
Master's	54.7
Post Master's	2.9
Missing	16.9
Major race/ethnic population served	
Asian	3.7
Black	22.6
Hispanic	18.0
Native American	2.4
White	51.4
Other	1.0
Primary payment source	
HMO	22.1
Medicaid	45.6
Medicare	2.3
Private insurance	18.2
Self-pay	7.2
Other	5.0

Table 3.2.2 Midwives' preferences and characteristics of their midwifery practices ($n = 234$)

Variable	%
Are there differences in the amount your practice is reimbursed based on the number of prenatal visits attended?	
Yes	26.5
No	45.2
Don't know	27.8
Visit schedule followed for typical low-risk primiparous women?	
ACOG	88.1
Reduced frequency	5.47
Other	6.55
Are you familiar with reduced frequency prenatal visit schedules?	
Yes	73.7
No	26.3
Are you familiar with the research on reduced frequency prenatal visit schedules?	
Yes	50.2
No	49.8

Only 7.1% of midwives reported use of the reduced frequency schedule for multiparas. An even smaller number (5.5%) used some form of reduced scheduling with primiparous clients, and even fewer (1.6%) stated that they used the RFVS with pregnant adolescent women. When polled on the number of visits they felt were required to receive adequate low-risk prenatal care, respondents' answers ranged from four to 20 visits for primiparous women and from three to 14 visits for multiparous women. Fifty-nine percent of participants indicated the minimum number of visits needed for a low-risk multiparas was eight or less (mean = 8.6, SD = 2.2), whereas 64% of midwives reported the minimum number of visits required for primiparous women was 10 or less (mean = 10.25, SD = 2.3).

Student t-tests were conducted to compare midwives who were familiar with the reduced visit schedule ($n = 170$) with those that were not familiar ($n = 62$) against the five factors. Midwives in the familiar group were significantly more satisfied with its quality ($t = -6.29, df = 230, P < 0.0001$), more able to manage their practice ($t = -2.97, df = 229, P = 0.003$), perceived increased patient satisfaction with reduced frequency scheduling ($t = -3.18, df = 230, P = 0.002$), and thought structural barriers were less of an issue in implementing the RFVS ($t = -2.89, df = 229, P = 0.004$).

In evaluating the two study aims – (1) to explore midwives' attitudes toward a reduced frequency prenatal care visit schedule and (2) to evaluate midwives' use of a reduced frequency prenatal care visit schedule – the analyses revealed that midwives agreed they could give effective prenatal care by using reduced frequency scheduling (71%), but few respondents actually used it in practice.

The statements with which the midwives agreed most strongly were that it would be cost-effective for low-risk women to attend care using the RFVS (75.5%) and that midwives could provide effective prenatal care using the RFVS (71%). Other statements with which midwives agreed strongly were that the CNM had the ability to control or change the visit schedule in their practice (60.5%) and that the traditional visit scheduling was not based on sound scientific evidence (52.8%). In addition, although almost half of the midwives (48.4%) thought that they would not lose women from their practice if they used reduced scheduling, about the same number were unsure if this were true (42.1%) – see Appendix A.

Discussion

This descriptive study used a convenience sample of midwives attending the 1999 ACNM Annual Meeting. Therefore, results cannot be generalized to the entire population of midwives, although those who participated represented 42 of the 50 states, and their practice demographics were not dissimilar to those in the randomized sample of midwifery practices reported by Paine et al. (1999).

Results from this study reveal that midwives are familiar with and have positive attitudes toward the effectiveness of a reduced frequency prenatal visit schedule for pregnant women of low obstetric risk. Not surprisingly, midwives who used and/or were familiar with the schedule indicated satisfaction with the quality of care provided by the RFVS both from their perspective as providers as well as perceived satisfaction from clients.

The pregnant woman's level of empowerment or self-care abilities when using the RFVS was also viewed as positively affected by those who used and/or were familiar with the reduced schedule. Active listening, empowerment, and quality care are all essential components of midwifery care and may in fact improve compliance rates for prenatal care visits (Berglun & Lindmark, 1997), thereby making the use of the RFVS a good fit with midwifery care. These findings were comparable to those of Clement et al. (1996), which suggested that women who were satisfied with reduced visit schedules were more likely to have a caregiver who encouraged them to ask questions and would listen if they wanted to talk about their pregnancy and their feelings.

Midwives who used and/or were familiar with the reduced visit schedule also had positive attitudes about their ability to manage their own practice and their ability to overcome barriers to instituting a reduced frequency prenatal visit schedule. However, although 59% of the midwives surveyed indicated a minimum number of eight visits or less was necessary to provide effective prenatal care, only 17% of participants actually reported following a reduced frequency visit schedule for prenatal care. Even though most midwives responded that the minimum prenatal visit schedule should consist of equal or fewer visits than is recommended in the reduced frequency schedule, this survey was not able to explain the reason for the low percentage of midwives actually making use of the schedule. Some clues as to this discrepancy may lie in the fact that midwives who were familiar with and/or used the RFVS also perceived that they had more control over their practice and fewer barriers to overcome in implementing the schedule. In other words, those who are not using it may have less control in the management of their practice and more perceived barriers toward implementing it in their practice environments.

For women of low obstetric risk, it is most likely the content of the prenatal visit and not the quantity of visits that promotes healthy outcomes. However, it is of interest to note that the exact number of prenatal visits needed to promote healthy outcomes is still undetermined. A growing number of studies (Binstock & Wolde-Tsadik, 1995; Sikorski et al., 1995a; McDuffie et al., 1996; Munjanja et al., 1996; Berglun & Lindmark, 1997; Walker & Koniak-Griffin, 1997; Villar et al., 2001) have reported no significant differences in perinatal outcomes between the traditional and RFVS. Although some of these studies also demonstrated that there were no differences in perinatal outcomes, women who followed the reduced visit schedule were referred less often for hypertensive disorders (Munjanja et al., 1996), had fewer ultrasounds, and experienced fewer prenatal inpatient hospital admissions (Sikorski et al., 1995a; Berglun & Lindmark, 1997). Despite these findings, most midwives surveyed continue to adhere to the use of the traditional prenatal care schedule, even though more than half (52.8%) agreed with the statement that this schedule is not based on sound scientific research. When queried about familiarity with research on RFVS, the study sample was almost equally divided between those that were familiar with the research (50.2%) and those that were not (49.8%).

Midwives care for women from vulnerable populations who may be considered at higher risk for poor pregnancy outcomes, and they may believe these women need more frequent prenatal visits. A significant but low negative correlation was found between midwives' perceived satisfaction with the quality of care afforded with RFVS and a higher proportion of black clients served. This may suggest that the respondents believe the quality of care would diminish in this population if an RFVS was instituted. Previous studies have documented that black women have more prenatal complications, such as hypertension, infection, and preterm births, and infants with lower birth weight than those of white women (Anonymous, 1996a, b; Davis & Collins, 1997; Adams et al., 2000). Knowledge of these studies may lead the prenatal care providers to recommend more frequent prenatal visits for black women and feel less comfortable in using RFVS. This cautious attitude may or may not be warranted, and further research in this area is needed. In addition, this conservative stance may not apply to all minority groups. One study (Walker & Koniak-Griffin, 1997) demonstrated low-risk Hispanic pregnant women whose funding source was primarily Medicaid experienced no differences in perinatal outcomes using the RFVS. Furthermore, the women in the RFVS group were significantly more satisfied with both the prenatal care received and the provider (Walker & Koniak-Griffin, 1997).

A weakly positive, although significant, correlation was found between respondents' perception of the quality of care afforded with RFVS and caring for a Medicaid population. This finding may suggest that midwives believe the women receiving Medicaid will benefit from following a reduced prenatal visit schedule. A reduced frequency schedule might be easier for women using Medicaid to follow if there are barriers, such as transportation, child care, or time constraints, in accessing prenatal care. Although some prenatal care providers advocate more frequent visits for women from a lower socio-economic status, a 1995 study by Marsh suggested that they may actually be happier with reduced schedules than women from a higher socio-economic status. In the study by Clement et al. (1996), women who were satisfied with reduced schedules were more likely to be living in rented accommodation. A more detailed evaluation is needed to discern which subgroups among the vulnerable populations are appropriate for reduced frequency visit scheduling and which are not. In addition, the type of visit may be important for optimizing outcomes in vulnerable populations. For example, some women may need more WIC/dietitian, social worker, or public health nursing visits and fewer clinician visits.

Most midwives surveyed did not respond to the questions on cost or billing aspects of their prenatal practices, nor did many report if reimbursement was different when women attended fewer prenatal visits. There were very few responses to the questions related to the financial aspects of reimbursement and costs of prenatal care, making it difficult to link reimbursement issues to the use of an RFVS. Within managed care systems, finances may have less direct influence on providers' scheduling considerations. However, when billing nonmanaged care insurance, providers generally bill globally for prenatal care. Only when providers bill for less than the total (global) OB package are there differences in charges for the quantity of visits attended. In a practice in which a midwife only provides prenatal care and the births are attended by another provider, there may be pressure to see women more frequently during their pregnancies to bill at the higher rate, and this could present a potential barrier to using the RFVS.

The survey tool had its limitations but provided acceptable reliability for the first use of the instrument. Continued psychometric evaluation is necessary.

Results of this study provide many potential avenues for further research. More research is necessary to assess the reasons why midwives feel positive about and support the RFVS in principle yet continue to adhere to the traditional visit schedule for provision of prenatal care to women of low obstetric risk. Barriers to the implementation and dissemination of not only these research findings, but others as well, in midwifery practices may also provide fruitful avenues of inquiry. Additional research may also examine ways to discern which women from vulnerable populations may be better served by using a reduced frequency prenatal visit schedule.

Women's satisfaction with the RFVS has also been mixed, as reported by the current body of research. The understanding of women's perceptions of the RFVS would also be a beneficial avenue for further exploration. One way to institute change to a new model of care may be to create consumer demand, similar to the natural childbirth movement in the 1960s, by pregnant women requesting fewer visits during their prenatal care. For this to occur, women's views would require further exploration, and additional education as to the benefits and safety of the RFVS would be important.

Conclusion

More than 10 years have passed since the USDHHS recommended that a reduced frequency visit schedule may be effective for low-risk women while preserving the quality of prenatal care (Public Health Service Expert Panel on Prenatal Care, 1989). However, it is evident from this study that although most midwives surveyed were familiar with reduced frequency scheduling, they

are not using it. Requiring healthy women to attend 14 prenatal care visits during their pregnancy, when similar perinatal outcomes may be achieved with fewer visits, may be an undue burden for the health care system as well as for pregnant women in time, money, and other factors. In addition, research has demonstrated that women who are seen more frequently may be subjected to higher rates of unnecessary interventions with no differences in perinatal outcomes (Munjanja et al., 1996; Berglun & Lindmark, 1997).

On the basis of the available evidence about RFVS, clinicians now have more choices to offer women for prenatal visit scheduling. Offering women a choice of schedules is congruent with midwifery care. Unless the RFVS is contraindicated, midwives should tailor schedules of care based on the best evidence related to prenatal visit scheduling and the individual preferences of clients.

Acknowledgements

The authors gratefully acknowledge the receipt of funding from Rho Chapter, Sigma Theta Tau International, which partially supported the work of this project.

REFERENCES

Adams MM, Elam-Evans LD, Wilson HG, Gilbertz DA. 2000. Rates of and factors associated with recurrence of preterm delivery. J Am Med Assoc, 283: 1591–1596

American College of Obstetricians and Gynecologists, American Academy of Pediatricians. 1997. Guidelines for Perinatal Care. American Academy of Pediatrics and American College of Obstetricians and Gynecologists, Elk Grove Village, IL. American College of Obstetricians and Gynecologists, American Academy of Pediatricians, Washington, DC

Author Anonymous. 1996a. Hypertension among pregnant black women contributes to poor birth outcomes. Res Act, 194: 4–5

Author Anonymous. 1996b. Increased risk of preterm birth among pregnant black women may be due in part to a higher rate of vaginal infections. Res Act, 197: 7–8

Berglun AC, Lindmark GC. 1997. Health services effects of a reduced routine programme for antenatal care: an area-based study. Eur J Obstet Gynecol Reprod Biol, 77: 193–199

Binstock MA, Wolde-Tsadik G. 1995. Alternative prenatal care: impact of reduced visit frequency, focused visits, and continuity of care. J Reprod Med, 40: 507–512

Clement S, Sikorski J, Wilson J, Das S, Smeeton N. 1996. Women's satisfaction with traditional and reduced antenatal visit schedules. Midwifery, 12: 120–128

Davis RJ, Collins JW. 1997. Differing birth weight among infants of US-born blacks, African-born blacks and US-born whites. New Engl J Med, 337: 1209–1214

Carroli G, Villar J, Piaggio G, Khan-Neelofur D, Gulmezoglu M, Mugford M et al. 2001. WHO systematic review of randomized controlled trials of routine antenatal care. Lancet, 357: 1565–1570

Jewell D, Sharp D, Sanders J, Peters TJ. 2000. A randomized controlled trial of flexibility in routine antenatal care. Br J Obstet Gynecol, 107: 1241–1247

Marsh G. 1985. New programme of antenatal care in general practice. BMJ, 29: 646–648

McDuffie RS, Beck A, Bischoff K, Cross J, Orleans M. 1996. Effect of frequency of prenatal care visits on perinatal outcome among low-risk women: a randomized controlled trial. J Am Med Assoc, 275: 847–851.

Munjanja SP, Lindmark GC, Nystrom L. 1996. Randomized controlled trial of a reduced-visits programme of antenatal care in Harare, Zimbabwe. Lancet, 348: 364–369

Paine LL, Lang JM, Strobino DM, Johnson TR, DeJoseph JF, Declercq ER et al. 1999. Characteristics of nurse-midwife patients and visits, 1991. Am J Public Health, 89: 906–909

Public Health Service Expert Panel on Prenatal Care. 1989. Caring for Our Future: The Content of Prenatal Care. US Department of Health and Human Services, Washington, DC

Sanders J, Somerset M, Jewell D, Sharp D. 1999. To see or not to see? Midwives' perception of reduced antenatal attendances for "low-risk" women. Midwifery, 257–263

Sikorski J, Wilson J, Clement S, Das S, Smeeton N. 1995a. A randomized controlled trial comparing two schedules of antenatal visits: the antenatal care project. BMJ, 312: 546–553

Sikorski J, Clement S, Wilson J, Das S, Smeeton N. 1995b. A survey of health professionals' views on possible changes in the provision and organization of antenatal care. Midwifery, 11: 61–68

SPSS. 1997. SPSS for Windows, Rel. 8.0.0. SPSS Inc., Chicago

Villar J, Khan-Neelofur D. 2000. Patterns of routine antenatal care for low-risk pregnancy. In: The Cochrane Database of Systemic Reviews, Vol. 4. The Cochrane Library.

Villar J, Ba'aqeel H, Piaggio G, Lumbiganon P, Belizan JM, Farnot U et al. 2001. WHO antenatal care randomised trial for the evaluation of a new model of routine antenatal care. Lancet, 357: 1551–1564

Walker DS, Koniak-Griffin D. 1997. Evaluation of a reduced-frequency prenatal visit schedule for low-risk women at a free-standing birthing center. J Nurse Midwif, 42: 295–303

Walker DS, McCully L, Vest V. 2001. Evidence based prenatal care visits: when less is more. J Midwif Women's Health, 46: 146–151

Appendix A

Midwives' responses to individual questionnaire items (n = 234; 1 = Strongly Disagree to 5 = Strongly Agree)

Item	Mean (SD)	%
Subscale: Quality of Care of the RFVS (Cronbach's α = 0.85)	3.40 (0.77)	
The number of visits in the ACOG prenatal visit schedule are not necessary for high-quality prenatal care.	3.25 (1.11)	5. Strongly Agree: 7.6 4. Agree: 46.8 3. Unsure: 16.9 2. Disagree: 20.7 1. Strongly Disagree: 8.0
Scheduling women more frequently in the prenatal period does not ensure better outcomes.	3.32 (1.08)	5. Strongly Agree: 8.9 4. Agree: 45.1 3. Unsure: 21.7 2. Disagree: 17.4 1. Strongly Disagree: 6.8
I feel I would not miss a complication if women attended prenatal care less often than the ACOG visit schedule.	3.33 (1.00)	5. Strongly Agree: 3.4 4. Agree: 23.1 3. Unsure: 16.4 2. Disagree: 51.7 1. Strongly Disagree: 5.5
I could give effective prenatal care to women seen on an RFVS.	3.72 (0.93)	5. Strongly Agree: 15.7 4. Agree: 54.9 3. Unsure: 17.4 2. Disagree: 9.4 1. Strongly Disagree: 2.6
The ACOG guidelines for visit scheduling are not based on sound scientific evidence.	3.63 (0.95)	5. Strongly Agree: 20.7 4. Agree: 32.1 3. Unsure: 38.4 2. Disagree: 7.2 1. Strongly Disagree: 1.7
Reduced frequency scheduling allows me to form a close bond with pregnant women.	3.19 (1.03)	5. Strongly Agree: 5.1 4. Agree: 41.9 3. Unsure: 25.8 2. Disagree: 20.8 1. Strongly Disagree: 6.4
Subscale: Women's Empowerment/Self-care with RFVS (Cronbach's α = 0.72)	2.92 (0.57)	
Women who attend prenatal care on the reduced frequency schedule feel more empowered.	2.83 (0.74)	5. Strongly Agree: 0.4 4. Agree: 15.1 3. Unsure: 55.0 2. Disagree: 25.6 1. Strongly Disagree: 3.8

Appendix A – continued

Item	Mean (SD)	%
Attending prenatal care on the RFVS enhances women's self-care skills.	2.95 (0.80)	5. Strongly Agree: 1.3 4. Agree: 21.9 3. Unsure: 50.6 2. Disagree: 22.8 1. Strongly Disagree: 3.4
Women attending care on the RFVS will not make other contacts (phone call, drop-in visits, ER visits, etc.) more frequently than if using the ACOG schedule.	2.93 (0.91)	5. Strongly Agree: 2.2 4. Agree: 26.3 3. Unsure: 38.4 2. Disagree: 28.4 1. Strongly Disagree: 4.7
I believe that women who attend prenatal care using the RFVS are more satisfied with their care.	2.96 (0.66)	5. Strongly Agree: 5.5 4. Agree: 48.7 3. Unsure: 25.4 2. Disagree: 19.1 1. Strongly Disagree: 1.3
Subscale: Management of Practice (Cronbach's α = 0.62)	3.52 (0.68)	
It would be cost-effective for women to attend visits on the reduced frequency schedule.	3.81 (0.84)	5. Strongly Agree: 16.0 4. Agree: 59.5 3. Unsure: 13.5 2. Disagree: 11 1. Strongly Disagree: 0
It would be cost-effective for my practice to see women using the RFVS.	3.38 (0.98)	5. Strongly Agree: 8.1 4. Agree: 45.8 3. Unsure: 25.8 2. Disagree: 16.5 1. Strongly Disagree: 3.8
Seeing low-risk women on an RFVS allows more time to see women who are at higher risk for poor pregnancy outcomes.	3.38 (0.90)	5. Strongly Agree: 5.5 4. Agree: 48.7 3. Unsure: 25.4 2. Disagree: 19.1 1. Strongly Disagree: 1.3
Subscale: Patient's Satisfaction (Cronbach's α = 0.66)	3.25 (0.67)	
Women do not complain about the number of visits they are scheduled to attend when using the RFVS.	3.32 (0.74)	5. Strongly Agree: 6.1 4. Agree: 28.1 3. Unsure: 58.3 2. Disagree: 6.1 1. Strongly Disagree: 1.3
If I use RFVS, my patients will feel they are receiving adequate care.	3.01 (1.04)	5. Strongly Agree: 4.7 4. Agree: 33.5 3. Unsure: 27.1 2. Disagree: 28.0 1. Strongly Disagree: 6.8
I will not lose women from my practice if I use the RFVS.	3.44 (0.78)	5. Strongly Agree 6.4 4. Agree: 41.7 3. Unsure: 42.1 2. Disagree: 8.9 1. Strongly Disagree: .9
Subscale: Structural Barriers (Cronbach's α = 0.37)	3.41 (0.88)	
In my practice, the CNM can control or change the visit schedule.	3.51 (1.34)	5. Strongly Agree: 28.3 4. Agree: 32.2 3. Unsure: 12.2 2. Disagree: 17.0 1. Strongly Disagree: 10.4
Reimbursement is not a barrier to using the RFVS.	3.32 (0.86)	5. Strongly Agree: 6.0 4. Agree: 35.9 3. Unsure: 46.2 2. Disagree: 8.1 1. Strongly Disagree: 3.8

Journal of Midwifery and Women's Health 2002; 47(4): 269–277

Australian women's stories of their baby-feeding decisions in pregnancy

Athena Sheehan, Virginia Schmied, Margaret Cooke

Objective: to describe the baby-feeding decisions of a group of Australian women prior to birth.

Design, setting and participants: a qualitative study using face-to-face, in-depth interviews was undertaken with 29 women. All interviews were audiotape recorded and transcribed verbatim. Data were analysed using thematic analysis.

Findings: the women observed and sought information from a variety of sources, as well as exploring their own understandings of themselves and their breasts. Based on this knowledge the women made their antenatal baby-feeding decisions. These baby-feeding decisions grouped into four thematic groups, 'assuming I'll breast feed'; 'definitely going to breast feed'; 'playing it by ear' and 'definitely going to bottle feed'. Each of these standpoints was associated with, and precipitated, a number of behaviours and strategies.

Implications: the findings of this research highlight the need for antenatal educators and midwives who provide care in pregnancy to acknowledge a range of experiences and expectations of women and to provide diverse educational opportunities to meet a range of needs. There is a need for further research to identify how midwives can encourage and assist women to explore and challenge their assumptions about breast feeding as they relate to other aspects of their lives.

Introduction

Breast feeding is recognised and recommended globally as the optimum means of baby feeding, conferring benefits to both the mother and baby. As a consequence of this, many research efforts have been aimed at identifying factors that predict breast-feeding initiation and duration or breast-feeding attrition. In a review of the literature of factors associated with the initiation and duration of breast feeding, Scott and Binns (1999) found that in recent studies employing multivariate analysis there was a strong and consistent association with demographic factors such as maternal age and level of education, and a less consistent association with factors such as marital and socio-economic status. Similarly, associations that had previously been identified between breast feeding and biomedical factors, such as parity, method of delivery and baby health, were less consistent in multivariate studies. The authors also identified a consistent negative association between maternal smoking habits and breast-feeding duration and evidence to suggest that fathers play an important role in

the breast-feeding decision and that intended duration is a strong predictor of actual duration (Scott & Binns, 1999).

It can be argued that many studies consider or assume that the decision to breast feed is largely a matter of individual choice and rational decision-making. Breast-feeding decisions and experiences are, however, complex, and rather than being an individual act, baby-feeding decisions are constructed and practised within the social milieu in which women live (Dettwyler, 1995). It has been found that factors such as a woman's physical health, the health of her baby, the needs of her other children and family members, the family's living conditions and other demands on the woman's time and energy will all influence a woman's baby-feeding decision (Carter, 1995; Hoddinott & Pill, 1999; Murphy, 1999).

Health professionals have predominantly studied the biophysical aspects of breast feeding and it can be argued that this focus habitually fails to recognise just how interdependent, and complex, the whole breast-feeding experience is (Dignam, 1995). Consequent to this, it is not surprising that professional practices and understandings around breast feeding are often incongruent with the understandings and experiences of breast feeding for women (Schmied & Barclay, 1999). There is, however, a growing body of research studies interested in women's actual experiences of breast feeding. These studies have highlighted the emotional and social significance that breast feeding may have for women (Bottorff, 1990; Hills-Bonczyk et al., 1994; Dignam, 1995; Hoddinott & Pill, 1999; Schmied & Barclay, 1999).

The aim of this study was to explore the physical, social and emotional experiences influencing women's baby-feeding decisions by investigating women's own decision-making processes and what they perceived influenced these decisions. The purpose of this article is to present findings from this study that looked at women's experiences of baby-feeding decisions before birth.

Methods

Participants in this study were drawn from a larger research study that surveyed the postnatal outcomes of women. The purpose of the postnatal outcomes study was to examine the social, physical and psychological health outcomes of women in the first six months postpartum. The study was conducted in three public hospitals in one area health service in Sydney during 1999–2000. Women were recruited to the study during pregnancy when they were between 28 and 36 weeks gestation. If women gave informed written consent to the larger study they were then asked if they would also be willing to consent to participate in a face-to-face interview with a researcher about their baby-feeding experiences. If the woman was willing to participate in an interview she was then required to sign a separate consent form. Women who gave consent to participate in the face-to-face interview were then purposively sampled according to the answers they gave to breast-feeding questions asked in the larger study questionnaires. These questionnaires were administered antenatally and then at two weeks, six weeks, three months and six months postnatally. Purposive sampling was chosen in order to obtain a variety of baby-feeding experiences and socio-demographic characteristics such as age, parity, socio-economic status, based on income, breast-feeding intention, reasons for breast feeding and experience with breast feeding. Ethics approval to conduct this study was granted to the researchers by the participating Area Health Service Ethics Committees and the University of Technology Sydney, Human Research Ethics Committee.

Data collection and analysis

Ultimately 29 women were interviewed. Twenty-nine women were included in the sample because we found this number provided sufficient variation in socio-demographics and feeding experiences. Our previous work has also found that between 25 and 30 participants provides sufficient details, through interviews on aspects of an experience, to generate enough data for rigorous analysis.

In-depth semi-structured interviews were used to collect data. Interviews were conducted at a mutually agreed and convenient place and time, usually the participant's home. Interviews were tape recorded, then transcribed verbatim. Prompts such as, 'Tell me about your decisions regarding baby feeding', 'What has influenced your decision to breast feed?', 'How do you feel about your decision?', 'Who have you discussed your decisions with?' and 'What do you think it will feel like feeding your baby?' were used to stimulate the woman's own accounts. Data were analysed using descriptive thematic analysis. Transcripts were initially coded to identify concepts in the data using a process based on the precepts of grounded theory (Strauss & Corbin, 1998). These concepts were then grouped to form broad themes that centred on the women's decisions, factors that influenced their decisions, and the consequences of these factors and decisions.

Narrative has been chosen to present these data because it is an evocative and highly personalised way of presenting women's experiences (Richardson, 1994). Four stories have been written using the women's own words to illustrate each of the four identified decision categories. Although each story has been given a single name, each story is an amalgamation of a number of women's experiences whose stories were typical of the decision category that they come within. Each category included the stories and decisions of women who were both multiparae and primiparae.

Findings

Nineteen women were primiparae and 10 women were multiparae. Twenty-three women were married; three were in a de facto relationship, one woman identified herself as single and two women as divorced or separated. The age range of the participants was 20–41 years and the mean age was 31 years. Two women of the sample had private health insurance; all other participants were covered by Australian public health cover. Five women stated that they received a government pension. In terms of highest completed level of education, 16 women in the sample had completed a diploma or degree, five had completed secondary school to year 12 and eight had completed secondary school < year 12.

Analysis of the women's accounts revealed that many gave considerable thought to their decision regarding baby feeding. The decisions women made in relation to baby feeding before birth were in four thematic groups. These groups were: 'assuming I'll breast feed'; 'definitely going to breast feed'; 'playing it by ear'; and 'definitely going to bottle feed'. Each of these decisions appeared to be based on a number of influences and were associated with a number of other behaviours. Women in this study sought information from health professionals such as midwives, naturopaths and homeopaths, as well as friends and family. The women also observed, listened to and talked to other mothers, read books, pamphlets and searched the Internet. In addition to this, some women had previous experiences of breast feeding that they drew from. After making their decisions, the women committed to, and planned for, their decisions and some of them, who believed that their decision might be socially unacceptable, hid their decisions. These are their stories.

Belinda: Assuming I'll breast feed

Belinda just assumed she'd breast feed. She said:

I just assumed I'd breast feed yes ... well it's just part of having a baby you know, you get pregnant, you have a baby and you breast feed. That's what breasts are there for. Just having a baby you'd automatically breast feed.

Belinda did not even question it. There was no choice, there was no:

... shall I breast feed, shall I bottle feed. Maybe it's because mum breast fed all of us or just that my breasts are part of my body, part of being a woman. I don't know it was part of having a baby.

Belinda was not aware of any external pressure to breast feed and so she certainly did not consider that breast feeding could be problematic, and she made no specific plans regarding breast feeding, she thought it would just happen:

I thought ... naturally it would be part of it ... it went with the pregnancy, it was part of the parcel. I don't think we ever discussed it, it was more, you know, 'my breasts are getting bigger oh wow' you know buying the next bra size up and then before he was born buying a couple of feeding bras, so it was never under discussion, it was always going to be part of it.

Following her baby's birth Belinda stated, 'I didn't even think about it ... I'd planned to breast feed but I never really put any thought into it'.

Emily: I'm definitely breast feeding

In contrast to Belinda, Emily had thought a lot about how she was going to feed her baby. While some of the reasons given for breast feeding were similar to Belinda's for example, 'breast feeding was what breasts were for', Emily differed from Belinda in that she had given considered thought to why she wanted to breast feed. Emily was definitely going to breast feed. She said:

I've always intended to breast feed. I've always seen breast feeding as the way you do it. I just grew up with everybody tit out. That's how you feed a baby.

Emily saw breast feeding as primitive and instinctual:

It's what they did hundreds and hundreds of years ago. The baby looks for it. It's their first instinct; their eyesight is from here to your breast, that's the only instinct they know. The natural thing is to breast feed, not to shove a bottle in its mouth. Even as a child I thought bottle feeding didn't look right.

Emily also stated that she knew breast was best and she wanted to be able to give her baby:

... a good chance and build up the immunity and make sure he was well nourished.

In addition to this, Emily was convinced that breast feeding was more comforting for the baby and crucial to bonding:

I think breast feeding just makes the bonding that bit stronger, it gels the trust. You know he's crying, he's hungry, so you just drop your body closer and then a nice, privileged moment together, a privilege for both of us.

Emily was sure her partner would expect her to breast feed, to do the best for their baby.

Despite being sure she would breast feed, Emily was aware that breast feeding might not be easy, but this did not appear to affect her resolve, instead Emily set about committing herself to her decision and making plans to ensure that she would be successful:

I don't necessarily think breast feeding is going to be easy. Some people I know have tried ... they've given it a go and for whatever reason it just wasn't working. In fact people say to me you'll be disappointed if you can't breast feed. Well that won't be me. I am determined to breast feed. I'm going to give it a one hundred per cent shot. I'm not going to be one of those people. I'm going to drink dill tea; it's good for the milk and well my homeopath has given me a kit. I've been assured everything is fixable. And I really believe if you have the confidence in yourself you'll be able to breast feed. Everyone has horror stories about mastitis and cracked nipples and biting and things like that! So I am a bit concerned that it's going to hurt and I am going to end up with mastitis, but some people in my family had problems; it took a few weeks but they got over them. You know I think it's all in the mind really; if you are confident then you'll be able to breast feed.

Emily was conscious that feeding in public was not always looked on positively and although she felt she would have no problems feeding in public, stating that if your baby needs food then you should just 'flop it out and feed', she did qualify this by saying 'but I wouldn't do it in front of my father-in-law though, because he was taught not to show affection. It would embarrass him'.

Emily was aware also that there was a pressure to breast feed, although she herself was not experiencing any pressure. She said:

You know, there's a lot of pressure on women to breast feed and a lot of negativity about people that choose not to breast feed. I haven't actually had that pressure I guess because I've expected that I'm going to breast feed.

Emily highlighted that because of the pressure to breast feed she knew some women were unwilling to disclose their decision to bottle feed. She said:

Do you realise a lot of women who choose not to breast feed just say they are going to breast feed.

Melanie: I'm going to play it by ear

Melanie had decided that she was going to 'play it by ear'. Like Emily she had invested a lot of thought into her decision. Emily identified two main reasons for her decision and these were because she was not sure she would cope with the physical sensations related to breast feeding, and because she had seen other women encounter problems with breast feeding and as a consequence felt there could be a lot of difficulties and stress connected to breast feeding. Melanie talked about her feelings relating to the actual act of breast feeding and also to her feelings about her breasts in terms of being touched. She said:

You know, I don't feel very comfortable with the thought of breast feeding. The thought just makes me feel like a big cow. I know some women feel so womanly but I feel less than a woman, less attractive. My breasts have never been a very sensual part of my body. I don't even like them being touched with sex.

Melanie talked about observing women who had difficulties with breast feeding. Melanie had friends who tried to breast feed but could not for various reasons and she had friends who had really persevered. Melanie saw that there was resultant stress in either persevering or having difficulties. She said:

I've seen other friends also when things go wrong or become difficult or are not as they expected it's going to be, they get absolutely distraught; in fact, most of the stress that I've seen in my friends is because of breast feeding.

This knowledge, that breast feeding could be difficult and stressful, made Melanie fearful and added to her concerns about breast feeding.

Melanie was very aware of the benefits of breast milk, however, and stated:

I'm not unintelligent; I am very aware of the benefits of breast feeding … and ultimately I know that's the best thing I can do for my baby.

But this knowledge contributed to an underlying concern that if she did not breast feed she would not be doing the best for her baby and would consequently feel guilty:

But I'm sure I will still have feelings of guilt if its not working and I decide to bottle-feed. I'll think, 'Oh my God I'm doing the wrong thing by my child'.

Melanie felt these feelings were exacerbated by an 'incredible pressure' she felt was exerted on women to breast feed. Melanie had experienced this pressure from her family, friends and professionals. She said:

I've found there's incredible pressure out there to breast feed. You know when I told my sister I was thinking I might not breast feed she was aghast! And when I asked the midwife at the hospital whether I will encounter any problems with the staff if I don't breast feed she said 'yes' and those ads, you know, telling you and it is telling you not … it doesn't feel like it's ever advising that breast feeding's best and how could you not.

As a result of this pressure Melanie had chosen to keep her concerns regarding her decision to herself. She said:

So I just haven't brought it up again, and even if I was going to bottle feed I wouldn't do it in hospital, I'd wait until I got home.

Melanie felt the pressure to breast feed had made her feel like she was not a good mother, stating:

They're the kind of undertones that you get all the time, you're being the worst mother in the world by not breast feeding.

She was concerned that a woman's right to make a decision was somehow manipulated and that a woman's individual choices were not respected:

I don't think they respect you as an individual person, a person in your own right who has feelings and whatever as well. You tend to get caught up in the machinery of 'this is what you should be doing'.

Melanie talked about needing support for her decision:

I suppose in the whole process you're really searching for someone to say it's okay to feel like that and what you decided is good and it's a good thing for you and that's great.

This was despite the fact that she felt she had the support of her partner, who had said 'Whatever you want, whatever is most comfortable and easiest for you'. Ultimately, Melanie sets limits, she was willing to start with breast feeding but she was not prepared at this stage to persevere if problems arose.

In terms of feeding in public, Melanie stated that she would not feel comfortable feeding in public or in somebody else's home with other people:

So that there's my personal thing. I just don't feel comfortable with it, I don't look at women who do it and think 'how revolting', I don't, you know. I think 'I wish I could be

...' but it's just ... it's not something that I feel comfortable with. Some women are very comfortable with just breast feeding wherever but I'm just not like that.

Alexia: I'm going to bottle feed

Finally, Alexia's story illustrates the decision to bottle feed. Alexia had also put a lot of thought into her decision to bottle feed, stating that she knew as soon as she became pregnant that she was never going to breast feed. One of the reasons given for this perspective was based on her feelings about her breasts:

It sort of like repulses me and the idea of having a baby sucking on them is oh ammm.

Alexia felt that these feelings of revulsion would affect her relationship with her baby. Another major reason that Alexia gave for her decision to bottle feed was that she felt she wanted her body back. She stated:

... and besides I think by the end of nine months of being pregnant, I just want my body back.

Finally, Alexia viewed breast feeding as very demanding of herself and her time, possibly problematic and as a result stressful.

Alexia also had inverted nipples and felt this would make it even more difficult for her to breast feed. She had observed that 'even people with really healthy nipples still have trouble feeding'. Her mother had also confirmed that breast feeding with inverted nipples was problematic. While Alexia was aware that there were 'these awful things to suck them out' she was not prepared to go through this. She talked about the midwives' suggestion that she see a lactation consultant who would just look on her nipples as a challenge. Her response to this was:

Well she's not going to look on mine as a challenge. It is my body, just leave it alone.

She felt:

It's almost like you as a person are gone and we need your body and we need those breasts and we need those nipples out.

Alexia also talked about the disapproval she received from some of her friends and family, as well as health professionals, if she voiced her decision to bottle feed. As a consequence of this disapproval she had chosen to hide her decision to bottle feed.

Anyway, I just decided I wouldn't say anything about not breast feeding until, you know, I get a bit further into the pregnancy. I just won't say anything until I get to about 38 weeks.

Alexia felt that while it is not actually said, there was an assumption that if you were not breast feeding then you were not being a good mother.

Alexia stated there was an enormous pressure to breast feed. She felt that everyone just assumed you would breast feed and that 'at all costs' you were to breast feed, and that this was done in such a way that if you did not breast feed there was enormous guilt. As she described:

Even the education campaign is all really done on a guilt basis. You're told if you don't breast feed you know your child is going to get sick because it is not going to have any immunity and your child is going to get an allergy. The doctor told me 'Your child will have a better chance of going to university if you breast feed'.

Alexia felt that her decision was not always respected and that in all this promotion of breast feeding, the woman just got lost in amongst it all:

It seems to me that the medical profession is too stuck on what the WHO says and forgets that people are people, they do things differently, they have different temperaments and stuff.

In spite of acknowledging the benefits of breast milk, Alexia talked about observing friends with young children who were bottle fed and who looked well:

But you know many of my friends they use bottle feeding and their babies are all healthy and look good and have no problems at all.

Alexia talked about comparing children who were bottle fed with breast-fed children and felt:

A lot of babies survive and thrive on formula.

Alexia recognised that although artificial milk might not be as good as breast milk, formula was still very good. She stated:

... and you can't tell me in this day and age that if you can clone people and sheep that you can't get something that's pretty darn close to breast milk. I'll get that milk with the added oil.

Although Alexia was quite clear that she would not feel comfortable feeding in public, she was also compelled to let it be known that she would not be put off or repulsed by seeing other people feed in public.

Discussion

The purpose of this research was to describe the baby-feeding decisions made prior to birth by a group of women in Sydney, Australia. One of the limitations of this research is that it describes the experiences of a specific, small group of women and therefore the degree to which the findings apply to the breast-feeding population cannot be estimated. It does, however, add to the growing knowledge base of other qualitative studies that have endeavoured to provide a deeper understanding of the complexity of baby-feeding experiences for women. The findings of this study demonstrate that, apart from the women who assumed they would breast feed, women put a lot of thought into their breast-feeding decision during pregnancy. They observed and listened to other women and reflected on their own needs and experiences both in relation to breast feeding, as well as their feelings about their breasts and understandings of themselves. They also read and sought information and planned for their decision. Contrary to other research findings (Scott & Binns, 1999), the father did not appear to play an integral role in the breast-feeding decisions of the women in this study, although it could be argued that there was an implicit need for the husband's approval in some of the quotes. For example, Emily was sure her husband would expect her to breast feed. The decision to breast feed was made either prior to pregnancy, during pregnancy or for some women they were waiting to decide until after the birth of their baby. A number of actions appeared to occur as a result of these women's decisions that were related to specific responses and plans.

A number of themes were identified in this study that appeared to influence the baby-feeding decision. One of the most dominant themes affecting the decision was the embodied expression of breast feeding. 'Embodiment' can be explained as describing both the conscious and unconscious physical and emotional sensations and perceptions of the body. Embodiment is a term that recognises the body not just as a physiological entity, but as a sensual, emotional and social entity that has conscious and unconscious needs, desires and boundaries (Merleau-Ponty, 1962). Some women in this study expressed this embodied experience as a nurturing, natural experience that provided a continued connectedness between them and their baby that was a benefit and privilege to both of them. Other women identified that, for them, the thought and experience of breast feeding was uncomfortable and repulsive and that even touching the breasts was difficult for them.

Schmied and Barclay (1999) identified that breast feeding was an embodied experience that women found difficult to articulate. In their study, they identified that, for some women, this embodied experience was 'connected, harmonious and pleasurable', while for others it was 'disruptive, unpleasant and violent' (p. 325).

In this study, when women expressed a strong sense of embodiment in relation to breast feeding, they also related how this would affect their relationship with their baby. Women who felt strongly that breast feeding was nurturing and natural expressed how breast feeding would translate into a strong bond between the mother and her baby. Women who voiced a strong sense of repulsion with breast feeding were concerned that this embodied reaction could affect their relationship with their baby, but in a negative way. This effect on relationship was extremely important to both perspectives.

Another dominant theme articulated by these women was that breast feeding could be difficult and problematic. The only exception to this was the group who just assumed they would breast feed. The perception that breast feeding could or would be difficult appeared to create a sense of fear amongst the women and, depending on the woman's decision, this knowledge had two main responses. Women who were 'definitely going to breast feed' responded to the fear of breast-feeding difficulties by committing themselves to breast feeding and making plans for possible difficulties. Those who were 'playing it by ear' set limits to how much they would persevere with breast feeding if they experienced difficulties, stating they would not persevere if, for example, either they or their baby were not enjoying it, or if they were experiencing difficulties.

Other researchers have recognised the concept of 'commitment' to breast feeding. In her phenomenological study, Bottorff (1990) found commitment to be important to persistence in breast feeding, arguing that the more a woman commits herself to breast feeding, the more she will be able to do so, even in the face of difficulties. Alternatively, in their quantitative study, Lawson and Tulloch (1995) found no relationship between commitment and confidence as a predictor of breast-feeding duration. This could be because their sample only comprised of primiparous women (Lawson & Tulloch, 1995) and, as Bottorff (1990) explains, a mother will not know the reality of breast feeding until she begins to breast feed and it is 'only in the execution of the action that our inner strength and intentions are put to the test' (p. 203).

Using discourse analysis, Hoddinott and Pill (1999) also identified that commitment and confidence were important to breast-feeding decisions and used these terms in the classification of respondents into baby-feeding groups. Our findings, however, appear to be somewhat different to the findings of Hoddinott and Pill (1999) in terms of commitment. In their study, 'committed breast feeders' did not spontaneously bring up anticipated problems, whereas in this current study, the women who said they were definitely going to breast feed and committed themselves to it did mention possible difficulties with breast feeding. Commitment to breast feeding in this study appeared to be as a result of knowing that there could be potential problems.

There are no clear definitions to explain the concept of commitment in relation to breast feeding in any current research. It can be argued that the concept of commitment to breast feeding needs to be more fully explored in order to fully understand its implications and effect on breast-feeding decisions and outcomes, and whether it is a modifiable concept. The following gives an interpretation of what commitment meant to the women in this particular study.

The women in the 'definitely breast feeding' group talked about their commitment to their decision, about giving breast feeding a 100% shot and not changing their mind. Commitment appeared to be a result of making the decision to breast feed in the face of the reality that breast feeding is not always easy and, in fact, can be problematic. For the women in this study, commitment extended to ensuring they had things in train should there be difficulty with breast feeding, such as homeopathic aids and/or consuming galactagogues, such as dill tea. Commitment was also seen as needing to be prepared mentally for the experience of breast feeding – that is, needing to believe and feel confident that they could successfully breast feed.

The women in all groups appeared to know the benefits of breast feeding, but not all the women felt that breast was always best for mother and baby. Women in the 'definitely going to breast feed' group appeared to use the information that 'breast is best' to confirm and justify their decision to breast feed. For some women in the 'playing it by ear' and the 'definitely bottle feeding' groups they used this information to compare and observe bottle-fed babies and breast-fed babies, and then questioned the validity of 'breast is best' in terms of the everyday, arguing that babies can obviously survive and thrive on artificial milk. Women in the 'play it by ear' and 'definitely bottle feeding' categories also felt that information promoting 'breast is best' contributed to the pressure to breast feed. They felt health professionals saw breast is best for the baby as pre-eminent over the mother's needs, or problems leading some women to feel that they needed to feed at all costs and if they did not, their babies would be disadvantaged and they would be considered or feel bereft as a mother. These feelings resulted in a sense of guilt for some women. Other researchers have also identified that women express feelings of guilt and self-doubt when they are unable to breast feed (McNatt & Freston, 1992; Sheehan, 1999).

In response to the 'breast is best' mantra, a number of women in the 'playing it by ear group' and the 'definitely bottle feeding' group were quite adamant that breast feeding was not always good for the mother and that it could cause, amongst other things, high levels of distress and disrupt their relationship with their baby and their partner. Even one of the women in the definitely breast-feeding group readily acknowledged that breast feeding was not for all women and that in fact women should be given a choice in baby feeding without prejudice.

In this study, it appeared that some women chose to hide their decisions about bottle feeding. It could be argued that this was done in order to maintain some sense of control over their decision, rather than being subjected to the need to explain their decision and the concomitant disapproval that would result in their decision not to breast feed. Maushart (1997) also found that in certain groups of women it is almost unacceptable to relate why one stopped breast feeding.

Murphy (1999) argues that 'infant feeding decisions are as much about morality as they are about nutrition' (p. 225) and that a woman's baby-feeding decisions call for her to establish her goodness, not only as a mother but also as a partner and woman. Women in this study expressed the need for support even if they chose to bottle feed. Interestingly, over 80% of women in Australia currently choose to initiate breast feeding (Donath & Amir, 2000) and a significant proportion (5–8%) will cease breast feeding prior to discharge from hospital (Fetherston, 1995; Scott et al., 2001), with approximately a further 9% discontinuing in the first two weeks postpartum (Scott et al., 2001). It could be hypothesised that at least some of these women may have decided that they would not breast feed prior to birth but went through the motions to prevent condemnation.

One other important issue that was raised in this study was the issue of feeding in public. Even women who had chosen to 'definitely breast feed' raised this issue and had considered strategies for overcoming perceived difficulties with this. Strategies included deciding who they would not feed in front of, and where they would feed in public, or timing their feeding to not occur when they were out. This is not surprising given that in Western cultures the breast is largely fetished as a sexual object and one of the reasons given for not breast feeding is embarrassment (Morrow, 1995; Dykes & Griffiths, 1998).

Conclusion

While the stories have been aggregated into four major antenatal baby-feeding decision groups, this research demonstrates the complexity of the baby-feeding decisions and the differing needs of women making these decisions. This has implications for midwives caring for women in the antenatal period and particularly childbirth educators who are encouraged to provide antenatal breast-feeding education. These findings highlight the need for acknowledging a range of experiences and expectations of women, and providing diverse educational opportunities to meet a range of needs. More research is required to identify how midwives can encourage and assist women to explore and challenge their own feelings and assumptions about breast feeding as they relate to other relevant aspects of their lives, including without feeling guilty, rather than simply providing breast-feeding advice about the benefits and/or the 'how to' of the breast-feeding process. These findings also highlight the importance of describing and theorising the complexity of women's breast-feeding experiences.

REFERENCES

Bottorff J. 1990. Persistence in breastfeeding: a phenomenological investigation. Journal of Advanced Nursing, 15: 201–209

Carter P. 1995. Feminism, Breasts and Breast-feeding. Macmillan Press, Houndmills

Dettwyler K. 1995. Beauty and the breast: the cultural context of breastfeeding in the United States. In: Stuart-Macadam P, Dettwyler K (eds), Breastfeeding Biocultural Perspectives. Walter de Gruyter, New York

Dignam D. 1995. Understanding intimacy as experienced by breastfeeding women. Health Care for Women International, 16: 477–485

Donath S, Amir LH. 2000. Rates of breastfeeding in Australia by state and socioeconomic status: evidence from the 1995 National Health Survey. Journal of Paediatrics and Child Health, 36: 164–168

Dykes F, Griffiths H. 1998. Societal influences upon initiation and continuation of breastfeeding. British Journal of Midwifery, 6(2): 76–80

Fetherston C. 1995. Factors influencing breastfeeding initiation and duration in a private Western Australian maternity hospital. Breastfeeding Review, 3(1): 9–14

Hills-Bonczyk SG, Tromiczak KR, Avery MD et al. 1994. Women's experiences with breastfeeding longer than 12 months. Birth, 21(4): 206–212

Hoddinott P, Pill R. 1999. Qualitative study of decisions about infant feeding among women in East End of London. British Medical Journal, 318(7175): 30–34

Lawson K, Tulloch M. 1995. Breastfeeding durations: prenatal intentions and postnatal practices. Journal of Advanced Nursing, 22: 841–849

Maushart S. 1997. The Mask of Motherhood. Vintage, Sydney

McNatt M, Freston M. 1992. Social support and lactation outcomes in postpartum women. Journal of Human Lactation, 8(2): 73–77

Merleau-Ponty M. 1962. Phenomenology of Perception (Smith C, transl.). Routledge & Kegan Paul, London

Morrow M. 1995. Barriers to Breastfeeding, Vol. Set VII. Lactation Resource Centre, Melbourne

Murphy E. 1999. 'Breast is Best': infant feeding decisions and maternal deviance. Sociology of Health and Illness, 21(2): 187–208

Richardson L. 1994. Writing a method of inquiry. In: Denzin NK, Lincoln YS (eds), Handbook of Qualitative Research. Sage Publications, Thousand Oaks, CA

Schmied V, Barclay L. 1999. Connection and pleasure, disruption and distress: women's experience of breastfeeding. Journal of Human Lactation, 15(4): 325–334

Scott JA, Binns CW. 1999. Factors associated with the initiation and duration of breastfeeding: a review of the literature. Breastfeeding Review, 7(1): 5–16

Scott JA, Landers MC, Hughes R et al. 2001. Psychosocial factors associated with the abandonment of breastfeeding prior to hospital discharge. Journal of Human Lactation, 17(1): 24–30

Sheehan A. 1999. A comparison of two methods of antenatal breast-feeding education. Midwifery, 15: 274–282

Strauss A, Corbin J. 1998. Basics of Qualitative Research: Techniques and Procedures for Developing Grounded Theory. Sage Publications, Thousand Oaks, CA

Midwifery 2003; 19(4): 259–266

The big pregnancy brain mush myth

Sara Wickham

Researchers at a recent British Psychological Society conference claim to have refuted the 'myth' that women's mental capacities diminish during pregnancy (HMG Worldwide Ltd, 2003). Their small study investigated whether there was any justification in the idea that pregnant women tend to suffer from impaired memory and concentration. They found that, although the pregnant women felt that their memory and concentration were reduced, there were no differences in the cognitive abilities of the pregnant and non-pregnant women studied.

The authors clearly feel these results are very positive. They have shown that pregnant women score just as well on intellectual tests as non-pregnant women. They feel we can now be rid of the 'myth' that women have different cognitive capabilities during pregnancy. The authors are also keen to debunk another 'myth' – that women have different cognitive abilities at different stages of their menstrual cycle. Hooray! Women, even pregnant and menstruating ones, are just as 'rational' as men.

But is rationality what we really desire during pregnancy? I don't have any real doubt that women can be rational and intellectual during pregnancy, if that is their choice. I suspect that might have been the (possibly subconscious) choice of the pregnant women in this study, who may well have seen value and personal reward in proving their cognitive capabilities in tests against the scores of non-pregnant women. But I am not convinced that this is a route we should allow psychologists to take pregnancy down, at least not without first engaging in the debate.

I suppose, in questioning the value of this research, I could be seen as one of the midwives criticised by the study for perpetuating the idea that the brain is different in pregnancy. But I don't do this to denigrate pregnant women, and I don't want to insist that pregnancy leads to automatic cognitive impairment. If anything, I am trying to hold a space for pregnant woman where it is acceptable to feel different, and where that does not lead to negative consequences, sarcastic comments or assumptions about the value of their abilities. I want it to be okay for all pregnant women to experience whatever it means for them to be pregnant. If that means they want to carry on and be as rational as possible, perhaps staying in an intellectually demanding job until they give birth, then let's support that as their choice. But if they want to know it's also okay to be in a less-than-rational space for part or all of their pregnancy, then I'd like to support that possibility too.

Cultures that place a high value on rationality are usually characterised by male-based society and religion, and have tended to suggest that menstruating and sometimes pregnant women should be segregated because they are less than clean. Even today, while menstruating women are not segregated in the UK, we are still bombarded with adverts which offer products to help us hide the fact that we are menstruating and enable us to carry on with our everyday roles. Yet older, female-based philosophies enabled women to set themselves apart, so that they could experience and enjoy their 'differentness' (Eisler, 1995). In some circles, the menstruating (and menopausal) woman is still perceived as especially magical and wise, and value is given to her increased ability to be intuitive, rather than taken from her decreased desire to be rational.

Some very experienced midwives have talked about the value of not being rational during pregnancy, and how this enables the woman's hormones and body to lead her in her journey towards birth and motherhood (Wickham, 1999; Gaskin, 2002). We clearly needed to move on from the image of the helpless and dependent middle-class Victorian woman in claiming the rights of women as equal and valuable community members, but it is quite another thing to find that we are in danger of ending up in a position where we deny difference. My fear is that, by setting out to prove that pregnant women are no different from non-pregnant ones, or from men, we will lose the little space that women do have to explore what female rites of passage mean for them.

I don't know whether the 'big pregnancy brain mush myth' is a myth or not. I don't know whether all women have the potential to experience a different kind of reality during menstruation, pregnancy and menopause, or whether this idea has developed as a way of simply allowing women more space at this time. I do know, both rationally and in my heart, that to continue to extol the rational as better than other ways of being and knowing is not going to take us nearly as far as if we stay open to the possibilities and stop trying to deny or remove difference.

REFERENCES

Eisler R. 1995. The Chalice and the Blade, 2nd edn. HarperCollins, New York

Gaskin IM. 2002. Spiritual Midwifery, 4th edn. TNL The Book Publishing Company, Summertown

HMG Worldwide Ltd. 2003. Women 'not mentally affected' by pregnancy. http://uk.news.yahoo.com/030314/103/dvfzg.html (accessed 27 March 2003)

Wickham S. 1999. Reclaiming the art in birth. Midwifery Matters, 83(Winter): 6–7. Republished at: www.midwifery.org.uk

The Practising Midwife 2003; 6(5): 41

A body of knowledge – body image in pregnancy and the role of the midwife

Lorna Davies

Pretty women wonder where my secret lies
I'm not cute or built to suit a model's fashion size
But when I start to tell them
They think I'm telling lies.
I say
It's in the reach of my arms
The span of my hips
The stride of my steps
The curl of my lips.
I'm a woman
Phenomenally
Phenomenal woman
That's me.
(Angelou, 1995)

How many of us truly feel the pride apparent in this wonderful poem by Maya Angelou in relation to our appearance? How many of us are really happy with how we look, the size of our breasts and bellies, the cellulite on our hips and thighs? Women are under constant pressure to buy into, as Naomi Wolf (1994) accurately phrases it, 'The Beauty Myth'. We are barraged by the image of the body beautiful by the beauty, fashion and dieting industries, and are urged to aspire to this, in order to achieve a resemblance to a Western industrialised culturally shaped definition of 'beauty'. The truth is that if we stop for a moment and reflect on what is traded as the current body ideal, the youthful, curvy yet toned, fresh faced, symmetrically featured fashion model, we know in our hearts that we are, to use a proverbial expression, being sold a pup.

In this article I intend to explore what effect perceived body image may have on women during pregnancy, how these perceptions are manifested following the birth of their baby, and how the midwife can help to promote a positive attitude by exploring their own feelings about their own bodies.

As a facilitator, I run a session on body image which I begin by getting the group to use a self-reflection tool. The tool consists of the following questions. The participants are informed that the questions refer only to their physical state and not to their personalities.

- How do you see or picture yourself?
- How do you feel others perceive you?
- What do you believe about your physical appearance?
- How do you feel about your body?
- How do you feel in your body?
  (International Eating Disorder Referral website)

The questions are presented one at a time, and the participants are given some time to contemplate the questions on their own. They then get into pairs and then groups of four to discuss the questions and, if they so wish, their own responses. It is always an emotionally charged session where voices increase in volume and pitch and normally quiet group members become animated during the process. A box of tissues is always readily available, as sometimes there are tears. I wander around the groups and ask them if everything is OK and invariably the responses that I receive vary little between groups. The women (I have only ever carried this out in the presence of women; I feel that the presence of men would create a very different dynamic) almost unanimously make negative comments about the way that they picture themselves. These negative comments, as you may have guessed, usually focus around their weight (sometimes under, more often over) followed by comments about age. The question about how they feel that others perceive them is usually met with a mixed response. Some of the group members, who had previously made disparaging comments about their size, acknowledge that others might perceive them as 'relatively slim' or 'quite attractive', whereas others feel that the outside world identify them as negatively as they perceive themselves. The third question, asking them what they really believe about their bodies, can be very illuminating, as some of the group members acknowledge that they actually only made disparaging comments about their appearance in order to be contradicted, and really deep down, they are not desperately unhappy about how they look. In essence they are seeking approval. Responses to the fourth question echo those of the first question, and they use terms like 'repulsed' and 'disgusted'. The final question is, in my opinion, probably the most revealing because quite a large number of the women find that in spite of previous negative thoughts around being fat, they do not actually feel uncomfortable in their body. In fact, they quite like the way that they feel within their body. I think of this as the 'Damascene' moment, as these women suddenly realise that they are what they are and that they actually don't dislike their bodies as much as they thought that they did. I would like to think that perhaps for some it is a turning point.

Many of the trends that emerge in this challenging session have been mirrored in studies exploring the issue of women and body dissatisfaction over the past few decades. Lamb et al. (1993) used a silhouette scale and asked women to identify which silhouette represented their current shape and their ideal shape. It emerged that the women, regardless of their age, presented an ideal that was far slimmer than their perceived actual state. Pinhas et al. (1999) discovered that women's moods would change for the worse and that their self-esteem appeared to have lessened when they were exposed to photographs of fashion models.

Cohen (2001) argues that we are all born into a culture, which could be defined as a set of shared ideas about the nature of what is right and what is wrong and what is positive and desirable and what is negative and undesirable. She states that the desirability of a specific body image has varied across time and culture, from the waif to the voluptuous, with many ideals in between. However, I feel that at this point in time there are several factors that change the landscape somewhat from other periods in history, and which have made the desire for the body ideal *the* most important feature for many women in Western society today. I would hypothesise that this is linked to the materialistic society in which we live. Consumerism encourages greed and an 'I must have' mindset, which applies to all areas of life. There is more than ever before and yet it would seem that we are no happier than we ever have been, if not less (Schumacher, 1993). The advertising world bombards us from every corner of our lives, creating dissatisfaction because most of us cannot hope to achieve the perfect world that the advertising moguls

would have us live in. This applies equally to how we are expected to look. As Susan Conheim (2003), one of the founding mothers of the Real Women Project, eloquently states:

When it comes to women, self-hate is capitalism's love child. There is a lot of money to be made upon the backs of women not liking who they are and not valuing their diversity (http://www.judithstock.com/Life_Lines_by_Judith_Stock/Real_Women/real_women.html)

In a recent television documentary entitled *The Trouble with Women*, a group of 11-year-old girls were interviewed about what would make them 'successful' in life. The girls unanimously felt that being beautiful was the most important marker on the road to success. One of the group did say that she thought that being nice might help her to become successful. However, when the presenter pressed her to decide which was more important, being beautiful or being nice, the little girl thought for a moment and sadly reflected that being beautiful was probably more important than being nice. At the tender age of 11 our daughters are already indoctrinated into believing that beauty is the most important attribute in terms of 'success'. In fact, we know from a number of studies that the indoctrination begins at a very early age, long before puberty (Wood et al., 1996; Cohane & Pope, 2001).

In the image-obsessed world of the 21st century, the message that beauty equals success is suffocating us and causing us to lose sight of sensibility and reason. It is stifling our self-worth and self-esteem, and creating an epidemic of eating disorders (Lamb et al., 1993; Fear et al., 1996; Barker & Galambos, 2003).

It would seem that the most important indication of beauty for women in Western societies is the prevailing ideal of thinness. This belief results in the desire of many women to acquire an unrealistically thin body shape. Certainly a range of different methodologies shows that the majority of women and girls perceive themselves as too fat and are dissatisfied with their body shape (Wardle & Beales, 1986; Lamb et al., 1993; Cash et al., 2004).

Rogan (1999) suggests that the emphasis on thinness oppresses women by serving as a form of social and psychological control. If this is so, then I would advocate that the issue of body shape and size takes on a particular significance during pregnancy, where the issues of control may create huge problems for many women.

Bordo (1995) argues that the body ideal is a body that is completely under control, tight and contained. In pregnancy, however, the woman has little control over her physical state, and it is unlikely to remain in a tightly controlled state. Her baby is going to grow, her body is going to grow her baby and consequently her body shape will change, perhaps for just a given period, perhaps forever.

Additionally, from the onset of her pregnancy, the woman will usually find that her body is under the regulation of external agencies that may remove her own sense of control even further. Bordo (1995) argues that the control of pregnant women is not simply exerted by the involvement of medical practitioners, but also more subtly in the ubiquitous and continuous promotion of self-restraint. We only need to consider the enormous list of the things that a pregnant woman is expected to do and not to do, what to eat and what not to eat in order to comply with the defined normative values of how a woman should behave during pregnancy.

What effect does this have on her response to her body image and her eating habits? One might imagine that a perceived loss of autonomy may have a negative impact on self-perception during pregnancy, but other than women who have serious eating disorders, such as anorexia nervosa and bulimia, this would not necessarily appear to be the case, at least during pregnancy.

In a 1994 study, Davies and Wardle evaluated the body image, body satisfaction and dieting practices of women during pregnancy, which they felt was a stage of life when social pressures for slimness might be expected to be relaxed. They discovered, by using an inventory to explore the 'drive for thinness' levels of an individual, that women had lower scores than their non-pregnant counterparts. They also ascertained that when body mass index was controlled for, the pregnant participants had significantly lower body dissatisfaction scale scores. They also rated themselves as less overweight in terms of body size and attempted to lose weight less. However, what the study also unearthed was that there was no evidence that pregnancy was associated with any relaxation of body image ideals. That is, that pregnant women would continue to choose a similar size of figure to non-pregnant women as their ideal. The authors reported that these results might suggest that the state of pregnancy may be associated with reduced weight concern despite an increased body size. This may be because they feel that there is greater social acceptability of their fatness during pregnancy, and the belief that they are 'eating for two'.

Another study which leads us to reflect on this possibility was carried out by Fox and Yamaguchi (1997). These researchers examined the relationship between pre-pregnant body weight and body image change in primigravid women. They found that women who were overweight before pregnancy were more likely to have a positive attitude to their changed body during pregnancy than women of a weight perceived to be within the 'normal' range. However, in spite of the fact that they felt better about themselves in pregnancy, overall the overweight women had a greater number of body concerns than the normal range group. Once again, was it the freedom from pressure that made women feel better about themselves during pregnancy? If this was the case, how would they cope with their bodies in the postpartum period?

The work of Carter et al. (2000) alleges that the positive behavioural and attitudinal changes that are seen to be associated with regard to eating and weight during pregnancy may not be borne out in the postnatal months. It would appear that this period is a vulnerable time for those with weight concerns. In the early weeks and months following birth, many women are carrying more weight than they did prior to conception and, in contrast to pregnancy, they may no longer attribute the weight gain to the positive aspects of nurturing their developing baby. A number of studies concur in their findings that the postnatal period is rife with concerns about the weight gained during pregnancy (Hisner, 1986; Baker et al., 1999). The work of all of these studies suggest that associations between eating attitudes, body mass index, and depression and anxiety are different in pregnancy compared with the postpartum period.

So where does this information leave us as midwives. Is there anything that we can or need to do in order to promote a positive body image during pregnancy that may help women to develop a more positive attitude during the postnatal period and beyond?

I would like at this juncture to return to the sessions that I facilitate on body image. What I didn't mention at the beginning of the article is that the sessions have all been held with groups of midwives and student midwives, who clearly carry the same hang-ups and negative feelings about their bodies as any other group of women. The activity makes the group aware of what negative baggage we carry around with us about our own bodies. What sort of messages are we then conveying to the women that we meet in our professional lives? I would suggest that if we promote a positive message about our own body image when meeting with pregnant women during the antenatal period, then we effectively provide a positive role model. In the evaluation of the session we revisit the 'Damascene' moment, when they realised that they do actually quite like their bodies, in spite of the fact that they do not necessarily meet the idealised body beautiful, and analyse how liberating that moment actually felt. How equally therapeutic could that be for the women that they work with in practice?

After the group members have finished discussing the issues and have reconvened, I ask one of the group if they would mind sitting in a chair at the front of the group. I explain that I am going to ask some of the remaining group members to offer a positive statement about the physical attributes of the chair occupier. Anyone in the group may raise their hand to make a contribution, but the person in the chair chooses just two or three people to speak, in order to allow everyone the chance to occupy the chair. In my experience the vast majority of the group will, after initial reticence, opt to sit in the chair, and the comments that are made will occasionally embarrass them, but equally thrill them and sometimes reduce them to tears. We are not very good at accepting praise in our busy lives, particularly praise relating to our physical state. The exercise serves to remind the group members how little attention they actually pay to themselves in their everyday lives.

Once again a point has been made which we can then relate to, the importance of getting the women that they meet in pregnancy to feel positive about themselves, and the importance of the comments that they make as midwives. Positive affirmation may turn a negative mindset into a positive one and could mean the difference between a woman who feels that she cannot cope with the overwhelming expectations of motherhood and a woman who has self-belief and knows that she can cope with support.

If we start the process by exploring our own feelings about our own bodies, we may gain greater insight and understanding into how women may be feeling during pregnancy and in the first months of motherhood. If, as the research suggests, women feel generally more positive about their bodies during pregnancy, then perhaps we should capitalise on that and use that period to give positive affirmation about the amazing job that she is doing in growing her baby and about how fabulous that she looks, and as we know many women, particularly in the middle months of their pregnancy, do look amazing. If she doesn't feel fabulous because of morning sickness, heartburn, piles and any other of the so-called minor problems of pregnancy, then we should inform her of why these things are occurring physiologically. For example, the fact that her body is producing plenty of progesterone, causing some discomfort but anchoring the pregnancy and preparing the body for birth. Just knowing that there is a sound physiological reason for most of these perceived negative episodes may make them more tolerable and may make her feel better about herself.

We need to unpack the much cited 'getting back to normal'. What is normal? Do we mean the pre-pregnancy state, which is certainly not 'normal' once a woman has been through pregnancy and childbirth? She has been through an amazing and transformative experience, to the centre of the labyrinth, and life will never be the same again. When in pregnancy do we really address the issue of the body after birth? In parent education sessions the use of a 'What I am looking forward to most after having my baby' activity will invariably lead to someone in the group saying 'I can't wait to get back into my jeans'. This is a golden opportunity to talk positively about the changes that may occur as she crosses the bridge from maiden to mother. This is doubly valuable if her partner is present, because they are the key person in making her feel loved and beautiful regardless of her changing shape and size during this time. We should remember that men are equally exposed to the ideal of the Beauty Myth and may well benefit from unpacking the issues as much as women.

Clearly, there are many other things that we could discuss with regard to promoting a more positive body image for women during pregnancy, such as being given a greater opportunity to establish stronger relationships by changing working practices to case loading, etc. Also at a societal level we could do much more to negate the damage wrought by the promotion of the body ideal, starting by making weight prejudice unacceptable, encouraging the value of diversity and encouraging citizens to take pride in developing a healthy lifestyle with a focus on healthy eating and healthy activity every day, with an emphasis on healthy living and not on looking more attractive.

However, if we begin by critically acknowledging our own hang-ups and act to address them, then we may be better placed to encourage pregnant women and make new mothers feel positive if not proud of their bodies regardless of the size and shape, before during and after pregnancy, and remember that:

Women need the power that comes from being at ease within their own bodies.

(Counihan & Van Estrik, 1999)

REFERENCES

Angelou M. 1995. Phenomenal Woman: Four Poems Celebrating Women. Random House, New York

Baker CW, Carter AS, Cohen LR, Brownell KD. 1999. Eating attitudes and behaviors in pregnancy and postpartum: global stability versus specific transitions. Annals of Behavioral Medicine, 21: 143–148

Barker, ET, Galambos, NL. 2003. Body dissatisfaction of adolescent girls and boys: risk and resource factors. Journal of Early Adolescence, 23: 141–165

Bordo S. 1995. Unbearable Weight: Feminism, Western Culture, and the Body. University of California Press, Berkeley

Carter A, Wood Baker C, Brownell KD. 2000. Body mass index, eating attitudes, and symptoms of depression and anxiety in pregnancy and the postpartum period. Psychosomatic Medicine, 62: 264–270

Cash TF, Morrow JA, Hrabosky JI, Perry AA. 2004. How has body image changed? A cross sectional investigation of college women and men from 1983 to 2001. Journal of Consulting and Clinical Psychology, 72: 1081–1090

Cohane GH, Pope HG. 2001. Body image satisfaction, dieting beliefs, and weight loss behaviors in adolescent girls and boys. Journal of Youth and Adolescence, 20: 361–379

Cohen B. 2001. The Psychology of Ideal Body Image as an Oppressive Force in the Lives of Women. http://www.healingthehumanspirit.com/pages/body_img.htm

Counihan C, Van Estrik P. 1999. Food and culture. A reader. Sociology of Health and Illness, 21(1): 124

Davies K, Wardle J. 1994. Body image and dieting in pregnancy. Journal of Psychosomatic Research, 38(8): 787–799

Fear JL, Bulik CM, Sullivan PF. 1996. The prevalence of disordered eating behaviours and attitudes in adolescent girls. New Zealand Journal of Psychology, 25: 7–12

Fox P, Yamaguchi C. 1997. Body image change in pregnancy: a comparison of normal weight and overweight primigravidas. Birth, 24(1): 35–40

Hisner P. 1986. Concerns of multiparas during the second postpartum week. J Obstet Gynecol Neonatal Nursing, 16: 195–203

International Eating Disorder website, http://www.edreferral.com/

Lamb CS, Jackson LA, Cassiday PB, Priest DJ. 1993. Body figure preferences of men and women: a comparison of two generations. Sex Roles, 28: 345–358

Pinhas L, Toner BB, Ali A, Garfinkel PE. 1999. The effects of the ideal of female beauty on mood and body satisfaction. International Journal of Eating Disorders, 25: 223–226

Rogan S. 1999. Body Image. Routledge, London

Thirty Minutes. 2005. The Trouble with Women. Channel 4 News, UK

Schumacher EF. 1993. Small is Beautiful: Study of Economics as if People Mattered. Vintage Press, London

Wardle J, Beales S. 1986. Restraint, body image and food attitudes in children from 12 to 18 years. Appetite, 7: 209–217

Wood KC, Becker JA, Thompson JK. 1996. Body image dissatisfaction in preadolescent children. Journal of Applied Developmental Psychology, 17: 85–100

Wolf N. 1994. The Beauty Myth. Vintage, London

www.market-research-report.com/datamonitor/DMCM1820.htm

Where might we go from here?

In her article on pregnancy and body image, Lorna Davies highlights how important it is for midwives to explore these issues, and describes the sessions she runs on 'body image'. If you wrote (or reflected on) the questions at the beginning of this section before reading her article, you might like to go back over what you wrote and explore it in the light of the article.

Lorna raised a number of issues relating to the way our culture views women's bodies, and pregnancy can raise these issues for women. I'll leave you with a reiteration of one of the questions raised in her article as an invitation for further debate:

Where does this information leave us as midwives? Is there anything that we can or need to do in order to promote a positive body image during pregnancy that may help women to develop a more positive attitude during the postnatal period and beyond?

Focus on...
Building Communities of Women

SECTION CONTENTS

4.1

Being used? Motive for user involvement

Beverley A Lawrence Beech

User involvement in maternity care has a long history. Individual women who questioned the quality of maternity care soon realised that their voices were stronger when they were representing a group. So, in the 1960s both the Association for Improvements in the Maternity Services (AIMS) and the National Childbirth Trust (NCT) were established. These groups work at many levels, empowering individual women to argue their case, assisting members to be effective committee members and responding to 'consultations' from a huge range of official bodies.

The 'ignorant' user

There was a time when user involvement in maternity care was viewed with amusement and, at times, horror. Women admitted to hospital were expected to consent to whatever the staff wanted to do and not worry their pretty little heads about the decisions that were being made. As the Medical Defence Union (1974) put it:

… When she enters hospital for her confinement it can be assumed that she assents to any necessary procedure, including the administration of a local, general or other anaesthetic.

Nor was it uncommon for the users to be dismissed as ignorant (Barrie, 1985):

It has to be pointed out that she has no medical or nursing qualifications, nor any form of recognised paramedical or scientific training … She cites literature she cannot possibly evaluate.

In 1974 Jean Robinson's article in *The Times* (Robinson, 1974) about unnecessary inductions of labour highlighted the harm that women were saying inductions caused, despite obstetricians' claims that induction of labour was a good thing.

Having failed to persuade obstetricians to listen to what women were saying, Robinson approached a social scientist, Ann Cartwright, and encouraged her to carry out a study of women's views of maternity care. Her research was the first major study of patients' views of hospital care. Users were realising that if obstetricians could not be persuaded to change, then other disciplines could be approached to provide scientifically based data to support the anecdotal accounts the user groups were hearing.

A growing voice

The National Perinatal Epidemiology Unit (NPEU) in Oxford was the first maternity organisation to involve users properly in its activities. Its director, Professor Sir Ian Chalmers, vigorously supported user involvement and from its inception in 1981 the NPEU invited users to its planning meetings.

In 1985 Professor Martin Bobrow, from the Paediatric Research Unit at Guys Hospital in London, invited AIMS to bring together interested maternity groups to discuss setting up a randomised controlled trial into chorionic villus sampling compared with amniocentesis. The meeting resulted in user groups assisting Professor Bobrow in producing an information leaflet that properly informed women about this trial, and was successfully distributed to the trial participants.

Use or abuse?

The next section highlights the increasing levels of user involvement instigated by government, hospitals and clinicians. On the face of it, such developments appear to be a positive move forward. However, levels of effectiveness vary and many different motives are at work.

Maternity Services Liaison Committees

Following a House of Commons Social Services report in 1980, the Government established Maternity Services Liaison Committees (MSLCs) in 1982. Their objectives were to monitor the effectiveness of procedures as they apply to individual women, and enable an integrated group of specialists and users to work together to improve maternity care. But while some MSLCs provided an effective way of including users in the planning and monitoring of services, many were used merely as 'talking shops' and were set up in a way that nobody was compelled to listen or act on their decisions.

The work of one committee does stand out. The recent House of Commons Select Committee Report on Choice in Maternity Services highlighted the evidence of Elizabeth Key, a north-west Lancashire MSLC member. Together with local midwives and mothers, this MSLC provided a factual, research-based information leaflet for local women. However, the Health Authority would not fund it, the primary care trusts refused to support it and the GPs would not distribute it because they 'were not happy' with the wording – and were not prepared to supply specific examples or alternatives. It is believed that the mention of 'home birth' and emphasis on the role of the midwives were enough to ensure GP opposition.

Hospital 'questionnaires'

Hospitals are keen to publicise examples of happy clients. Many do this by devising inadequate questionnaires designed to produce positive results.

Questionnaires are given to women before they leave hospital, they are not anonymised, they invariably ask simplistic multiple-choice questions, and a limited number of selected women are approached. The responses are then used to claim client satisfaction. Such 'pseudo' research is commonplace and rightly criticised by consumers, who want qualitative research to be carried out by social scientists who understand the issues.

Consultation overload

During the 1990s clinicians began to realise that excluding users from decisions about the provision of maternity care could be counter-productive. Users were developing an extensive network of like-minded individuals and organisations, and were producing their own books, leaflets and videos, and professionals were beginning to take the view that it was probably 'safer' to have users on the inside rather than the outside. There then developed a fashion of 'consultation'.

It seems that no self-respecting report can today be published without seeking user comments. As a result, childbirth groups are deluged with paperwork or, even worse, invitations to download reports from the Internet. This neatly ensures that postage is saved and the user groups bear the printing costs, which are not insubstantial. For example, the latest consultation document that AIMS has been invited to comment on is

260 pages long. Furthermore, the organisations producing these lengthy documents expect sensible comments, but they refuse to finance the time involved in considering such a document, and they usually set a very short deadline so that any comment is often rushed and not subjected to in-depth consideration.

Informed vs 'real' users

Although organisations involved with childbirth have remained lay and lay-dominated, their knowledge is increasing, they are often better informed than professionals, can make far more robust criticisms and give parents a different point of view to help them assess professional opinions. Professional bodies today recognise this, and it is now almost obligatory to have a token user representative to demonstrate willingness in involving and respecting user opinions.

However, an informed user is scary and, having found one in their midst, some professionals look for 'real' users – that is, the woman who has just had a baby. These women are perceived as being more willing to appreciate the 'professional' view and, because they have only their own, preferably recent, experience of childbirth, are likely to be unaware of the wider issues.

While there are examples of effective user involvement, such as the leaflet 'Planning a caesarean birth' written by users, obstetricians and midwives and given out to all women who are being offered an elective caesarean section at London's St George's Hospital, Tooting, these initiatives are not commonplace.

Conclusion

If users' goodwill is to continue, then professionals need to respect their views and seriously address the issues they raise. Unfortunately, as we have seen, the majority of users are asked to respond to a pre-set agenda rather than assisting in setting the agenda. When they are invited to contribute, then often only one user per project is permitted. Unless these issues are addressed, users will become increasingly dissatisfied and turn their attention elsewhere.

REFERENCES

Barrie H. 1985. Faculty News, 5(April): 4
Cartwright A. 1977. Mothers' experiences of induction. British Medical Journal, 2(6089): 745–749
Medical Defence Union. 1974. Consent to Treatment. Medical Defence Union, London
Robinson J. 1974. A time to be born, a time to be born. The Times, 12 August

The Practising Midwife 2003; 6(8): 12–13

Powerful sharing?
Creating effective user groups

Julie Wray

Involving service users in a participatory and meaningful way can be a real challenge. One of the prime concerns can be deciding what term to use or which label to attach. A favoured term is 'people'; 'consumer' was, latterly, frequently applied internationally; and debates have also focused on the merits of 'citizens', 'partners in health' or 'clients'. In maternity care 'woman' or 'women', sometimes prefixed by 'antenatal', 'labouring' or 'postnatal', are most commonly used.

However, the real goal concerns getting users involved, so that effective dialogue, information exchange and collaboration between professionals and service users can take place. In 1994 Bastian wrote in detail about consumer participation within the Cochrane Collaboration and the far-reaching benefits of sharing knowledge to improve the quality of care. She highlighted that professional views of the world can become unbalanced and incomplete and, in so doing, they can create distances from the rest of the population which may or may not be consistent with public interest. Processes that seek to harmonise this position through public participation are required so that a body of knowledge is put together based on the realities of people's lives. In addition, Kelson (1997) provided a guide to developing effective user involvement strategies in the NHS to enable joint planning, monitoring and development of health services.

The development of user groups

Since Bastian and Kelson's work, much has been written on why user involvement is important, but very little has emerged on 'how to do it', and even less on how to sustain active involvement in a meaningful way that moves beyond the rhetoric. It appears, then, that establishing and sustaining participation and involvement is a real challenge. Yet maternity care has a

rich history of being committed to seeking the views of, and engaging with, service users.

For example, Maternity Services Liaison Committees (MSLCs) were set up in the 1980s as a framework for involving users and local women in maternity services, with the Department of Health offering specific guidance for supporting MSLCs (NHS Executive, 1996). However, their success varied in different geographical locations; some were not appropriate, functional or supported locally, while others were very successful. Professionals tended to dominate committees, in quantity more than anything else, and as such impinged on user participation in its fullest sense. Nevertheless, scope existed to debate and discuss matters of shared concern.

The current climate

The present context of health policies – prolific as they are – reminds us of the significance of listening and responding to service users within the health service. For example, the NHS plan outlines explicitly, under the heading 'Changes for patients', steps to ensure that health provision is shaped around the convenience and concerns of patients, and that patients have more say in their treatment and more influence over the way the NHS works (Department of Health, 2000). A framework of reforms is outlined to give patients new rights and roles within health services, including more choice, greater information, a new patients' advocacy service and improved ways to obtain patients' views.

Again, these are not new messages for midwives and maternity services. Listening to women and their families, offering choice and encouraging women to play an active role in decision-making is an integral part of 'being with women'. Participation on an individual level is what midwives seek to achieve; after all, it is grounded in midwifery philosophy.

Overcoming obstacles

But problems do exist, in particular in forming, sustaining and supporting user groups. A wide variation of experience exists across many parts of the UK. Despite the many challenges or problems that we face, the reality is that we need to overcome them in order to be inclusive and deeply committed to hearing and responding to the voices of service users. This will ensure that a relevant body of knowledge is developed that guides practice alongside a range of sources, while including the realities of women's experiences.

Think local

Midwives need to be aware of what is happening in their own practice area. More importantly, they must have insight into how women's views are being recorded locally about maternity care and their realties of using the services. Women's own knowledge and experiences of childbirth and their usage of services should be captured, heard, valued and integrated into service provision.

Interestingly, a dedicated resource pack was developed and made widely available to maternity services that sought to help health professionals and user representatives ask users for their views, in order to enable and build a responsive maternity service (Craig, 1998). Is this resource being used? If not, why not? If it is being used, what are midwives' experiences and how useful has it been?

A success story

One local maternity unit in the north-west of England that represents a diverse urban population set up a user group a few years ago. Although small in numbers, the group has taken time to form and achieve effective dialogue and interaction. More recently, the group suggested key topics for evaluation and participated in designing a survey of women's views about care after birth (Wray, 2002). The group has been consistently supported by the same midwifery manager and is reliant on this support for its functioning.

Conclusion

Setting up effective user groups is not straightforward and there are many pitfalls. Barriers to participation can include professionals, which is why structures need to be in place to ensure that proper consideration and consultation take place to enable effective user participation to emerge and to be sustained. As shown here, it really does takes time and effort to build up trust and successful dialogue.

We need to move away from selective listening – hearing only what we choose to hear – and be responsive to and respectful of women's experiences and views of the service. For those who are on the fringe, having access to services and resources can be a further challenge. Exploring ways to engage actively with them is therefore even more central, as capturing the missing voices adds depth and breadth to service provision.

If the primary goal of focusing on women's needs is to develop and encourage relationships between professionals and the communities they serve, then active participation is crucially the aim rather than a passive endeavour. How far have we moved towards powerful sharing or a weak undertaking?

REFERENCES

Bastian H. 1994. The Power of Sharing Knowledge: Consumer Participation in the Cochrane Collaboration. UK Cochrane Collaboration

Craig G. 1998. Women's Views Count: A Resource Pack to Help Health Professionals and User Representatives Ask Service Users Their Views. College of Health, London

Department of Health. 2000. NHS Plan. Stationery Office, London. http://www.doh.gov.uk/nhsplan/

Kelson M. 1997. User Involvement: A Guide to Developing Effective User Involvement Strategies in the NHS. College of Health, London

NHS Executive. 1996. Maternity Services Liaison Committees: Guidelines for Working Effectively. Department of Health, Leeds

Wray J. 2002. Care after birth: views of Salford and Trafford mothers – a baseline evaluation. Main Report, The University of Salford, ISBN 0902896431

The Practising Midwife 2003; 6(8): 18–19

An evaluation of a support group for breast-feeding women in Salisbury, UK

Jo Alexander, Tricia Anderson, Mandy Grant, Jill Sanghera, Dawn Jackson

Objective: to evaluate a newly set-up breast-feeding support group.

Setting, participants, design and analysis: lay 'Bosom Buddies' were trained, and ran a weekly drop-in group with a breast-feeding counsellor and a midwife in a socio-economically disadvantaged housing estate. During the first 31 weeks, 53 breast-feeding women attended and consent was sought to send an anonymous postal questionnaire six weeks after their first attendance. Content analysis and descriptive statistics have been used.

Findings: the response rate to the questionnaire was 87% (45/52), with 76% of respondents (34/45) reporting that they were still breast feeding. Only four women had discontinued for the reason for which they had initially attended the group. While the greatest value of the group was considered by the women to relate to its function in supporting breast feeding, 46% (141/305) of the aspects identified by them as being 'good' related to issues of a predominantly psychosocial nature. Of the women sent questionnaires, 38% (20/52) came from areas with high or medium unemployment.

Key conclusions: this group appears to be highly successful in supporting women to continue to breast feed for at least six weeks following their first attendance. It also appears to provide psychosocial benefits.

Introduction

The health advantages of breast feeding are well known (Howie et al., 1990; Saarinen & Kajosaari, 1995; Wilson et al., 1998), but the majority of women discontinue during the first few postnatal weeks. It is also known that in the UK women from lower occupational groups are less likely than other women either to start to breast feed or to continue long enough to enhance the health of their babies (Hamlyn et al., 2002). It has been suggested that, in view of the public health importance of breast feeding, there is a need to develop some form of supplementary support strategy (Sikorski & Renfrew, 2000).

A support group run by lay 'Bosom Buddies', a midwife and a breast-feeding counsellor, has been set up to try to address some of these issues. The group is held in a socio-economically disadvantaged housing estate in Salisbury (UK). It was built upon a model previously successfully developed in a relatively affluent area, also in the South of England (Anderson & Grant, 2001), in the belief that it would be transferable and in the light of some evidence (Jones & West, 1985) suggesting that supportive interventions are most successful in increasing continued breast feeding among women from lower socio-economic groups.

Over recent years there has been an upsurge in initiatives involving a variety of modes of counsellor support of breast feeding. These have included initiatives both in the UK (Wright, 1996; Timms, 2002) and the USA (Kistin et al., 1994; Long et al., 1995; Schafer et al., 1998; Morrow et al., 1999).

In their systematic review of support for breast-feeding mothers, Sikorski et al. (2002) concluded that lay support was effective in sustaining exclusive breast feeding, while the strength of its effect on the duration of any breast feeding was uncertain. Prior to this, despite a relative lack of evidence from randomised controlled trials, it had still been argued that the breadth of evidence indicated that support programmes offered by experienced and trained peers might increase the numbers of women breast feeding and could be further developed (NHS Centre for Reviews and Dissemination, 2000). That bulletin also stressed that the impact of such programmes needed to be monitored and women's views on their acceptability explored. Strategies depending mainly on face-to-face support appear to be more effective than those relying primarily on phone contact (Sikorski et al., 2002) and these considerations are relevant to the work reported below.

Women interested in the first peer support training programme were recruited via local midwives, health visitors and advertisements in the local press and radio. Eleven 'Bosom Buddies' completed the six-week course in February 2001 and the weekly two-hour drop-in support group was launched in March. There were a further 16 women on the second Bosom Buddy training programme in October. The 27 Bosom Buddies help the breast-feeding counsellor at the weekly group on a rotational basis. There is close liaison with local midwives and health visitors. Details of the course and the running of the group are as described in relation to the earlier initiative (Anderson & Grant, 2001).

Methods

A letter was distributed to mothers attending the previously mentioned similar but long-standing support group, inviting them to attend a focus group to discuss what was good about the group and what might be better. The information gained was used to inform the development of a questionnaire.

Those attending the newly formed support group in Salisbury for the first time were given a letter explaining the evaluation and requesting their written consent for the questionnaire to be posted to them six weeks later. The questionnaires were anonymous but numbered and one reminder was sent after a further two weeks as necessary. They were returned by post to JA, who was not involved in running the group. At their first attendance, their consent was also gained to the completion of a data sheet giving some demographic details and identifying their reason for coming.

Content analysis and descriptive statistics have been used. ACORN profiles for the postcodes of those who agreed to be sent questionnaires were used in order to describe their geodemographic characteristics; these profiles are available via CACI Information on the website www.upmystreet.com. The different profile types represented within the data were then grouped according to whether unemployment was described as being high, medium or low.

As the women were attending a support group run by a lay organisation it was not possible, at this time, to access the Local Research Ethics Committee; however, the University's IHCS Research Committee provided the services of ethical scrutiny.

Findings

During the first 31 weeks that the support group was running, a total of 53 breast-feeding women attended. An average of 8.5 breast-feeding women attended each week (range 3–15; SD 2.7); an average of 3.9 'helpers' also attended (range 1–11; SD 2.1). The term 'helpers' includes the Buddies, the breast-feeding counsellor and any midwives who attended. Ninety-eight per cent (52/53) of the women gave consent for their initial data sheet to be used for this evaluation and for the questionnaire to be posted to them six weeks after their first attendance. The mean age of the mother at first attendance was 30.7 years (range 17–38; SD 5.27) and of the baby 10.7 weeks (range 1–53; SD 11.9). One further baby was two years and four weeks at first attendance. Six babies were more than six months old when they first attended the group. The majority were first-time mothers; for further characteristics on first attendance, see Table 4.3.1. In addition, there were 18 pregnant women who attended the group but, for the purposes of this paper, they have been excluded from the analysis.

The 20 different ACORN geodemographic profile types represented within the postcode data were grouped according to whether unemployment was described as being high, medium or low (see Table 4.3.2). Ten of the women (19%) came from a postcode in which it was high, 10 (19%) medium and 32 (61%) low. Thus, 20 women (38%) came from a postcode in which there was high or medium unemployment.

Table 4.3.1 Characteristics of breast-feeding women on first attendance at the group

	Mean	Range	SD
Maternal age (years)	30.65	17–38	5.27
Baby's age (weeks)	10.65	1–53	11.9
Type of birth	Number	%	
Normal	34	65	
Forceps	3	6	
Ventouse	8	15	
Caesarean	6	11	
Missing	1	2	
Total	52	100	
Born < 37 weeks	5	10	
Primiparous women	39	75	
Multiparous women not breast fed before	2	4	
Multiparous women breast fed before	11	21	
Total	52	100	

Table 4.3.2 Unemployment by geodemographic profile type

ACORN profile type no.	Unemployment	No. of people in group	No. with high/med/low (totals)
43	High	4	
33	High	3	
41	High	2	
25	High	1	10
37	Med	5	
34	Med	3	
31	Med	2	10
29	Low	9	
3	Low	4	
2	Low	3	
6	Low	3	
27	Low	2	
5	Low	2	
12	Low	2	
13	Low	2	
1	Low	1	
10	Low	1	
15	Low	1	
28	Low	1	
30	Low	1	32
			52

The reasons for first attendance were recorded by the group leader (see Table 4.3.3), the commonest reasons being advice related to breast feeding (42) and the social benefits of attending (22).

The methods by which the women had heard about the group are shown in Table 4.3.4. The commonest methods were through contact with the health services (26), via a friend (11) or the National Childbirth Trust (7).

The overall response rate to the questionnaire sent six weeks after their first attendance was 87% (45/52). The mean age of the baby at the time of questionnaire completion was 18.7 weeks (range 7–90; SD 16.11). One further reply was received from a mother whose baby was two years and four months old.

Of those who responded to the questionnaire, 76% (34/45) were still breast feeding. Of the 11 women who had discontinued, only four reported having done so for the same reasons that prompted them to first attend the group. Of those who had discontinued, seven did so before the baby was 16 weeks of age (range 3–15) and four did so between 21 and 47 weeks.

The reasons given for discontinuing breast feeding are shown in Table 4.3.5. The commonest reasons cited (each being given by four women) were having breast fed for as long as intended, that breast feeding took too long and insufficient milk.

Table 4.3.3 Reason for attending the group (more than one reason could be given)

	No. of women
Social/company	22
Difficult feeding patterns	7
Low weight gain	6
Thrush	5
Sore nipples	5
Very disturbed nights	4
Suspects milk insufficiency	4
Wants to be a buddy	3
Using nipple shields	2
Mastitis	2
Other	9

Table 4.3.4 Where women heard about the group

	No. of women
Friend	11
Hospital	9
Health visitor	8
NCT	7
Midwife	6
Flyers	4
Newspaper	3
Antenatal classes	2
GP/surgery	1
Group leader	1
Total	52

Table 4.3.5 Reasons for discontinuing breast feeding (more than one reason could be given)

	No. of women
Had breast fed for as long as intended	4
Took too long	4
Insufficient milk/baby seems hungry	4
Returning to work	3
Painful breasts or nipples	3
Hard to judge how much baby had drunk	2
Not convenient	2
Baby could not be fed by others	2
Domestic reasons	2
Baby was ill	2
Mother was ill	2
Baby lost interest	1
Stress	1

The respondents reported a mean of 3.3 attendances at the support group (range 1–8; SD 2.14).

Their views concerning what was good about the group are given in Table 6. Five aspects were identified by more than half of the women: that they were able to talk about breast-feeding problems ($n = 43$), the enthusiasm of those running the group ($n = 36$), access to videos and books ($n = 37$), that it increased their confidence in breast feeding ($n = 26$) and that they received consistent advice about breast feeding ($n = 24$). Fifty-three per cent (163/305) of the aspects identified by the women related specifically to breast feeding; the remainder related mainly to issues of a psychosocial nature, such as being able to talk about other problems ($n = 22$) and making new friends ($n = 21$).

Twenty-four (53%) of the respondents identified issues that were 'less good' about the group, each identifying one issue only. The majority of these ($n = 12$) were that the accommodation became overcrowded. Two women felt that more reassurance was needed that it was all right to discontinue breast feeding, two that the location was inaccessible and two that hot drinks posed a safety problem. The remaining issues were each raised by one woman only: advice differed from that given by health care professionals; toddlers were breast feeding; women attending from out of the local area; location difficult to find; unsuitable time; not enough for toddlers to do.

Discussion

It could be considered that the lack of a control group constitutes a weakness in this work; however, the study was set up as a service evaluation and consequently the conclusions drawn from it have to be viewed with suitable caution. However, unlike some earlier work (NHS Centre for Reviews and Dissemination, 2000), this study has sought women's appraisal of a peer-support programme. In order to allow comparisons with the UK triennial infant feeding reports (Foster et al., 1997; Hamlyn et al., 2002), it might have appeared desirable to report on the proportion of babies breast feeding at specific time points postnatally. However, at the time of setting up the evaluation, it was known from the experience of the already existing Bosom Buddy group that the age of the baby at first attendance was likely to be highly variable and, therefore, it was decided instead to send out the evaluation questionnaire six weeks after the first attendance.

In this questionnaire the mothers were simply asked whether they were still breast feeding their baby and no detail was sought as to whether this was full or partial breast feeding. In view of this limitation, it is not safe to assume that all the babies were being fully breast fed. However, even given this caveat, it appears that the level

Table 4.3.6 Aspects of the group that women considered good (more than one aspect could be given)

	No. of women
Able to talk about breast-feeding problems	43
Enthusiasm of those running group	36
Access to books and videos	37
Increased confidence in breast feeding	26
Getting consistent advice about breast feeding	24
Being able to talk about other problems	22
Making new friends	21
Having somewhere I can take a new baby	19
It is led by mothers	18
Seeing breast feeding happening	16
Increased confidence in parenting	14
Seeing older babies breast feeding	11
Increased confidence in general	7
Having access to a buddy	4
Other	7
Total	305

of breast-feeding success achieved by women attending this group was remarkable. Seventy-six per cent of those who returned the questionnaire sent six weeks after their first attendance were still breast feeding. Even taking the most pessimistic approach possible by presuming that the one woman who declined to be sent a questionnaire and those who did not respond had discontinued, and adding them to the respondents who reported having done so, 64% of those who attended were still breast feeding.

Only four women reported discontinuing for the reason that had originally caused them to attend the group. Only seven of the women who had discontinued breast feeding reported doing so before their baby was four months of age and thus earlier than the Department of Health (1994) recommended. In contrast, in 2000 in the UK, 56% of those who were breast feeding at birth had discontinued by four months postnatally (Hamlyn et al., 2002). Figures relating to the Primary Care Trust in which the support group was run, and gathered for children attending routine developmental screening appointments, indicated approximately 52% of all babies to be receiving breast milk at six weeks and 26% at eight months (Siderfin, personal communication).

While the options given in the question asking why breast feeding had been discontinued were the same as those reported in the 1995 triennial national infant feeding survey (Foster et al., 1997), the sample size is too small to allow a meaningful comparison. However, it is important to note that four of the 11 women who had discontinued stated that they had breast fed for as long as they had intended.

Despite the increase in recent years of initiatives involving peer counsellor support of breast feeding, information about the acceptability of such interventions to the women themselves has previously been limited (NHS Centre for Reviews and Dissemination, 2000). While the greatest value of the group was considered by the women to relate to its function in supporting breast feeding, 46% (141/305) of the aspects identified by them as being 'good' related to issues of a predominantly psychosocial nature. For example, 31% ($n = 14$) of the women stated that the group had increased their confidence in their parenting. Likewise, in her personal account of the group that she ran, Timms (2002) stated that one of the main reasons that women attended was for friendship and support from other breast-feeding women. Forty-two per cent ($n = 22$) of the women in this evaluation gave the desire for social contact or company as one of their reasons for attending and 40% ($n = 21$) having made new friends as one of the things that they subsequently found to be good about their experience of attending. This appears to support the view of Hoddinott and Pill (1999) that taking a more socio-cultural approach to the promotion of breast feeding than has been taken in the past is probably desirable.

It is known that conflicting advice relating to breast feeding remains an important problem (Dykes & Williams, 1999) and it is salutary to note that 53% ($n = 24$) of the women specifically identified the consistent advice that they received at the group as being one of its positive facets. This suggests that they had not always received consistent advice before going to the group.

It is perhaps surprising that only four of the women identified having access to a Buddy as a positive aspect; however, this question did not specify whether this access was within the group meeting or outside it, and may not have been interpreted consistently. Forty per cent ($n = 18$) of the women specifically praised the fact that the group was run by mothers and it is perhaps salutary that Timms (2002) observed that it appeared easier for the women at her group to talk to other women about breast feeding than to a health care professional. Likewise, in a quasi-randomised controlled trial of predominantly telephone-based peer support in Canada (Mongeon & Allard, 1995), 71% of women in the intervention arm felt that a nurse would not have been able to support them any better than the volunteer had.

Thirty-six per cent ($n = 16$) identified that it had been beneficial for them to see other mothers breast feed at the group. From their interviews with mothers in a deprived area of London who were expecting their first babies, Hoddinott and Pill (1999) similarly found that regularly seeing relatives or friends breast feed increased the women's confidence and commitment to breast feeding, and the likelihood of them succeeding. They also found

that it was important that other people present during such an experience did not make negative remarks and it seems likely that coming to the support group provided similar 'embodied knowledge' (Hoddinott & Pill, 1999) in a very positive atmosphere. In fact, the enthusiasm of those running the group was its second most commonly cited attribute.

Relatively few negative comments were made about the group. The commonest was that the room became overcrowded. The large numbers that sometimes attended had not been anticipated and in this the group became a victim of its own success.

The issue of the optimum duration of exclusive breast feeding has been much debated (Kramer & Kakuma, 2002) and, as discussed earlier, unfortunately it is not known whether respondents exclusively breast fed or mixed breast fed. At first attendance at the group, 12% (6/52) of the babies were more than six months of age and the focus group data suggested that the group provided something of a haven for these women. This was also borne out by the 24% (11/45) of respondents who identified that seeing older babies breast feed was one of the aspects that they particularly valued about the group. However, one mother identified this as something that she disliked.

ACORN profiles were used in preference to other potential sources of geodemographic information as they are based on information that is more recent than the 1991 census. They also provide data relating to postcode which cover on average 15 addresses (Martin, 1996) rather than the larger geographical areas (wards) described by census data. The increased accuracy provided by this latter characteristic was felt to be particularly important.

Despite the fact that the breast-feeding support group is held on a socio-economically disadvantaged housing estate, 62% of the women came from areas where unemployment was low. This appears to suggest that women from affluent areas feel a considerable need to find additional breast-feeding support and will travel some distance to gain it. However, 38% of women came from areas with high or medium unemployment. Evidence from two non-randomised controlled trials conducted in the USA (Kistin et al., 1994; Shaw & Kaczorowski, 1999) also suggest that peer counsellor support can be effective in increasing both the initiation and continuance of breast feeding among less affluent women. Other evidence from Dublin has also shown that experienced mothers can deliver a health promotion programme effectively within a disadvantaged community (Johnson et al., 1993). This seems particularly important as women from lower occupational groups are less likely to continue to breast feed than other women (Hamlyn et al., 2002) and as their babies are at greater risk of ill health.

Conclusion

This group appears to be highly successful in supporting women to continue to breast feed for at least six weeks following their first attendance. It also appears to provide psychosocial benefits.

Acknowledgements

Without the enthusiastic involvement of the women attending and of those running the group, this evaluation would not have been possible. One year's funding was received from the Department of Health in order to set up, run and evaluate this group.

REFERENCES

Anderson T, Grant M. 2001. The art of community-based breastfeeding support. The Blandford Breastfeeding Support Group, incorporating the 'Blandford Bosom Buddies'. MIDIRS Midwifery Digest, 11(Suppl. 1): S20–S23

Department of Health. 1994. Weaning and the weaning diet. Report of the working group on the Weaning Diet of the Committee on Medical Aspects of Food Policy. Report on Health and Social Subjects 45. HMSO, London

Dykes F, Williams C. 1999. Falling by the wayside: a phenomenological exploration of perceived breast-milk inadequacy in lactating women. Midwifery, 15(4): 232–246

Foster K, Lader D, Cheesbrough S. 1997. Infant Feeding 1995. The Stationery Office, London

Hamlyn B, Brooker S, Oleinikova K et al. 2002. Infant Feeding 2000. The Stationery Office, Norwich

Hoddinott P, Pill A. 1999. Qualitative study of decisions about infant feeding among women in east end of London. British Medical Journal, 318: 30–34

Howie PW, Forsyth JS, Ogston SA et al. 1990. Protective effect of breastfeeding against infection. British Medical Journal, 300: 11–16

Johnson Z, Howell F, Molloy B. 1993. Community mothers' programme: randomised controlled trial of non-professional intervention in parenting. British Medical Journal, 306: 1449–1452

Jones DA, West RR. 1985. Lactation nurse increases duration of breast feeding. Archives of Diseases in Childhood, 60: 772–774

Kistin N, Abramson R, Dubline P. 1994. Effect of peer counsellors on breastfeeding initiation, exclusivity and duration among low-income urban women. Journal of Human Lactation, 10(1): 11–15

Kramer MS, Kakuma R. 2002. Optimal duration of exclusive breast feeding (Cochrane Review). In: The Cochrane Library, Issue 1. Update Software, Oxford

Long DG, Funk-Archuleta MA, Geiger CJ et al. 1995. Peer counselor program increases breastfeeding rates in Utah Native America WIC population. Journal of Human Lactation, 11(4): 279–284

Martin D. 1996. Geographic Information Systems – Socioeconomic Applications, 2nd edn. Routledge, London

Mongeon M, Allard R. 1995. Essai controle d'un soutien telephonique regulier donne par unc benevole sur le deroulment et l'issus de l'allaitment. Revue Canadiennne de Sante Publique, 86(2): 124–127. Cited in: Sikorski J, Renfrew MJ. 2000. Support for breastfeeding mothers (Cochrane Review). In: The Cochrane Library, Issue 3. Update Software, Oxford

Morrow AL, Guerrero ML, Shults J et al. 1999. Efficacy of home-based peer counselling to promote exclusive breastfeeding: a randomised controlled trial. Lancet 353(9160): 1226–1231

NHS Centre for Reviews and Dissemination. 2000. Promoting the initiation of breastfeeding. Effective Health Care Bulletin, 6(2): 10

Saarinen UM, Kajosaari M. 1995. Breastfeeding as prophylaxis against atopic disease: prospective follow-up study until 17 years old. Lancet, 346: 1065–1069

Schafer E, Vogel MK, Viegas S et al. 1998. Volunteer peer counselors increase breastfeeding duration among rural low-income women. Birth, 25(2): 101–106

Shaw E, Kaczorowski J. 1999. The effect of a peer counseling program on breastfeeding initiation and longevity in a low-income rural population. Journal of Human Lactation, 15(1): 19–25

Sikorski J, Renfrew MJ. 2000. Support for breastfeeding mothers (Cochrane Review). In: The Cochrane Library, Issue 3. Update Software, Oxford

Sikorski J, Renfrew MJ, Pindoria S et al. 2002. Support for breastfeeding mothers (Cochrane Review). In: The Cochrane Library, Issue 4. Update Software, Oxford

Timms M. 2002. What are Osmaston and Allenton Sure Start doing towards community based breastfeeding support? A midwife's story. MIDIRS Midwifery Digest, 12(2): 278–279

Wilson AC, Stewart Forsyth J, Greene SA et al. 1998. Relation of infant diet to childhood health: seven year follow-up of cohort of children in Dundee infant feeding study. British Medical Journal, 316: 21–25

Wright J. 1996. Breastfeeding and deprivation – the Nottingham peer counsellor programme. MIDIRS Midwifery Digest, 6(2): 212–215

Midwifery 2003; 19(3): 215–220

The Birth Resource Centre: a community of women

Fiona Armstrong, Lyssa Clayton, Jane Crewe, Nadine Edwards, Andrea St Clair,

Lee Seekings-Norman, Sara Wickham

This article has been woven together from the words and stories of a group of women who have been pivotal in the creation and development of the Birth Resource Centre (BRC), a community-based project in Edinburgh which seeks to offer 'practical and emotional support to enable all women and their families to experience pregnancy, birth and parenthood with confidence and dignity'. The BRC 'provides antenatal and postnatal classes focusing on movement and relaxation, one-to-one and group support, sharing experiences, information, advocacy and child-centred activities in a warm and welcoming environment' (from the BRC Identity Statement, 2003).

The BRC started in 1985, when Nadine Edwards began to run groups for women during pregnancy. They wanted to come back afterwards, so she started doing postnatal groups as well. The BRC evolved and grew out of that network of women: women who understood the value of the relationships and support that were developed through the groups. In time, its growth was further enhanced when Nadine was joined by Andrea St Clair, and together they developed what we now call the Birth Resource Centre.

Nadine explains:

I really saw the value in women getting to know each other, talking about things they wanted to talk about, sharing their experiences and knowledge, rather than me telling them about things, and I suppose that's what fostered the relationships antenatally, which then went on postnatally. I think it was the fact that women could understand the importance of that way of working and being in the community themselves that enabled the BRC to come into being. The people who then started to have input as volunteers, coordinators, directors and helpers were people who had experienced that community and valued what we were doing.

The BRC is still evolving: it moved from Nadine's sitting room to a community centre and then to its own premises in 2004. It now provides a range of classes, day workshops and events for women at all stages of the childbearing journey, and for their partners and families. The BRC community links with the wider midwifery and birthing community via the publication of *Birth and Beyond* magazine three times a year.

Women's own stories are central to the BRC's philosophy: sharing experiences is a key part of the classes, and giving space to personal stories in women's own words is one of the roles of *Birth and Beyond*. We therefore begin with the stories of two women whose experiences of pregnancy, birth and parenting were enriched through the BRC.

Jane's story

For many years, I suffered from severe mental illness. I was suicidal and would regularly self-harm. I was offered beds in psychiatric wards in three different health authorities as we travelled about the country: offers we never accepted.

We wanted a child so, contrary to advice from the medical profession, we accepted the so-called risks and decided to start trying. I was approaching 35 years old and we felt we had wasted too much time simply waiting for me to get better. I continued to take medication for my illness, although we knew it was potentially dangerous, but I think neither my husband nor I believed I would ever become pregnant.

It happened surprisingly quickly. I immediately stopped taking the tablets, and wanted to know if taking medication for the first three weeks of my pregnancy could have caused any problems. Nobody seemed to know (or care).

As I entered the second trimester, my mood began to sink lower and lower. Severe antenatal depression set in. I was seeing a succession of different people for my antenatal appointments and care was based around the physical aspects of pregnancy. How could I begin to unpack my mental health history to a complete stranger?

Things became so bad that the GP and psychiatrist recommended that I go back on the medication. They believed my mental state was more threatening to myself and the baby than the risks of abnormality from the drugs. With support from my husband, I refused, although every day felt like a lifetime and I just wanted to escape from my own mind.

During this time I began attending NHS parenting classes. I will never forget the tone of the first class. It went like this: birth hurts, *really hurts*, this is what we can do about it... drugs leaflet handed round. Someone asked about natural childbirth and was informed that only hardy, stalwart individuals did that. At the end of the session I spoke to one of the midwives and explained a little of my situation. She suggested I opt for a nice easy birth with an epidural, as traumatic birth has been shown to increase the risk of postnatal depression. This made sense to me and I decided to take the advice.

I did discover at these sessions that health visitors were available to support women antenatally. No one had offered me anything other than drugs before. This was to be my turning point. My health visitor had previously worked as a midwife and gave me a whole afternoon of her time every two weeks. When I was 26 weeks pregnant, she brought me a flyer for the Birth Resource Centre. 'I think you should do some classes here,' she said. 'The yoga would be good for you, I think it would help.'

Nervously, I called the number and began to attend class every Wednesday morning. At each class we began by introducing ourselves, then we performed gentle yoga-based exercises and relaxation, as our facilitator gently told us to listen to our bodies, do what felt right and tune in to our babies. After this, we had tea and talk. Someone in the class usually had a question, an issue to discuss or a parenting book they had read, and we learned from each other while the facilitator skilfully and imperceptibly deepened knowledge or dispelled myths. Women who had given birth returned to show off their babies and tell their stories. They were eagerly questioned and their experiences added to our knowledge.

Gradually I realised that I was relaxed and happy during these classes. I was beginning to trust my body and my baby, and it was then that I realised that an epidural as first resort would not be right for me. I had learned of the risks associated with epidurals: how could I spend months trying to protect my baby to then expose him to unnecessary intervention?

With this revelation came the need to birth in an environment where natural birth was supported and valued. Our maternity hospital had a normal delivery unit staffed only by midwives. I spoke to my GP and said I wanted to be booked there. I was informed I was too

old and I could have a normal delivery on the main labour ward. With my new-found confidence I phoned the normal delivery unit myself. I spoke to a midwife who said she would be delighted to book me there. With my husband's full support and belief in my ability to birth my baby, I began to feel calmer and, as 40 weeks approached, I felt serene, powerful and whole.

My labour was calm and beautiful. I couldn't stop smiling as I welcomed each contraction. We were really going to have a baby. We drove to the hospital and, in the normal delivery unit, with soft lights and a single midwife, I travelled to my innermost being and birthed our first baby in consciousness and strength.

And the power of this glorious birth has achieved what no doctor could. I now have three beautiful children and have never since taken any medication for mental illness.

The BRC was crucial, in that I would not have had that birth without the BRC, and without it, it's impossible to predict what would have happened. I feel that I've got my whole family to thank the BRC for. The support I had from the BRC compared to the support I had from the system was huge. It helped my relationship with my baby, with my husband, with my whole life. This community of women has always been there for me, validating me and valuing me.

Fiona's story

I first went to the Birth Resource Centre when I was expecting my first daughter, Caroline, who is now five years old. I had picked up a leaflet in my GP's surgery, and immediately felt it would be the right place for me. I had been doing yoga for three years so I felt the yoga for pregnancy would be perfect, and I was really attracted to a place which focused on both pregnancy and the postnatal period, as I was somewhat at sea with the experience of my first pregnancy. None of my friends had children, and I had never held a baby, yet I was to have one of my own. The Birth Resource Centre was to become my anchor.

I loved the yoga classes and never missed a single one. They were the highlight of my pregnant week. The exercise and relaxation were wonderful, but the tea and chat at the end were the key. Information was acquired almost by osmosis – there was no set 'curriculum' but through conversation and questions and answers, those of us at the class found out what we needed to know to help us on our journey through our pregnancies into motherhood.

I thought of the birth rather as a bridge that would take me from my present life to my new life with a child. I was excited, but also rather apprehensive about what I would find on the other side. One of the important things for me about the BRC was that there was a wide range of postnatal sessions as well as the antenatal classes, so I would have somewhere to go back to with my new baby. I did not intend to return to my old job after I had had my baby, so I knew I needed to make new friends and forge a new life around being a mother, and the BRC felt like a community to which I could belong. That was exactly what it proved to be for me.

I went to lots of sessions after my baby was born: baby music, postnatal yoga, the postnatal get-togethers and baby massage. My week was structured around these, which gave me a good grip on my new life. I made some good friends, most of whom are still very close now – our relationships have evolved over the years, just as our children have developed and new babies have been born. I still feel held within the network of relationships that I first established through the BRC, and my life would have been infinitely poorer without it.

Circles of community

Community is a focus for those involved with the BRC; it changes and evolves over time and with developments such as moving to the BRC's own premises.

Now that we have a venue that's not Nadine's house, we're increasingly aware that things like drop-in social and open sessions, which help build community, actually take a lot of planning and commitment. And of course you have to consider people's energy levels and time, availability, family and other commitments; most people are involved on a voluntary basis, and they fit it into their lives. But there's a sense in which that can be really hard. Community building takes work!

There are groups of parents still meeting together who first met through the BRC groups back in the 1980s. These relationships have played an important part in people's parenting journeys and have provided a source of sustenance. The BRC is not just one community, it is actually several interrelated communities, overlapping circles of community. Women pregnant at the same time connect with each other antenatally and that continues postnatally; others find the BRC as new parents and join in some of these communities.

Then there is the management committee that oversees the running of the centre and plans for its future development. This is made up of directors, who are part of the larger community of women on the committee, some of whom are or have been users of the centre and some not. There are the facilitators, some of whom are members of the Scottish Birth Teachers Association, a community which is separate from but linked to the BRC.

Birth and Beyond further involves people who might not get to the centre, and it highlights what is happening elsewhere in the world as well. It has published articles about birth and midwifery in Nepal, Canada and Australia. *Birth and Beyond* has also been a developing entity, and over the last few years has become a forum for printing women's stories of pregnancy, birth and parenting, as well as information and discussion.

Receiving women's stories always feels like a real honour. The first time I was pregnant, that was how I discovered about birth – by reading other women's stories and thinking, I could do that, or there's no way I would let that happen ... So it is wonderful when a woman is happy to send her story. It's about accepting whatever the story is; it's not about just one kind of experience. Over the last few issues one of the other things we've developed is to ask a midwife to write some kind of commentary about a story, to get a midwifery perspective, or highlight the options in a particular area. We always check that back with the woman who's written the story before we publish it; that's really important to us, and we do a lot of thinking and talking about the many subjects that arise as we pull each issue together.

The BRC communities mean different things to different people, not just in terms of whether they are a mother, a volunteer or a facilitator, but what they look to the BRC for. In the words of a current facilitator:

I get two things out of it. First is the satisfaction of being able to help parents and babies at what can be a vulnerable time and to help them find a sense of strength and joy as a parent. The other is a connecting with people which gives me a sense that I'm not on my own with what I'm doing and with my perspective. It's not that we're all the same, but we're all into enabling people rather than telling them, helping them to grow and flower but not be a guru.

Come as you are...

An integral feature of the BRC is the emphasis placed on welcoming and accepting people exactly as they are, as expressed in the 'Values' statement (2003).

People can come absolutely as they are ... Parenting is wonderful but it can also be hard, pushing you to your wits' end. In our society it's hard to say 'actually I'm having a shitty time' because people don't want to hear that. We try to help people come and be themselves however this is, and to feel able to express this if they want, simply to be heard. So many people try to tell parents how they should do everything, so we don't automatically respond with advice unless it really seems to be wanted – that's one reason we use the word facilitator rather than teacher or leader.

Having a child with learning difficulties, I get so much support from the BRC and one of the most important things is them being OK with who I am and who he is.

The thing I feel most strongly about the BRC is its ability to bring together a wide range of people from different backgrounds and with various philosophies on life and create links rather than divisions. Many organisations claim to value difference and to embrace diverse opinions, but in the BRC I have seen this brought to life and made real. The way the organisation functions also demonstrates the positive way women in particular are able to work together, through listening and valuing the views of everyone and reaching workable solutions through consensus.

I meet people through the BRC and you just accept people as they come in, then you find out that amazing things have happened to them as a result of their involvement, because of someone they've met there or something someone has said. It's hard to quantify that when you talk to funders or when people want evidence. It's intangible. We don't ask women for evaluation; women come how they come, they show us what they want us to see and we respect them for that.

Expanding options

Although the BRC very much focuses on accepting and honouring people for who they are, there is also an emphasis placed in classes, personal contacts and in *Birth and Beyond* on offering information and discussion on different choices, where women are interested in that:

My main interest is letting women know different options for doing different things. You so often hear women say, 'my baby's like this but he'll grow out of it', or 'my pelvis is causing me problems but I know I'll just have to live with it' – the examples are endless. A woman may be struggling physically or emotionally with the huge transformations of becoming a mother but doesn't know there are other sources of support and help. I have my own biases through long-term use of homoeopathy and cranio-sacral therapy, and suggesting contact with La Leche League. What's important is to offer information about different things and say, 'These are some of the things that might be interesting to you for your family's health.' Again this is where reading about other women's choices can be enlightening and informative.

Often women's experience of care during pregnancy, labour, birth and the postnatal period is very focused on physical checks and is quite cold in a way, with birth seen as medicalised and mechanised. What we're trying to provide is a more holistic experience that acknowledges and nurtures the emotional and spiritual, because they are needs that women say aren't being met. There's no room for birth to be experienced emotionally and spiritually within a very fragmented, time starved, efficiency-based service.

Often people are as stuck for a range of information with a new baby as when they're pregnant; they get information from the health visitor but that's just one source and one view. Our classes expand the range of what they can choose from and give practical skills and support. For example, one woman was at her wits' end, exhausted from being up with her baby, and her health visitor wanted her to try 'controlled crying'. The woman really didn't want to do that, so we talked about how the yoga we do for babies might help. In cultures where babies are carried all the time, babies get lots of physical contact and

passive movement which satisfies their needs, whereas in our culture, where prams, car seats and other baby seats and carriers are the norm, babies may not have enough of their movement and touch needs met, without this being realised. So we talked about all of this, and this particular mother went away and tried giving her baby more touch and movement, including making more use of the yoga and massage we'd been doing in the class. When she came back, she said she'd had a totally different week. The baby seemed so much happier and settled and didn't have wakeful hours in the night. She had totally turned the situation around. I find that really exciting.

'The tea and chat were the key'

Tea and chat are an important part of the BRC community. They are an integral component of groups and sessions, as discussions over tea are one of the key ways of sharing information in community.

One of the things that I always think about and I know that people don't always understand easily is that a lot of the knowledge exchange and the skills exchange and the way that people develop happens in quite an informal way. It really struck me, years ago, when I had two visiting student midwives in the class. We went through relaxation and yoga and there was a woman with an older daughter so we got to talking about children being at birth. It raised a lot of issues about what birth means, then someone wanted to talk about prenatal screening and we had a really in-depth discussion about how each individual woman faces those kind of choices and that responsibility and how it makes a difference as to whether you would consider a termination and so on, and then this led to another equally profound discussion on something else. Afterwards, the student midwives said, 'I see you just do the exercises, you don't provide information', and I thought that was really fascinating; that they hadn't 'seen' the discussion as information and knowledge sharing because I hadn't been telling the women about this subject and that subject!

I think my whole philosophy is that we mainly have the knowledge within ourselves and all I'm doing is facilitating that and helping women to get in touch with the knowledge that they have or find the knowledge that they need. When people who have been to BRC classes go to NHS classes, they often say, 'actually I had all that information but I didn't realise it till I got there ...'

The continuing evolution of community

There can be no real conclusion to an article which is about an evolutionary process and which is composed of the stories of women who are continuing on their journey. In lieu of a conclusion, we offer a few current thoughts on the importance of this community in women's lives.

Of course, community needs time and nurturing. I was talking with someone recently about how we often end up having so many meetings about important agenda items and things like what's going in Birth and Beyond. *Recently, Nadine's book was launched and it was a really lovely get-together, and we said we'll have to do this again; have nurturing time for the people involved. That's the kind of thing that can get lost in women's busy lives; we all need to remember how important that is. It's not just light relief, it's actually essential if we are to maintain what we've created in all its integrity.*

The BRC is a beacon. It is hugely politically significant. If birthing autonomy is to remain a reality and not just a pie-in-the-sky concept, communities like the BRC need to be sustained – beacons need fuelling.

It's like when you watch images on television of the third world. It's always the worst cases that are shown, and that's important, because people don't take notice unless it's horrendous. But most people's lives aren't like that, so small things can make huge differences in people's lives, and it seems to me that that's what we're about – making differences. Not just for the women, but for their families, for a whole new generation of people growing up.

Box 4.4.1 Values

We welcome everyone, whatever their beliefs, background, choices and circumstances, and are open to different approaches, conventional and complementary.

We believe that people make the best choices for themselves and their families when they have balanced and comprehensive information, non-judgemental support and confidence in themselves.

We honour individuals and their different circumstances and choices around birth, and respect every unique experience.

We recognise the benefits of normal birth and of breast feeding, where possible and where these are what parents choose.

We acknowledge that parents have different needs and concerns before and after birth, so we aim to offer continuing support, friendship and activities throughout the process of becoming parents and raising children.

The Birth Resource Centre can be contacted at:
18 St Peter's Place
Edinburgh
EH3 9PH
Tel.: 0131 229 3667
www.birthresourcecentre.org.uk

Note. Future plans include changing the name of the BRC to Birth and Beyond, though at the time of writing these plans have not yet been implemented.

Questions for debate

Do you think it is important for women to be able to access sources of community, support and information which are independent of the local Trust?

Do you feel it is important for midwives to involve themselves in the regeneration of community, or do you feel that this is something that should ideally be set up by women who are not also midwives?

Labour and Birth

The questions in this section are the ones to which we are inviting responses! (In case you missed it, more details can be found in the introduction and at the back of the book.)

The question you might like to think about before you read the article is: have you ever experienced a situation where a woman's cervix seemed to 'go backwards' during her labour? For example, where a woman's cervix was found to be 7–8 cm dilated at one point, but on later examination was found to be 5 cm dilated? You may like to make a few notes on your own experience of this before you read that article and find out about others' experiences…

Current best evidence: a review of the literature on umbilical cord clamping

Judith S Mercer

Immediate clamping of the umbilical cord can reduce the red blood cells an infant receives at birth by more than 50%, resulting in potential short-term and long-term neonatal problems. Cord clamping studies from 1980 to 2001 were reviewed. Five hundred and thirty-one term infants in the nine identified randomized and nonrandomized studies experienced late clamping, ranging from three minutes to cessation of pulsations, without symptoms of polycythemia or significant hyperbilirubinemia. Higher red blood cell flow to vital organs in the first week was noted, and term infants had less anemia at two months and increased duration of early breastfeeding. In seven randomized trials of preterm infants, benefits associated with delayed clamping in these infants included higher hematocrit and hemoglobin levels, blood pressure, and blood volume, with better cardiopulmonary adaptation and fewer days of oxygen and ventilation and fewer transfusions needed. For both term and preterm infants, few, if any, risks were associated with delayed cord clamping. Longitudinal studies of infants with immediate and delayed cord clamping are needed.

After decades of discussion, debate, and dialog, there is little agreement about the optimal time to clamp the umbilical cord after birth. Similarly, consensus regarding the potential benefits or harm to the newborn infant that can be attributed to delayed cord clamping is lacking. Clear clinical guidelines based on solid data from research are thus needed.

In a recent survey of members of the American College of Nurse-Midwives, 35% of certified nurse-midwives (CNMs) and certified midwives (CMs) reported that they waited until pulsation stopped to clamp the cord (Mercer et al., 2000), whereas 26% reported that they clamp the umbilical cord before one minute. The reason stated for the delay was to promote optimal neonatal transition by providing oxygen, nutrients, and additional blood volume through the pulsating cord; the reasons given for immediate cord clamping were the beliefs that time makes no difference and/or that early cord clamping prevents jaundice and polycythemia. Most midwives offered few references for their beliefs and practices, indicating the lack of evidence-based practice and need for a current review of the literature. A 1950 survey of physician practices (the only one found) described most doctors as believing that cord clamping time was unimportant, although 24% reported milking the cord (McCausland et al., 1950). Does delayed cord clamping have any benefits for infants? Or does it cause harm such as neonatal jaundice or polycythemia? What is the evidence?

The purpose of this article is to evaluate the literature on cord-clamping practices published between 1980 and 2001 to provide the best possible foundation for clinical practice. The use of evidence-based research guidelines will allow clinicians to look beyond unsystematic clinical experiences, the pathologic emphasis on neonatal transition and institutional routines, and assist them to interpret the evidence obtained from clinical research (Albers, 2001).

Background

Over the last decade there has been a shift in how clinicians and researchers examine clinical questions – from relying on the opinions of experts or authorities (authority-based) to a careful critique of the completed research on the subject of interest. The latter approach, introduced by Dr Archie Cochrane (Sackett et al., 1997; Gray, 1997), has been labeled 'evidence-based medicine' or 'evidence-based practice'. Authority-based medicine continues to be an important component of clinical judgment when evidence is lacking and is not to be lightly discarded on the basis of a few studies. However, a careful review of the literature to establish the current best evidence offers the most defensible answers for the clinical questions faced by health professionals, when applied judiciously and conscientiously (Erickson-Owens & Kennedy, 2001).

Many practices in health care, especially in maternity care, were developed because of expediency, habit, or logic and were not subjected to the rigors of good science. The near abandonment of breastfeeding a few decades ago because of lack of knowledge about its benefits is a prime example.

Immediate clamping of the umbilical cord can reduce the number of red blood cells available to an infant by more than 50% (Yao et al., 1969), as seen in Figure 5.1.1. This practice originated with changes in obstetrics and the development of neonatology, and is just now beginning to receive the scientific review worthy of its potential impact on the neonate. Delayed clamping allows time for a transfer of the fetal blood in the placenta to the infant at the time of birth.

As Figure 5.1.1 shows, 'placental transfusion' can provide the infant with an additional 30% more blood volume and up to 60% more red blood cells, the only oxygen-carrying component in the body (Dixon, 1997). Both are lost with immediate cord clamping. What is debated is whether this transfusion is harmful or beneficial.

In the literature, it is common to find a theoretic association postulated between delayed cord clamping and symptomatic polycythemia with increased viscosity, hyperbilirubinemia, and transient tachypnea in term infants, although reference to specific well-designed studies (Blackburn & Loper, 1992; Werner, 1995; Fanaroff & Martin, 1997; Polin & Fox, 1998) is lacking. Benefits, such as less anemia (World Health Organization, 1996; American Academy of Pediatrics Work Group on Cord Blood Banking, 1999) and better cardiopulmonary adaption (Wardrop & Holland, 1995; Sweet & Tiran, 1997), are rarely mentioned, except in specialized reports (Wardrop & Holland, 1995; World Health Organization, 1996; Morley & Morley, 1998; American Academy of Pediatrics Work Group on Cord Blood Banking, 1999) and by way of the public media (Davis, 1987).

Figure 5.1.1 Percent change in blood volume and red cell volume caused by delayed cord clamping. BV = blood volume; RCV = red cell volume. Developed from data in Yao et al. (1969)

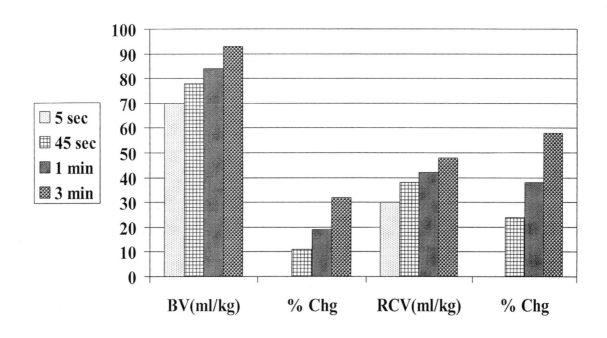

Selection criteria

This article will analyze the potential harms and benefits of delayed cord clamping by use of data obtained from randomized clinical trials and 'controlled trials'. A study done in which treatment groups were not randomized but were said to be indistinguishable before treatment will be considered a 'controlled trial'.

A literature review on umbilical cord clamping intervals was conducted using guidelines developed from evidence-based health care guidelines (Gray, 1997; Grimes & Atkins, 1998). For this review, only the randomized clinical trials for term (Nelson et al., 1980; Oxford Midwives Research Group, 1991; Geethanath et al., 1997; Grajeda et al., 1997) and preterm infants (Kinmond et al., 1993; McDonnell & Henderson-Smart, 1997; Narenda et al., 1998; Nelle et al., 1998; Rabe et al., 1998, 2000; Ibrahim et al., 2000) and well-designed controlled trials (Kliot & Silverstein, 1984; Linderkamp et al., 1992; Nelle et al., 1993, 1995, 1996) were included in the summaries found in Appendices A and B. Other studies, review articles, expert committee reports, and case studies are referred to as appropriate throughout the text.

Search strategy

The studies reviewed in this article were obtained through a variety of sources. Some references were available through the Cochrane Library, although a complete review has not been undertaken at the time of writing. Entering the key words *umbilical cord clamping* in the PubMed Database of the National Library of Medicine revealed a large number of articles on the subject. These articles yielded many secondary references. The four older review articles provided analyses and references of still older, but not necessarily unimportant, articles (Moss & Monset-Couchard, 1967; Yao & Lind, 1974a; Peltonen, 1981; Linderkamp, 1982).

Types of intervention

The primary study intervention examined was delayed clamping of the umbilical cord. In studies of delayed cord clamping for preterm infants, the term 'delayed' meant no longer than 30–45 seconds (Kinmond et al., 1993; McDonnell & Henderson-Smart, 1997; Narenda et al., 1998; Nelle et al., 1998; Rabe et al., 1998, 2000; Ibrahim et al., 2000). For term infants, the 'delay' ranges from three minutes (Oxford Midwives Research Group, 1991; Linderkamp et al., 1992; Nelle et al., 1993, 1995, 1996) to cessation of any pulsations in the cord (Nelson et al., 1980; Oxford Midwives Research Group, 1991; Grajeda et al., 1997) or up to 10 minutes (Kliot & Silverstein, 1984). The definitions used for 'early' cord clamping

ranged from immediate (Linderkamp et al., 1992; Nelle et al., 1993, 1995, 1996; Geethanath et al., 1997; Grajeda et al., 1997) to before one minute (Nelson et al., 1980; Oxford Midwives Research Group, 1991; Rabe et al., 2000) for term infants. For preterm infants, most studies defined 'early' cord clamping as immediate (Nelle et al., 1996, 1998; McDonnell & Henderson-Smart, 1997; Ibrahim et al., 2000); however, in two studies 'immediate' implied a 20-second delay (Rabe et al., 1998, 2000).

Other factors that have a significant impact on placental transfusion were also noted; these include the level at which the infant was held during the delay and the use of oxytocic medications for the mother after delivery. For example, variations range from holding the infant at the introitus or level of the placenta (Grajeda et al., 1997; Ibrahim et al., 2000), to placing the infant on the maternal abdomen (Nelson et al., 1980; Kliot & Silverstein, 1984; Oxford Midwives Research Group, 1991; Nelle et al., 1993, 1995, 1996; McDonnell & Henderson-Smart, 1997), to lowering the infant from 10 to 30 cm below the level of the placenta (Kinmond et al., 1993; Geethanath et al., 1997; Grajeda et al., 1997; Narenda et al., 1998; Nelle et al., 1998; Rabe et al., 1998, 2000). One study identified two placement levels (Grajeda et al., 1997).

Types of outcome measure

Outcome measures for all infants are highly diverse, preventing a meaningful meta-analysis at this time. For term infants, they include physiologic variables such as hematocrit and ferritin levels (Nelson et al., 1980; Kliot & Silverstein, 1984; Linderkamp et al., 1992; Nelle et al., 1993, 1995, 1996; Geethanath et al., 1997; Grajeda et al., 1997), bilirubin levels, time of cord separation, breastfeeding rates (Oxford Midwives Research Group, 1991), neonatal jaundice (Nelson et al., 1980; Oxford Midwives Research Group, 1991), and many variables that did not seem to differ between treatment groups. Examination of psychological and developmental variables were secondary efforts in two studies whose purpose was evaluation of the safety of a Leboyer birth (which includes delayed cord clamping) (Nelson et al., 1980; Kliot & Silverstein, 1984). These secondary variables included the Brazelton Neonatal Assessment and the mother's opinion at eight months postpartum as to whether the birth had influenced the infant's behavior (Nelson et al., 1980). Studies involving preterm infants looked at the need for transfusions (Kinmond et al., 1993; Nelle et al., 1998; Ibrahim et al., 2000; Rabe et al., 2000), hematocrit and blood pressures (Kinmond et al., 1993; McDonnell & Henderson-Smart, 1997; Narenda et al., 1998; Nelle et al., 1998; Rabe et al., 1998; Ibrahim et al., 2000), bilirubin levels (Kinmond et al., 1993; Ibrahim et al., 2000), and days of ventilation and oxygen use (Kinmond et al., 1993). The duration of any long-term follow-up of preterm infants was four to six weeks and included the number of transfusions received between birth and four to six weeks of life (Ibrahim et al., 2000; Rabe et al., 2000). All studies included can be found in Appendix A for term infants and Appendix B for preterm infants.

Methods

Participants were randomly assigned to treatment groups in each of the randomized clinical trials. All 'controlled trials' reported that there were no differences in the two groups at the beginning of the studies. Concealment of randomization or 'blinding' was not always addressed in cord-clamping studies and often is not possible, especially at preterm infants' births, when the presence of the neonatologist who will care for the infant is essential. However, the method of evaluating outcome measures after the birth was blinded whenever possible (Nelson et al., 1980). All patients were accounted for at the end of the trials, and most investigators specifically ensured that data were analyzed with subjects in their intended groups. Authors of two of the four randomized trials on term infants stated that they did not enroll parents who had a strong preference for delayed cord clamping (Nelson et al., 1980; Oxford Midwives Research Group, 1991).

Data analysis

A careful review of two issues of primary concern was conducted: (1) Is harm done to term or preterm infants by delaying cord clamping? (2) Are there real or potential benefits from delaying clamping for any infants? Alleged harmful effects examined include symptomatic polycythemia and/or increased viscosity (Blackburn & Loper, 1992; Fanaroff & Martin, 1997; Polin & Fox, 1998), increased incidence of jaundice and hyperbilirubinemia (Fanaroff & Martin, 1997; Polin & Fox, 1998), increased transient tachypnea for term babies (Fanaroff & Martin, 1997), and any adverse outcome for preterm infants.

Description of studies

The methodologic quality of the studies included ranged from satisfactory to rigorous. The search strategy revealed no published meta-analyses. One unpublished meta-analysis on preterm infants and cord clamping was found (Elbourne, 1991), but the results were extremely limited, because the studies differed widely on variables, methods, and conditions. Four randomized clinical trials involving term infants (Nelson et al., 1980; Oxford Midwives Research Group, 1991; Geethanath et al., 1997; Grajeda et al., 1997) and seven with preterm infants as

subjects were found (Kinmond et al., 1993; McDonnell & Henderson-Smart, 1997; Narenda et al., 1998; Nelle et al., 1998; Rabe et al., 1998, 2000; Ibrahim et al., 2000). In addition, there are five well-designed 'controlled trials' (without randomization) on term infants from the last decade (Kliot & Silverstein, 1984; Linderkamp et al., 1992; Nelle et al., 1993, 1995, 1996). Overviews of the randomized clinical trials and 'controlled trials' on cord clamping in term infants from 1980 to 2001 are presented in Appendix A. Current randomized clinical trials involving preterm infants follow in Appendix B. Older studies are cited in the narrative.

One randomized clinical trial offered poorly defined variables, listed no times of cord clamping, and did not state whether the investigator was present for the birth, but it is included because it was one of only four randomized clinical trials with term infants as subjects (Geethanath et al., 1997). Four review articles from 1967 to 1982 offer summaries of the research available before their dates of publication (Moss & Monset-Couchard, 1967; Yao & Lind, 1974a; Peltonen, 1981; Linderkamp, 1982). In addition, three expert opinion articles (Wardrop & Holland, 1995; Pisacane, 1996; Morley & Morley, 1998), two expert committee reports (World Health Organization, 1996; American Academy of Pediatrics Work Group on Cord Blood Banking, 1999), and two case studies were found (Cashore & Usher, 1973; Austin et al., 1997).

Essential physiologic parameters

Reasonable evaluation of the benefits or harms related to the timing of cord clamping requires a basic understanding of neonatal transitional physiology plus consideration of potential confounding factors. Approximately 110–115 ml/kg of blood are in the fetal–placental circulation at any point in time (Wardrop et al., 1996). Approximately 40% of the fetal cardiac output goes to the placenta per minute, whereas 8–10% goes to the fetus' lungs (Carlton, 1996; Lakshminrusimha & Steinhorn, 1999). The fetal lung is an organ of excretion producing up to 400 ml of amniotic fluid per day (Moore & Tipton, 1997). During labor, the production of fluid decreases but does not cease. Thus, at birth, the newborn's lung must make immediate dramatic changes in both function and structure. The lung function must change from a fluid-producing organ in the fetus to one of gas exchange in the neonate. The lung structure must change from the fluid-filled state in the fetus to that of open gas-filled alveoli with excellent capillary circulation (Jaykka, 1958; Mercer & Skovgaard, 2002).

These dramatic changes are precipitated by a massive increase in blood flow to the lung – from 8% of the cardiac output in fetal life to 45% immediately after birth (Lakshminrusimha & Steinhorn, 1999). The increased blood flow causes the pulmonary capillaries to become erect, thereby pulling open the alveoli and easing the entry of air (Jaykka, 1958; Mercer & Skovgaard, 2002). Immediate cord clamping limits access to the blood volume the infant needs to accomplish this huge task, because there is no reservoir within the body from which to draw (see Figure 5.1.1).

If the volume of blood in the capillary bed of the placenta is unavailable to the newborn because of early cord clamping, the necessary volume must be drawn from other organs, potentially causing their underperfusion. However, having lost placental support, all other organs must now function independently and need optimal perfusion as they begin vital functions essential for life. When the cord is not clamped, the umbilical circulation ceases when the umbilical arteries close and the cord stops pulsating. The umbilical arteries constrict spontaneously when oxygen levels in the infant's circulating venous blood rise to more than 36 mmHg, paralleling the changes noted between fetal levels and neonatal levels of oxygen (McGrath et al., 1986).

Table 5.1.1 provides an overview of the findings from several well-designed 'controlled trials' completed before 1980 that examined the physiologic effect of delayed cord clamping on the newborns' systems in the first few hours of life (Usher et al., 1963; Buckels & Usher, 1965; Arcilla et al., 1966a, b; Oh & Lind, 1966, 1967; Oh et al., 1966a, b, 1967; Pietra et al., 1968; Daily et al., 1970; Yao & Lind, 1971, 1977). Most of the differences result from increased vasodilation and perfusion, and include such findings as higher vascular pressures, higher peripheral temperatures, and increased renal blood flow. Many of these findings have been validated by the results from more recently completed trials.

Confounding factors in cord-clamping studies

Events that occur during labor and birth, as well as measurement factors, may confound the results of research on cord clamping. Four birth-related factors in addition to the timing of cord clamping influence the speed and amount of placental transfusion at birth. They include the level at which the infant is held (Yao & Lind, 1969), the type and method of delivery (Yao et al., 1967; Narenda et al., 1998), uterine contractions during third stage (Yao et al., 1968), and oxytocic use at birth (Yao & Lind, 1974b).

Problematic measurement factors in studies include the difficulty in measuring blood volume, inaccuracy of the hematocrit in reflecting blood volume in hypoxic babies, and effects of capillary leak syndrome (Faxelius et al., 1977; Wardrop & Holland, 1995). Other factors occurring during labor that might decrease a neonate's blood volume at birth, but are beyond the scope of this article, include hypoxia (Brace, 1986), nuchal cord (Cashore & Usher, 1973; Iffy & Varadi, 1994), and hypertonic uterine contractions.

Level infant is held

Delaying cord clamping and keeping the infant at the level of the introitus for 45 seconds results in an 11% increase in blood volume, but a 24% increase in oxygen-carrying red blood cells, as shown in Figure 5.1.1 (Yao et al., 1969). Raising the infant significantly (30–60 cm) delays placental transfusion and lowering the infant 30–60 cm speeds the transfusion of blood from the placenta from three minutes to one minute (Yao & Lind, 1969).

Table 5.1.1 Effects of delayed umbilical cord clamping on neonatal systems in the first hours after birth

Parameters	Change*	Parameters	Change*
Blood volume/components		**Other cardiac effects**	
Blood volume (Usher et al., 1963; Yao et al., 1969; Linderkamp, 1982)	↑	Heart rate (Buckels & Usher, 1965; Arcilla et al., 1966b; Yao et al., 1971)	=
Red cell mass (Usher et al., 1963; Yao et al., 1969; Linderkamp, 1982)	↑	Cardiac size (Buckels & Usher, 1965)	↑
Plasma volume (Usher et al., 1963; Yao et al., 1969; Linderkamp, 1982)	↑	Pre-ejection period (Yao & Lind, 1977)	↑
		Murmurs (Buckels & Usher, 1965)	↓
Hematocrit (Buckels & Usher, 1965; Oh & Lind, 1966)	=, ↑	**Renal function**	
Vascular pressures		Glomerular filtration rate (Oh et al., 1966a)	↑
Pulmonary artery (Arcilla et al., 1966a, b)	↑	Urine flow (Oh et al., 1966a)	↑
Atrial pressure (Arcilla et al., 1966a)	↑	Urinary sodium excretion (Oh et al., 1966a)	↓
Systolic blood pressure (Buckels & Usher, 1965)	↑	**Respiration**	
Blood flow		Respiratory rate (Buckels & Usher, 1965; Oh et al., 1966b, 1967)	↑, ↓
Renal blood flow (Oh et al., 1966a)	↑	Lung compliance (Oh et al., 1967; Daily et al., 1970)	↓
Cutaneous blood flow (Oh & Lind, 1967; Pietra et al., 1968)	↑	Function residual capacity (Oh et al., 1967; Daily et al., 1970)	↓
Systemic/pulmonary resistance (Oh et al., 1966b)	↑	Expiratory grunting (Yao & Lind, 1971)	↑, ↓

*↑ = increased; ↓ = decreased; '=' = no change found.

Vaginal vs cesarean birth

Because infants born by cesarean section tend to have lower blood volumes, the route of delivery must be noted in any study or review. Several authors have documented that placental transfusion occurs more successfully after vaginal birth than after a cesarean delivery (Yao et al., 1967; Narenda et al., 1998). Narenda et al. (1998) found increased blood volume with delayed cord clamping at all births, but there was a smaller increase when preterm infants were born by cesarean section than when they were born vaginally.

Uterine contractions

Uterine contractions after birth hasten the transfer of blood in the placenta to the baby (Yao et al., 1968). Occurring at regular intervals during third stage, they usually begin between one and three minutes postpartum (Caldeyro-Barcia et al., 1950).

Use of oxytocic drugs immediately postpartum

There are major differences in the use of oxytocics in the United States and Europe. Mothers in European studies are usually given oxytocic drugs immediately after delivery of the anterior shoulder (Oxford Midwives Research Group, 1991; Rabe et al., 2000) or after birth (Sweet & Tiran, 1997). In contrast, the usual practice in the United States is to wait until the placenta is delivered. The use of oxytocic drugs has been shown to speed up placental transfusion (Yao & Lind, 1974b) to the infant, making it inappropriate to compare these infants with those whose mothers were not given oxytocic drugs until after the placenta was delivered.

Method and speed of delivery

One birth practice common in the United States is to deliver the shoulders and body of the infant rapidly after birth of the head. This practice does not allow for the continued placental circulation that occurs while waiting for restitution and the next contraction. Delivering the shoulders and body immediately followed by rapid cord ligation results in significantly less placental transfusion at birth than the infant would receive with a slower, more physiologic birth.

Blood volume measurement

Currently, there is no direct, simple, accurate, and rapid way to measure blood volume. Blood volume has been measured by the tagging of one of its elements, such as albumin or red blood cells, with a tracer substance (Wardrop et al., 1996). Tagging red blood cells with nonradioactive chromium, or a similar substance, is the most accurate method; in fact, using red cell tagging,

Faxelius et al. (1977) found a 60% correlation between blood volume and hematocrit in more than 290 neonatal intensive care unit admissions. However, it requires specialized equipment and more than five days to analyze, making the test of little use for clinical decision making (Faxelius et al., 1977; Silver et al., 1998). Albumin tagging with radioactive substances such as iodine (^{125}I) was used in several older studies (Yao et al., 1969; Saigal et al., 1972; Saigal & Usher, 1977; Jones et al., 1990); however, the practice is no longer considered ethical, now that danger of exposure to radioactive substances is known.

Capillary leak syndrome

Capillary leak syndrome occurs when hypoxia causes vascular endothelial integrity to be compromised (Wardrop & Holland, 1995). Failure of the capillary endothelium allows components of plasma such as salt, water, and albumin to leak from the intravascular circulation. Albumin leakage raises the colloid osmotic pressure on the extravascular side of the capillary membrane, pulling fluid out of the circulation and resulting in hemoconcentration that elevates hematocrit. Capillary leak syndrome masks hemoconcentrated hypovolemia and, as a result, hematocrit can be an unreliable and misleading indicator of blood volume and adequacy of the blood for oxygen transport and tissue perfusion in the neonate (Jones et al., 1990; Wardrop & Holland, 1995).

Results

Issues of harm with delayed cord clamping

The concerns regarding delayed cord clamping include the possibility of precipitating polycythemia, hyperviscosity, hyperbilirubinemia, and transient tachypnea of the newborn. Each of these variables is discussed in detail.

Polycythemia

Saigal and Usher (1977) initially raised concerns about the potential for polycythemia with delayed cord clamping. They coined the phrase 'symptomatic neonatal plethora' to describe a subgroup of babies with various times of cord clamping who either had hypervolemia or elevated hematocrit develop and were symptomatic. Polycythemia is defined as a venous hematocrit level greater than 65–70% (Fanaroff & Martin, 1997; Polin & Fox, 1998) and has been associated with neurologic sequelae (Werner, 1995). Although clinical manifestations of polycythemia are nonspecific (Oh, 1986), Saigal and Usher (1977) reported such generalized symptoms as plethoric skin color, tachypnea, retractions, rales, cyanosis, grunting, hypotension, and hypoglycemia in addition to such neurologic symptoms as apneic spells, depression, and irritability. However, a randomized clinical trial found no differences in neurologic outcomes at 30 months when polycythemic infants and control infants returned for follow-up evaluation (Bada et al., 1992).

In the most extreme part of this protocol, term and preterm infants were held 30 cm below the introitus, and cord clamping was delayed for five minutes. Hematocrit and blood volume were measured using radioactive iodine-tagged albumin at four hours of age. Of this group, none of the preterm infants had polycythemia develop, but two of the term infants had hematocrit levels greater than 70 at four hours, and one became symptomatic. Eleven preterm infants and three term infants were labeled 'symptomatic', although only one of the term and none of the preterm infants had an elevated hematocrit. The diagnosis of 'hypervolemia' in the preterm infants was most likely due to capillary leak syndrome because the blood volumes listed for these infants were higher than plausible. This study is the only one found that suggests a link between delayed cord clamping and polycythemia, and lacks the methodologic rigor found in later studies. The results have not been replicated.

Other causes for polycythemia are better documented than delayed cord clamping. Pre-existing maternal conditions such as diabetes, pre-eclampsia, and hypertension increase the risk for chronic hypoxia in utero, and the resultant erythropoiesis may lead to polycythemia at birth. In a study of diabetic mothers, 5% of infants had polycythemia (Cordero et al., 1998). Kurlat & Sola (1992) found that the risk of polycythemia in appropriate-for-gestational-age infants of hypertensive mothers was 12.6-fold greater than that of the general population. Gruenwald (1969) found higher residual placental blood volumes, despite higher hematocrits, in infants of pre-eclamptic mothers, indicating that pre-existing hemoconcentration rather than placental transfusion was responsible.

Time of sampling and location of the blood draw may affect the results of hematocrit or hemoglobin studies. Shohat et al. (1984) assessed hematocrit over the first 16 hours in infants with cord clamping at 30 seconds and found a consistent elevation at four hours. However, all hematocrit levels returned to the birth level or lower by 16 hours. Oh and Lind (1966) found that peripheral hematocrit was lower when drawn from warmed heels and remained higher than venous or arterial measurements.

The data from the randomized clinical trials and the 'controlled trials' over the last two decades do not support the theory that delayed cord clamping causes symptomatic polycythemia, despite the fact that hematocrit levels are higher in late-clamped term and preterm infants. Symptomatic polycythemia was not found in the 531 late-clamped term infants in the studies or in any of the preterm infants. Only two infants, both asymptomatic, had hematocrit levels above 65%, and both had been lowered while clamping was delayed for three minutes (Grajeda et al., 1997). Other studies completed before 1980 reported no symptomatic polycythemia even when infants were held at the level of the perineum or lowered and cord clamping was delayed until pulsations ceased. One case report was found that attributed polycythemia to a water birth with delayed clamping (Austin et al., 1997). Because delayed cord clamping occurs routinely at water births, this singular report requires more investigation. Currently, the American Academy of Pediatrics (1993) does not recommend routine examination of newborn's hematocrit levels to check for polycythemia.

Hyperviscosity

Hyperviscosity, which often, but not always, accompanies polycythemia, is another concern raised by proponents of early cord clamping. Although earlier reports linked a hyperviscosity syndrome with poor neurologic outcomes (Drew et al., 1997), a later study failed to document any consistent pattern of damage (Bada et al., 1992). Blood transfusion and placental transfusion do increase whole blood viscosity in newborns. A marked rise in viscosity was found in late-clamped infants in two studies examining blood rheology (study of the flow of liquids and semisolids) (Linderkamp et al., 1992; Nelle et al., 1996). However, this increased viscosity was accompanied by a significant decrease in vascular resistance in the late-clamped newborn, resulting in increased pulmonary and generalized vasodilation – essential components of a normal transition. Principles of physics governing flow of liquid through a tube state that viscosity must increase for a fluid to dilate the 'tube' (in this case, arterioles and capillaries). Thus, an increased viscosity and a corresponding decrease in vascular resistance may be essential to effect the massive dilation of blood vessels required immediately after birth to adequately perfuse the lung and other organs. Examining only one parameter of blood rheology can be misleading, because checks and balances are essential to this intricate system.

Hyperbilirubinemia

Most infants experience some elevation of bilirubin. Elevated bilirubin levels are more common in preterm infants, whereas late-onset hyperbilirubinemia occurs frequently in term infants who are breastfed. Reports of hyperbilirubinemia from delayed cord clamping were found only in preterm infants in one older study (Saigal et al., 1972); however, inclusion of some infants who were probably small for gestation age confounded the finding. Of note are the 409 term infants in four randomized clinical trials with delayed cord clamping who showed no significant differences in bilirubin levels compared with the babies with early clamping (Nelson et al., 1980; Oxford Midwives Research Group, 1991; Geethanath et al., 1997; Grajeda et al., 1997). In two of the trials, bilirubin levels of 12 mg/dl or more occurred more frequently in the late-clamped infants but did not reach significance (Nelson et al., 1980; Oxford Midwives Research Group, 1991). The only trial to report any significantly elevated bilirubin levels was one of the 'controlled trials', which reported that three of 15 late-clamped babies had bilirubin levels greater than 15 mg/dl (Linderkamp et al., 1992); all infants in both groups were breastfed, but no other information on age of the infants at the time of diagnosis, treatment plan, or outcomes was offered. Even for preterm infants, no significant differences are noted in bilirubin levels between the 123 babies in the late-clamped groups versus the 124 babies in the early-clamped group in the seven randomized controlled trials (Kinmond et al., 1993; McDonnell & Henderson-Smart, 1997; Narenda et al., 1998; Nelle et al., 1998; Rabe et al., 1998, 2000; Ibrahim et al., 2000).

Transient tachypnea of the newborn
Transient tachypnea of the newborn occurs soon after birth and is diagnosed by mild cyanosis, grunting, retracting, flaring, and tachypnea (Fanaroff & Martin, 1997, p. 1046). The origin is believed to be from delayed reabsorption of lung fluid, because it is seen more commonly in infants born by cesarean section or after prolonged labor. The studies reviewed here show no indications of harm caused by transient tachypnea, although respiration rates are increased in babies with delayed cord clamping. The higher respiratory rates reported in late cord-clamped infants (Oh et al., 1966b, 1967) are thought to be a result of greater pulmonary vascular filling, necessitating more shallow rapid breathing. Yao et al. (1971) found increased grunting in seven of 33 late cord-clamped newborns but reported that it disappeared within three and a half hours in the infants without sequelae or treatment. It is important to note that these infants were observed away from their mothers and were not offered the opportunity to suckle during the first two hours of life, thus creating a less than ideal transition to extrauterine life. Allowing a newborn to suckle has been shown to improve oxygenation and

lowering of the heart rate (Shiao et al., 1997); thus, suckling should, theoretically, improve respiratory transition and reduce signs of grunting. Unfortunately, no studies on the effect of suckling on respiratory rates were found.

Beneficial effects of delayed cord clamping

Does delaying cord clamping at the time of birth lead to benefits for term or preterm infants compared with immediate or early cord clamping? Although most of the randomized controlled trials and 'controlled trials' involve small numbers of subjects and need replication, several important findings are suggested.

Hematologic benefits
Hematologic benefits were seen for delayed cord clamping in term and preterm infants. For term infants, improvements of higher hematocrit levels at two months of age and a trend toward increased ferritin levels are especially important findings (Geethanath et al., 1997; Grajeda et al., 1997). Anemia may have a larger impact on the normal development of infants than is currently realized. Lozoff and colleagues (Lozoff et al., 1998, 2000; Roncagliolo et al., 1998) report findings of altered central nervous system development in children who had iron deficiency anemia as infants. These results were evident in children as young as six months of age and persisted in these same children when re-evaluated at 10 years of age (Lozoff et al., 1998, 2000; Roncagliolo et al., 1998). Lozoff (2000) believes that iron is an important nutrient for myelination, which is occurring at a rapid pace during infancy and early childhood. Hematologic improvements for preterm infants include higher hematocrit and hemoglobin levels and a corresponding reduction in the need for transfusions in the first four to six weeks of life.

The World Health Organization expert committee report (1996), the American Academy of Pediatrics statement on cord blood collection (1999), and one expert (Pisacane, 1996) stress prevention of anemia as a reason to delay cord clamping. Even with the small numbers in the current study on anemia, the findings indicate a beneficial effect of delayed cord clamping and support the need for further study.

Cardiopulmonary benefits
Cardiopulmonary benefits of delayed cord clamping suggest better pulmonary and systemic vasodilation and higher red blood cell flow to the brain, body, and intestines for all babies (Nelle et al., 1995, 1998). For preterm infants, these findings support increased blood pressures (Nelle et al., 1998; Rabe et al., 1998; Ibrahim et

al., 2000), better cardiopulmonary adaptation with less need for oxygen and fewer days of ventilation (Davis, 1987), and decreased need for transfusions (Ibrahim et al., 2000; Rabe et al., 2000). Better capillary filling (Pietra et al., 1968), higher peripheral temperatures (Oh & Lind, 1967), and greater urine output (Oh et al., 1966a) have been documented in term infants because of increased perfusion from delayed cord clamping. Increased vasodilation accompanies increased perfusion and is especially important in the hemodynamics of neonatal lung adaptation. Lack of adequate vasodilation in the lungs of newborns is a characteristic of persistent pulmonary hypertension whose cause remains unknown. Increased vasodilation supports increased blood pressure, adequate peripheral perfusion, and improved perfusion of organ systems.

Potential behavior effects

An important potential behavioral effect from delayed cord clamping is suggested in the finding of increased early breastfeeding duration in the Oxford Midwives' study (1991). This study was the first to look at breastfeeding duration in delayed and early-clamped babies and did so only as a secondary dependent variable. More mothers in the delayed clamping group were still breastfeeding at 10–12 days postpartum ($p < 0.05$). It is important to note that of the 296 babies assigned to the delayed clamping in this study, 32 had early clamping because of intrapartum problems. Because the data were analyzed according to the intent-to-treat protocol, 32 babies with early clamping who were assigned to the late group were analyzed as part of the late group. This intent-to-treat analysis would reduce the significance of the differences in breastfeeding rates between groups.

This randomized controlled trial examined the differences in babies with cord clamping at one versus three or more minutes. At one minute, babies may have received 50% of their placental transfusion. The fact that the early group had cord clamping at one minute, and thus potentially more blood volume, would also decrease significance of effects from cord-clamping interval between babies in each group.

Based on a study that found better perfusion of and circulation to the gut after late clamping (Nelle et al., 1995), further study is warranted to assess whether the improved perfusion results in better digestion with less abdominal discomfort and less crying. If so, fewer mothers may abandon breastfeeding in the early stages.

In summary, hematologic benefits found in the studies reviewed earlier include findings of increased hematocrit and hemoglobin levels (Grajeda et al., 1997; Nelle et al., 1998; Ibrahim et al., 2000), blood pressure (Rabe et al., 1998), and blood volume (Narenda et al., 1998), and the reduced need for transfusions in the first four to six weeks in preterm infants (Ibrahim et al., 2000; Rabe et al., 2000); cardiopulmonary benefits consist of better adaptation with fewer days of oxygen and ventilation needed for preterm infants and higher red blood cell flow to vital organs in the first few days of life for all babies (Nelle et al., 1995, 1998); behavioral benefits suggested by the randomized controlled trials were increased duration of early breastfeeding for infants with delayed cord clamping of at least three minutes duration compared with early-clamped infants (Oxford Midwives Research Group, 1991).

Are there harmful effects of immediate clamping?

The studies reviewed did not reveal obvious or direct harm from immediate cord clamping in either term or preterm infants, except for an increase in anemia of infancy. It is important to note that none of the studies examined any long-term sequelae. The delay interval of 30–45 seconds in preterm infants may be too short to assess the full potential benefits and reduction of harm that may be achieved with a longer delay. A large multisite randomized controlled trial involving 300 preterm subjects has been completed in Europe (in Scotland; Wardrop, 2001, personal communication). This study's protocol involved a delay of 60–90 seconds with preterm infants lowered 30 cm. Analysis of the data will indicate whether a longer delay provides additional benefits. The analysis of the data should be completed and distributed by early 2002.

Does denial of 25% or more of an infant's blood volume create any damage? There is one study using an animal model that suggests harm from blood loss at birth. Rajnik et al. (2001) removed approximately 25% of newborn rat pup's blood volume immediately after birth. There was no other intervention. The authors reported finding proinflammatory cytokines in the lungs and liver at three hours of age in the rat pups who had blood removed; rat pups with no loss of blood had no cytokines present in their organs. Proinflammatory cytokines are important markers for tissue damage and, thus, indicated damage to the rat pup's lung and liver from removal of 25% of its blood volume. Figure 5.1.1 shows a reduction of approximately 30% in an infant's blood volume from immediately clamping. Proinflammatory cytokines have been found to be significantly higher in early blood samples from babies who later develop cerebral palsy (Nelson et al., 1998). Consequently, these cytokines may be important markers to use in examining the effect of various obstetric practices on infant outcomes. This study by Rajnik et al. (2001) documents that the denial of 25% of rat pup's blood volume alone, without any other intervention, elevated proinflammatory cytokines in the first three hours after birth. These findings lend support to the importance of re-examination of effects of immediate cord clamping in human infants.

Discussion

For all but the last 50–100 years of human existence, it is highly likely that the umbilical cord of a newborn infant pulsated until it closed spontaneously. Along with important advances in obstetrics and neonatology, the current practice of immediate cord clamping has evolved in many institutions without adequate study of its potential short-term and long-term effects. The literature contains many unsubstantiated references to the fact that delaying cord clamping leads to a variety of harmful effects. Currently, the belief that delayed cord clamping causes polycythemia is so prevalent that one often finds it stated in the literature as an accepted fact not needing scientific references (Oh, 1986; Blackburn & Loper, 1992; Fanaroff & Martin, 1997; Polin & Fox, 1998). The idea that delayed cord clamping is harmful is not supported by the findings from the 16 randomized controlled trials and five 'controlled trials' completed over the last two decades involving term and preterm infants and reviewed here (see Appendices A and B).

Implications for practice

Delayed cord clamping is consistent with gentle, physiologic birth. During the delay, the infant may be placed on the mother's abdomen with no obvious harm noted with a delay of three or more minutes (Nelson et al., 1980; Kliot & Silverstein, 1984; Linderkamp et al., 1992; Nelle et al., 1993, 1995, 1996). The trials verified that increased blood volume occurs even when the infant is placed on the maternal abdomen and cord clamping is delayed three or more minutes. Figure 5.1.1 shows that maximum transfusion occurs in three or more minutes. One other finding should be noted. A study was conducted in Israel to find how to maximize cord blood harvesting (Grisaru et al., 1999). The authors found that if the infant was placed on the abdomen and the cord was clamped in 30 seconds, 80 ml of cord blood could be collected. If the infant was placed on the obstetrician's lap (lowered), only 30 ml was obtained when the cord was clamped at 30 seconds. The authors implied that no harm was done, because hemoglobin levels were not significantly different at 24 hours. As stated earlier in the article, hemoglobin and hematocrit are not alone reliable indicators of harm or benefit from delayed cord clamping. However, if it is necessary to clamp the cord early and the CNM/CM wants to maximize the transfusion, then one should hold the infant lower than

the placenta for the brief interval involved. This study has implications for placement of distressed babies who may be in greater need of blood volume (Mercer & Skovgaard, in press). Any baby at risk for hypovolemia (very pale or mottled) can be lowered for 30 seconds to one minute before being placed on the abdomen or before the cord is clamped.

Implications for research

Whether delayed cord clamping influences breastfeeding duration or other behavioral outcomes is an important question that needs to be examined in more detail, and the findings need to be replicated. The benefits to infants and mothers from breastfeeding are significant. Every effort should be made to ensure that birth practices are not contributing to breastfeeding difficulties.

Replication of the study by Grajeda et al. (1997) showing an association between immediate clamping and anemia in early infancy is important, and longitudinal follow-up should be added. The studies by Lozoff and colleagues (Lozoff et al., 1998, 2000; Roncagliolo et al., 1998; Lozoff, 2000) revealing behavioral and development problems in older children who experienced anemia in infancy add urgency to the importance of repeating and lengthening this study to include examination of neurobehavioral development. Relatively noninvasive biologic research, such as measuring cytokines at birth, at three hours, and at later intervals in infants with immediate and delayed cord clamping, will tell us whether the rat pup's vulnerability is unique to that species or might affect our own.

All of the studies involving preterm infants have a relatively small number of subjects and need to be replicated and validated with larger samples of infants. Few deal with follow-up beyond four to six weeks. Studies examining progress and outcomes during the neonatal intensive care unit stay for preterm infants and follow-up beyond infancy are indicated on the basis of current findings.

Conclusions

Immediate clamping of the umbilical cord is an intervention that has developed in this country over the last century as birth moved into the hospital setting and represents the antipathy of the noninterventionist philosophy typical of midwifery care. None of the studies conducted before 1980 recommend immediate cord clamping – the most conservative recommendations were to delay one to one and a half minutes even for preterm infants (Arcilla et al., 1966b; Saigal et al., 1972). However, in our well-intended haste to transfer an infant to the pediatric staff, we may be denying the infant a significant part of his vital blood supply while placing him or her at risk of hypovolemia and resulting damage.

In this review of the literature, no cause for concern of harm is shown in more than 500 term infants enrolled in randomized controlled trials and 'controlled trials' whose cords were clamped between three and 10 minutes, or when pulsations ceased. Indeed, one finds that benefits are clearly documented for preterm infants and suggested for term infants. There is no evidence that early cord clamping is better, and evidence is lacking regarding long-term harm from immediate or delayed cord clamping. Until we have sufficient appropriate evidence showing otherwise, it is better to mimic nature than to interfere with the intricate, complex, and only partially understood design of the physiologic neonatal transition.

Acknowledgements

This article and related work was supported in part by grants from Sigma Theta Tau, Delta Epsilon Chapter, the University of Rhode Island Foundation, and the University of Rhode Island Research Committee. The author thanks Rebecca Skovgaard, CNM, MS, for a critical review of the manuscript.

REFERENCES

Albers L. 2001. "Evidence" and midwifery practice. J Midwif Women Health, 46: 130–136

American Academy of Pediatrics Committee on Fetus and Newborn. 1993. Routine evaluation of blood pressure, hematocrit, and glucose in newborns. Pediatrics, 92: 474–476

American Academy of Pediatrics Work Group on Cord Blood Banking. 1999. Cord blood banking for potential future transplantation: subject review. Pediatrics, 104(1, Pt 1): 116–118

Arcilla RA, Oh W, Lind J, Blankenship W. 1966a. Portal and atrial pressures in the newborn period. A comparative study of infants born with early and late clamping of the cord. Acta Paediatr Scand, 55: 615–625

Arcilla RA, Oh W, Lind J, Gessner IH. 1966b. Pulmonary arterial pressures of newborn infants with early and late clamping of the cord. Acta Paediatr Scand, 55: 305–315

Austin T, Bridges N, Markiewicz M, Abrahamson E. 1997. Severe neonatal polycythaemia after third stage of labour underwater. Lancet, 350: 1445

Bada HS, Korones SB, Pourcyrous M, Wong SP, Wilson WM III, Kolni HW et al. 1992. Asymptomatic syndrome of polycythemic hyperviscosity: effect of partial plasma exchange transfusion. J Pediatr, 120(4, Pt 1): 579–585

Blackburn S, Loper D. 1992. Maternal, Fetal, and Neonatal Physiology. WB Saunders, Philadelphia

Brace RA. 1986. Fetal blood volume responses to acute fetal hypoxia. Am J Obstet Gynecol, 155: 889–893

Buckels LJ, Usher R. 1965. Cardiopulmonary effects of placental transfusion. J Pediatr, 67: 239–246

Caldeyro-Barcia R, Alvarez H, Reynolds S. 1950. A better understanding of uterine contractility through simultaneous recording with an internal and a seven channel external method. Surg Gynecol Obstet, 91: 641–646

Carlton D. 1996. Pulmonary vasculature. In: Gluckman P, Heyman M (eds), Pediatrics and Perinatology, 2nd edn, pp. 820–825. Arnold, London

Cashore WJ, Usher R. 1973. Hypovolemia resulting from a tight nuchal cord at birth [abstract]. Pediatr Res, 7: 399

Cordero L, Treuer SH, Landon MB, Gabbe SG. 1998. Management of infants of diabetic mothers. Arch Pediatr Adolesc Med, 152: 249–254

Daily W, Olsson T, Victorin L. 1970. Transthoracic impedence: V. Effects of early and late clamping of the umbilical cord with special reference to the ratio air-to-blood during respiration. Acta Paediatr Scand, 207(Suppl.): 57–72

Davis E. 1987. Hearts and Hands: A Midwife's Guide to Pregnancy and Birth, 2nd edn. Celestial Arts, Berkeley

Dixon LR. 1997. The complete blood count: physiologic basis and clinical usage. J Perinatol Neonat Nurs, 11(3): 1–18

Drew JH, Guaran RL, Cichello M, Hobbs JB. 1997. Neonatal whole blood hyperviscosity: the important factor influencing later neurologic function is the viscosity and not the polycythemia. Clin Hemorheol Microcirc, 17: 67–72

Elbourne D. 1991. Early cord clamping in preterm infants. In: Chalmers I (ed.), Oxford Database of Perinatal Trials, Version 1.2, Disk Issue 6, Autumn, Record 5944

Erickson-Owens D, Kennedy HP. 2001. Fostering evidence-based care in clinical teaching. J Midwif Women Health, 46: 137–144

Fanaroff A, Martin R (eds). 1997. Neonatal–Perinatal Medicine: Diseases of the Fetus and Infant, 6th edn. Mosby, Boston

Faxelius G, Raye J, Gutberlet R, Swanstrom S, Tsiantos A, Dolanski E et al. 1977. Red cell volume measurements and acute blood loss in high-risk newborn infants. J Pediatr, 90: 273–281

Geethanath RM, Ramji S, Thirupuram S, Rao YN. 1997. Effect of timing of cord clamping on the iron status of infants at 3 months. Ind Pediatr, 34: 103–106

Grajeda R, Perez-Escamilla R, Dewey KG. 1997. Delayed clamping of the umbilical cord improves hematologic status of Guatemalan infants at 2 mo of age. Am Clin Nutr, 65: 425–431

Gray JAM. 1997. Evidence-based Healthcare. Churchill Livingstone, London

Grimes DA, Atkins D. 1998. The U.S. Preventive Services Task Force: putting evidence-based medicine to work. Clin Obstet Gynecol, 41: 332–342

Grisaru D, Deutsch V, Pick M, Fait G, Lessing JB, Dollberg S et al. 1999. Placing the newborn on the maternal abdomen after delivery increases the volume and CD34 cell content in the umbilical cord collected: an old maneuver with new applications. Am J Obstet Gynecol, 180: 1240–1243

Gruenwald P. 1969. The amount of fetal blood remaining in the placenta at birth. Exp Biol Med, 130: 326–329

Ibrahim HM, Krouskop RW, Lewis DF, Dhanireddy R. 2000. Placental transfusion: umbilical cord clamping and preterm infants. J Perinatol, 20: 351–354

Iffy L, Varadi V. 1994. Cerebral palsy following cutting of the nuchal cord before delivery. Med Law, 13: 323–330

Jaykka S. 1958. Capillary erection and the structural appearance of fetal and neonatal lungs. Acta Paediatr, 47: 484–500

Jones JG, Holland BM, Hudson IR, Wardrop CA. 1990. Total circulating red cells versus haematocrit as the primary descriptor of oxygen transport by the blood. Br J Haematol, 76: 288–294

Kinmond S, Aitchison TC, Holland BM, Jones JG, Turner TL, Wardrop CA. 1993. Umbilical cord clamping and preterm infants: a randomized trial. BMJ, 306: 172–175

Kliot D, Silverstein L. 1984. Changing maternal and newborn care. A study of the Leboyer approach to childbirth management. NY State J Med, 84: 169–174

Kurlat I, Sola A. 1992. Neonatal polycythemia in appropriately grown infants of hypertensive mothers. Acta Pediatr, 81: 662–664

Lakshminrusimha S, Steinhorn RH. 1999. Pulmonary vascular biology during neonatal transition [review]. Clin Perinatol, 26: 601–619

Linderkamp O. 1982. Placental transfusion: determinants and effects. Clin Perinatol, 9: 559–592

Linderkamp O, Nelle M, Kraus M, Zilow EP. 1992. The effects of early and late cord-clamping on blood viscosity and other hemorheological parameters in full-term neonates. Acta Paediatr, 81: 745–750

Lozoff B. 2000. Perinatal iron deficiency and the developing brain. Pediatr Res, 48: 137–139

Lozoff B, Klein NK, Nelson EC, McClish DK, Manuel M, Chacon ME. 1998. Behavior of infants with iron-deficiency anemia. Child Dev, 69: 24–36

Lozoff B, Jimenez E, Hagen J, Mollen E, Wolf AW. 2000. Poorer behavioral and developmental outcome more than 10 years after treatment for iron deficiency in infancy. Pediatrics, 105: E51

McCausland A, Holmes F, Schumann W. 1950. Management of cord and placental blood and its effect upon newborn. West J Surg, 58: 591–596

McDonnell M, Henderson-Smart DJ. 1997. Delayed umbilical cord clamping in preterm infants: a feasibility study. J Paediatr Child Health, 33: 308–310

McGrath JC, MacLennan SJ, Mann AC, Stuart-Smith K, Whittle MJ. 1986. Contraction of human umbilical artery, but not vein, by oxygen. J Physiol, 380: 513–519

Mercer J, Skovgaard R. 2002. Neonatal transitional physiology: a new paradigm. J Perinat Neonatal Nurs, 15(4): 56–75

Mercer JS, Nelson CC, Skovgaard RL. 2000. Umbilical cord clamping: beliefs and practices of American nurse-midwives. J Midwif Women Health, 45: 58–66

Moore T, Tipton E. 1997. Amniotic fluid and non-immune hydrops. In: Fanaroff A, Martin R (eds), Neonatal–Perinatal Medicine: Diseases of the Fetus and Infant, 6th edn, pp. 312–326. Mosby, Boston

Morley G, Morley GM. 1998. Cord closure: can hasty clamping injure the newborn? OBG Management, 7: 29–36

Moss AJ, Monset-Couchard M. 1967. Placental transfusion: early versus late clamping of the umbilical cord. Pediatrics, 40: 109–126

Narenda A, Beckett C, Aitchison T, Kyle E, Coutis J, Turner T et al. 1998. Is it possible to promote placental transfusion at preterm delivery? [abstract]. Pediatr Res, 44: 453

Nelle M, Zilow EP, Kraus M, Bastert G, Linderkamp O. 1993. The effect of Leboyer delivery on blood viscosity and other hemorheologic parameters in term neonates. Am J Obstet Gynecol, 169: 189–193

Nelle M, Zilow EP, Bastert G, Linderkamp O. 1995. Effect of Leboyer childbirth on cardiac output, cerebral and gastrointestinal blood flow velocities in full term neonates. Am J Perinatol, 12: 212–216

Nelle M, Kraus M, Bastert G, Linderkamp O. 1996. Effects of Leboyer childbirth on left and right systolic time intervals in healthy term neonates. J Perinat Med, 24: 513–520

Nelle M, Fischer S, Conze S, Beedgen B, Brischke EM, Linderkamp O. 1998. Effects of later cord clamping on circulation in prematures [abstract]. Pediatr Res, 44: 420

Nelson KB, Dambrosia JM, Grether JK, Phillips TM. 1998. Neonatal cytokines and coagulation factors in children with cerebral palsy. Ann Neurol, 44: 665–675

Nelson NM, Enkin MW, Saigal S, Bennett KJ, Milner R, Sackett DL. 1980. A randomized clinical trial of the Leboyer approach to childbirth. N Engl J Med, 302: 655–660

Oh W. 1986. Neonatal polycythemia and hyperviscosity. Pediatr Clin North Am, 33: 523–532

Oh W, Lind J. 1966. Venous and capillary hematocrit in newborn infants and placental transfusion. Acta Paediatr Scand, 55: 38–48

Oh W, Lind J. 1967. Body temperature of the newborn infant in relation to placental transfusion. Acta Paediatr Scand, 172S: 137–145

Oh W, Oh MA, Lind J. 1966a. Renal function and blood volume in newborn infant related to placental transfusion. Acta Paediatr Scand, 55: 197–210

Oh W, Lind J, Gessner IH. 1966b. The circulatory and respiratory adaptation to early and late cord clamping in newborn infants. Acta Paediatr Scand, 55: 17–25

Oh W, Wallgren G, Hanson JS, Lind J. 1967. The effects of placental transfusion on respiratory mechanics of normal term newborn infants. Pediatrics, 40: 6–12

Oxford Midwives Research Group. 1991. A study of the relationship between the delivery to cord clamping interval and the time of cord separation. Midwifery, 7: 167–176

Peltonen T. 1981. Placental transfusion: advantage and disadvantage. Eur J Pediatr, 137: 141–146

Pietra GG, D'Amodio MD, Leventhal MM, Oh W, Braudo JL. 1968. Electron microscopy of cutaneous capillaries of newborn infants: effects of placental transfusion. Pediatrics, 42: 678–683

Pisacane A. 1996. Neonatal prevention of iron deficiency. BMJ, 312: 136–137

Polin R, Fox W. 1998. Fetal and Neonatal Physiology, 2nd edn. WB Saunders, Philadelphia

Rabe H, Wacker A, Hulskamp G, Homig-Franz I, Jorch G. 1998. Late cord clamping benefits extrauterine adaptation [abstract]. Pediatr Res, 44: 454

Rabe H, Wacker A, Hulskamp G, Hornig-Franz I, Schulze-Everding A, Harms E et al. 2000. A randomised controlled trial of delayed cord clamping in very low birth weight preterm infants. Eur J Pediatr, 159: 775–777

Rajnik M, Salkowski C, Li Y, Thomas K, Rollwagen F, Volges S. 2001. Early cytokine expression induced by hemorrhagic shock in a non-resuscitated rat model. Pediatr Res, 49(4S): 44A

Roncagliolo M, Garrido M, Walter T, Peirano P, Lozoff B. 1998. Evidence of altered central nervous system development in infants with iron deficiency anemia at 6 mo: delayed maturation of auditory brainstem responses. Am J Clin Nutr, 68: 683–690

Sackett D, Richardson D, Rosenberg W, Haynes R. 1997. Evidence Based Medicine: How to Practice and Teach EBM. Churchill Livingstone, London

Saigal S, Usher R. 1977. Symptomatic neonatal plethora. Biol Neonate, 32: 62–72

Saigal S, O'Neill A, Surainder Y, Chua LB, Usher R. 1972. Placental transfusion and hyperbilirubinemia in the premature. Pediatrics, 49: 406–419

Shiao SY, Chang YJ, Lannon H, Yarandi H. 1997. Meta-analysis of the effects of nonnutritive sucking on heart rate and peripheral oxygenation: research from the past 30 years. Issues Compr Pediatr Nurs, 20: 11–24

Shohat M, Merlob P, Reisner SH. 1984. Neonatal polycythemia: I. Early diagnosis and incidence relating to time of sampling. Pediatrics, 73: 7–10

Silver HM, Seebeck M, Carlson R. 1998. Comparison of total blood volume in normal, preeclamptic, and nonproteinuric gestational hypertensive pregnancy by simultaneous measurement of red blood cell and plasma volumes. Am J Obstet Gynecol, 179: 87–93

Sweet B, Tiran D. 1997. Mayes' Midwifery: A Textbook for Midwives. Bailliere Tindall, London

Usher R, Shephard M, Lind J. 1963. Blood volume in the newborn infant and placental transfusion. Acta Paediatr Scand, 52: 497–512

Wardrop CA, Holland BM. 1995. The roles and vital importance of placental blood to the newborn infant. J Perinat Med, 23: 139–143

Wardrop CAJ, Holland B, Jones JC. 1996. Red cell physiology. In: Gluckman P, Heyman M (eds), Pediatrics and Perinatology, pp. 868–876. Arnold, London

Werner EJ. 1995. Neonatal polycythemia and hyperviscosity. Clin Perinatol, 22: 693–710

World Health Organization. 1996. Care in normal birth: report of the technical working group meeting on normal birth. WHO, Maternal Health and Safe Motherhood Program, Geneva

Yao AC, Lind J. 1969. Effect of gravity on placental transfusion. Lancet, 2: 505–508

Yao AC, Lind J. 1974a. Placental transfusion. Am J Dis Child, 127: 128–141

Yao AC, Lind J. 1974b. Blood flow in the umbilical vessels during the third stage of labor. Biol Neonate, 25: 186–193

Yao AC, Lind J. 1977. Effect of early and late cord clamping on the systolic time intervals of the newborn infant. Acta Paediatr Scand, 66: 489–493

Yao AC, Wist A, Lind J. 1967. The blood volume of the newborn infant delivered by caesarean section. Acta Paediatr Scand, 56: 585–592

Yao AC, Hirvensalo M, Lind J. 1968. Placental transfusion-rate and uterine contraction. Lancet, 1: 380–383

Yao AC, Moinian M, Lind J. 1969. Distribution of blood between infant and placenta after birth. Lancet, 2(7626): 871–873

Yao AC, Lind J, Vuorenkoski V. 1971. Expiratory grunting in the late clamped neonate. Pediatrics, 48: 865–870

Appendices

Appendix A: Literature on cord clamping in full-term infants randomized (4) and nonrandomized (5) controlled trials

Authors (year)	Study population	Cord management/placement of infant
Grajeda et al. (1997)	≥ 37 weeks, ≥ 2000 g, singleton vaginal deliveries, no GD, AP hemorrhage, CPD or other anomalies	EC: immediately LC: at end of pulsation, infant at level of placenta LC: after pulsations, infants held below introitus
Geethanath et al. (1997)	Term, vaginal births, mothers with Hgb > 10 g/dl	EC: immediately LC: after placenta in vagina; infant lowered < 10 cm
Oxford Midwives Research Group (1991)	37–42 weeks, vertex, vaginal delivery, no AP complications	EC: stat or ≤ 1 min LC: after 3 min or when pulsations stopped, infant on abdomen
Nelson et al. (1980)	Low OB risk, > 37 weeks, wanted Leboyer birth, would attend prenatal classes	EC: < 60 sec LC: after pulsations ceased, baby on maternal abdomen
Nelle et al. (1996)	30 FT neonates: from normal pregnancies and labors	EC: < 10 sec LC: > 3 min, infant on maternal abdomen
Nelle et al. (1995)	30 FT neonates: from normal pregnancies and labors	EC: < 10 sec LC: > 3 min, infant on maternal abdomen
Nelle et al. (1993)	Healthy, term, vaginal deliveries, pH ≥ 7.25, Apgar scores 9/10, all breastfed	EC: < 10 sec LC: > 3 min, infant on maternal abdomen (Leboyer method)
Linderkamp et al. (1992)	39–40 weeks, normal EFM, pH > 7.25, Apgars 9/10, AGA, 3390–3620 g	EC: < 10 sec LC: at 3 min, infant held at introitus
Kliot & Silverstein (1984)	Normal FT infants, from private practice	EC: < 60 sec LC: > 10 min on maternal abdomen Control: CC < 60 sec

AP = antepartum; BF = breastfeeding; BR = bilirubin; BV = blood volume; CC = cord clamping; CL = lung compliance; CPD = cephalopelvic disproportion; C/S = cesarean section; EC = early clamping; FT = full term; GD = gestational diabetes; GFR = glomerular filtration rate; Hct = hematocrit; HR = heart rate; LC = late clamping; PT = preterm; RBC = red blood cell; RPBV = residual placental blood volume; RR = respiratory rate; VD = vaginal delivery.

Sample size	Results	Comments
21 26 22	At 2 mo, 88% of infants with delayed CC had Hcts > 0.33 versus 42% in the early group ($p = 0.001$). No differences between two late groups.	Recommends delay in CC as a feasible low-cost intervention that can reduce anemia in developing countries. No differences in polycythemia or jaundice. Two babies with Hcts $> 65\%$ were asymptomatic.
48 59	Mean ferritin higher in LC: 73.6 vs 55.7 ng/ml, but did not reach significance level as set by PI.	Set difference for significance at 30 ng/ml of ferritin. Did not report other variables.
256 296	No significant difference in any variable except higher rates of continued BF at 10–12 days among mothers in LC group ($p = 0.05$).	Largest sample ever studied. No significant difference in jaundice. Highest BR levels = 12 mg/dl. 32 babies in LC group had early clamping (intent-to-treat analysis).
26 28	No differences in any variable except mothers' opinion at 8 mo that the birth influenced the child's behavior ($p = 0.05$).	Found that Leboyer method was not unsafe. Found no differences in polycythemia or jaundice.
15 15	Hcts were higher in LC ($p < 0.05$). Pre-ejection period ratios indicated higher systemic and pulmonary resistance on day 1 and same as EC babies on day 5.	Findings suggest more pronounced pulmonary vasodilation in the LC group in the first 5 days.
15 15	LC: BV 32% higher. Blood viscosity increased at 4 h by 32%; vascular hindrance 25% lower; RBC flow to brain and intestines 25% higher day 1 and 10% higher on day 5.	Higher viscosity offset by lower vascular hindrance (marked vasodilation). Authors state EC deprives infants of placental transfusions and increases risk of hypovolemia and anemia.
15 15	Residual placental blood volume higher in EC infants; Hct rose from 49% at birth to 58% at 2 h, 56% at 24 h, and 54% at 120 h. Viscosity increased by 32% in LC at 2 h with no further change.	Example: For 3-kg infant: EC = 135 ml in placenta, 210 ml in baby. LC = 75 ml in placenta, 270 ml in baby. See Nelle et al. (1995) for discussion of viscosity.
15 15	RPBV = 15 vs 47 ml/kg in EC; Hct increased at 2 h; blood viscosity at 2 h 40% higher; 3/15 with elevated BR over 15 mg/dl. All breastfed.	LC results in marked rise of blood viscosity caused by fluid shifting out of vascular space. No infants had any clinical symptoms. See Nelle et al. (1995) re: viscosity.
39 40	No significant difference in temperature, heart rate, Hct, BR, pH, Apgar scores, or other variables.	Completed random assignment to two Leboyer groups. Validated safety of Leboyer-type delivery.

Appendix B: Literature overview of cord clamping in preterm infants (randomized controlled trials: seven found)

Authors (year)	Study population	Cord management/infant placement
Ibrahim et al. (2001)	500–1250 g, 24–29 weeks, all vaginal births	EC: stat LC: at 20 sec; at introitus
Rabe et al. (2000)	Singleton, < 33 weeks	EC: 20 sec LC: 45 sec and lowered 20 cm + oxytocic
Nelle et al. (1998)	C/S, ≤ 1200 g, ≤ 30 weeks	EC: stat LC: at 30 sec; infants held 30 cm below placenta
Rabe et al. (1998)	< 33 wks	EC: 20 sec LC: 45 sec
Narenda et al. (1998)	24–31 weeks	EC: routine LC: ≥ 30 sec; lowered 30 cm, + oxytocic
McDonnell & Henderson-Smart (1997)	NVD and C/S, 26–33 weeks twins	EC: stat LC: 30 sec; on maternal abdomen
Kinmond et al. (1993)	SVDs 27–33 weeks	EC: routine, stat or early, < 10 sec LC: 30 sec; 20 cm below introitus

Journal of Midwifery and Women's Health 2001; 46(6): 402–414

Sample size	Significant results	Comments
16 16	LC: improved mean BP (0.01); less use of albumin (0.03); higher RBCs (0.003), Hct (0.01, mean = 50%), Hgb (0.0002); fewer transfusions (0.001) over 4-week period, higher 5-min Apgar scores.	No significant difference in BR in spite of higher Hct; decrease in transfusions is cost effective and safer. Study was of 4 weeks duration.
20 19	9 (LC) vs 16 (EC) transfused by day 42 ($p = 0.05$), OR 0.56 (CI 0.34–0.94).	All mothers got oxytocic immediately after delivery; concludes that anemia of prematurity can be decreased by delayed cord clamping.
8 11	LC = higher mean BP, systemic vascular resistance, Hgb, systemic and cerebral Hgb transport. EC group required more volume expansion in first 24 h.	LC resulted in sig. findings of most variables even with this small sample.
15 15	BP: 10 (66%) of EC and 6 (40%) of LC had BP < 30 mmHg in first 24 h.	LC can help prevent low BP and low microcirculation.
23 23	LC: BV increased by 8–19 ml/kg overall: vaginal births = 10–28.4 ml/kg increase; C/S = 2–16.4 ml/kg increase.	BV increased by 30 sec delay, most pronounced in VD. Analyzed by actual treatment, not intent-to-treat, subgroup of larger RCT.
24 22	Trend toward higher Hct in LC infants but did not reach statistical significance. Delayed CC at C/S feasible.	Recommends to delay CC for more than 30 sec in trials and that infants be lowered in relation to the uterus.
19 17	Initial PCV higher in LC (0.0013) and fewer RC Tfxs (0.03). In ventilated infants: higher A-a O_2 tension (0.02), less supplemental O_2 (0.009). No difference in bilirubin levels.	Study is being replicated, and results should be available mid 2002. Overlapping outliers in each group.

Perineal trauma: prevention and treatment

Rona McCandlish

This article examines two aspects of routine midwifery practice: management of the perineum at the end of the second stage of labor and management and repair of perineal injury. Although some aspects of perineal management and repair have been researched and there is reliable evidence on which to base practice, there remains a considerable and urgent collaborative clinical research agenda that midwives should actively pursue.

How does evidence-based care apply to midwifery?

Evidence-based care has been described as '... the integration of best research evidence with clinical expertise and patient values' (Sackett, 2000). These three components imply knowledge of valid, reliable evidence about care strategies, clinical competence to use this information, and consideration of the wishes and incorporation of the needs and values of the individual woman experiencing care.

The application of the principles of evidence-based care to routine midwifery practice has a large potential for fostering the most effective and sensitive maternity care for women and their families. Routine midwifery care, which has moderate or even small effects on an individual woman's health, has the capacity to have a substantial impact on the health of childbearing women overall. The corollary, that the apparently mundane practice may inadvertently do harm, should of course also be considered. The 'ordinary' matters!

Prevention, assessment, and treatment of perineal trauma associated with vaginal birth are examples of 'ordinary' core midwifery activities experienced by almost all women attended by midwives. This article will use two aspects of routine maternity practice to highlight the case for questioning the effectiveness of ordinary perineal care: (1) the use of manual pressure by the attending health professional on the woman's perineum and on the baby's head at the end of the second stage of labor, and (2) repair of perineal injury.

Both are the subject of contemporary debate, and the main aim here is to provide information to help establish whether there is high-quality evidence about the safety and effectiveness of care strategies and interventions used by midwives. This article discusses the incidence of perineal trauma and associated postpartum maternal morbidity; the background to the debate of whether to support the mother's perineum and manually control the speed of the birth of the baby at the end of second stage of labor; and the repair of perineal trauma; *that does not involve the anal sphincter*. Key studies on the effectiveness of midwifery interventions on these issues will be reviewed, followed by a discussion of how midwives can incorporate new evidence into their practice.

Perineal trauma: why is it important?

Many women who give birth vaginally experience some degree of perineal trauma (Albers et al., 1999; Hall & Popovic, 2000) either because of spontaneous tearing or episiotomy. Maternity care statistics for England for 1997–1998 were published recently and report that perineal laceration was the most common complication recorded during labor and birth (recorded in 31% of all births). Episiotomy was recorded separately in around 15% of births. This means that up to 57% of women birthing vaginally in a national context in which episiotomy was not routinely practised were recorded as having some level of perineal injury (Government Statistical Service, 2001).

Obviously, in contexts in which episiotomy is routinely used, few women who give birth vaginally escape perineal trauma. The evidence comparing liberal (routine) episiotomy with restricted episiotomy overwhelmingly demonstrates that there is no benefit to liberal episiotomy for either the mother or baby in the short term, and women who undergo episiotomy are at greater risk of serious tearing into the anal sphincter (Carroli & Belizan, 2001). Although there is no reliable evidence about most longer-term outcomes (such as uterine prolapse) associated with either policy, 'available evidence suggests that maternal pelvic floor damage is proportional to perineal trauma and that episiotomy does not prevent that damage' (Eason & Feldman, 2000). The weight of evidence clearly shows that the use of routine episiotomy is ineffective, unjustifiable, and should not be practised.

The assessment and classification of genital tract injury forms part of routine care immediately after birth. It is done to identify trauma that requires early intervention to stop bleeding, promote healing, and restore tissue function. Although there is no valid, reliable standardized classification system for perineal trauma, it is often recorded using the following ordered numeric categorization from least to most severe (Sultan et al., 1994; Sultan, 1999):

- First degree – perineal skin only
- Second degree – perineal muscle and skin, but not involving the sphincter
- Third degree – partial or complete disruption of the anal sphincter
- Fourth degree – complete disruption of the external and internal anal sphincter.

Perineal trauma is strongly associated with postpartum pain and morbidity, including bleeding and infection (Sleep, 1991; Albers et al., 1999). At least 20% of women experience some perineal pain during the first two weeks postpartum (Sleep et al., 1984; McCandlish et al., 1998a; Albers et al., 1999), and almost as many will continue to complain of some pain eight weeks after birth (Glazener et al., 1995). Such morbidity may interfere with normal activities, make breastfeeding harder because of difficulty in adopting a comfortable sitting position, affect bowel function, and adversely affect sexual activity (Sleep & Grant, 1987; Barrett et al., 2000). Perineal pain has also been identified as a contributor to disturbance of maternal postpartum mood, leading to changes in attitudes and behavior toward the baby (Reading et al., 1982). Although for most women, this pain resolves relatively soon after birth, as many as 7–8% continue to experience perineal pain three months after birth (Sleep et al., 1984; Glazener et al., 1995; Gordon et al., 1998; McCandlish et al., 1998a).

Perineal care at the end of the second stage of labor: hands on or hands poised?

During the late 1980s and early 1990s in England, new opportunities arose to support evaluation of common midwifery practices through large-scale, high-quality adequately funded research studies. The establishment of a program of research at the National Perinatal Epidemiology Unit (NPEU) in 1988, headed by a midwife researcher (Professor Mary Renfrew), provided a particular focus for these initiatives (Clarke, 2000).

Decreasing perineal trauma

Hands on or hands poised?

Perineal care had been a strong theme in the NPEU's research portfolio. For example, a pioneering randomized controlled trial (RCT) evaluating liberal and restricted use of episiotomy was led by a midwife (Jennifer Sleep) and conducted from the Unit (Sleep et al., 1984). In the early 1990s, when a new research agenda was being developed, Esther Floud, a midwifery student, contacted NPEU researchers for advice about a literature search on perineal care she was carrying out as part of her undergraduate education. Floud had observed considerable variation in routine perineal care used by midwives at the end of the second stage of labor and had identified this as an area in which research results might offer useful information on which to base practice.

Confusion and conflict in practice is prevalent in health care generally, and in maternity care these can be the source of dissatisfaction among women and their families and, even worse, can contribute to substandard and unjustifiable care (Garcia et al., 1998).

One particular conflicting aspect of care that Floud had observed was what an attending midwife did with her hands during second stage. Some midwives would instruct a student midwife to apply pressure to a woman's perineum with one hand and use the other to control the emergence of the baby's head. Once the baby's head was born the baby's body was to be supported out of the mother's vagina. Other midwives strongly disapproved of such intervention and insisted that there should be no touching the woman's perineum, baby's head, or body. Still other practitioners advocated a mixture of both practices during which the baby's head was 'allowed' to emerge without applying hands to head or perineum, and then the midwife's hands guided the baby's head and shoulders under the mother's pubic arch and out of her vagina. Another option was to apply light touch to the baby's head, but not touch the woman's perineum or the baby's head or body otherwise.

Floud published her literature reviews (Floud, 1994a–c); further systematic searches of the literature were then carried out by NPEU researchers (Renfrew et al., 1998) to clarify whether there was reliable evidence that any of the prevailing practices were better in terms of important clinical outcomes. The conclusion was that there was no evidence about the effectiveness of manual pressure to support the perineum and control the birth of the baby's head and shoulders.

The absence of reliable evidence on which to base such common care identified the need to carry out a large-scale evaluation, and so the NPEU midwifery research team designed an RCT of care of the perineum at delivery: the Hands-On Or Hands-Poised (HOOP) Study (McCandlish et al., 1998a). This study evaluated whether a policy of using the 'hands-poised' method would reduce perineal pain reported by women 10 days after birth compared with the 'hands-on' method (see Table 5.2.1).

HOOP involved almost 5500 women who gave birth attended by midwives in two large clinical centers in the south of England between 1994 and 1996. The primary outcome was perineal pain in the previous 24 hours as reported by women 10 days after birth. This outcome was selected because it was considered that pain, rather than the location and severity of any perineal trauma, was the outcome of greatest concern to women after birth. Extensive data about perineal trauma were collected from midwives who attended the births of all the women randomly assigned in the trial and have been reported (Albers et al., 1999).

Of the 5316 (97%) women who took part and contributed information about their experience of pain at 10 days after birth, 910 (34.1%) were in the 'hands-poised' group compared with 823 (31.1%) women in the 'hands-on' group, resulting in a relative risk of 1.10 (95% confidence interval (CI), 1.01–1.18) and an absolute difference of 3% (95% CI, 0.5–5%). There were no differences in the location and severity of perineal

Table 5.2.1 Description of the hands-on and hands-poised methods used in the HOOP Study

Hands on

With one hand, the midwife puts pressure on the baby's head to increase flexion, while using her other hand to support (guard) the woman's perineum. Once the baby's head is born, the midwife places her hand on either side of the head and uses lateral flexion to facilitate the birth of the shoulders by releasing them under the woman's pubic arch. She then supports the baby's body out of the woman's vagina.

Hands poised

The midwife keeps her hand poised, prepared to put light pressure on the baby's head in case of rapid expulsion but does not touch the head or perineum otherwise. The baby's shoulders and body are born spontaneously.

trauma between the groups. The only other statistically significant differences observed were in two secondary outcomes: episiotomy and manual removal of placenta. Episiotomy was lower among women in the 'hands-poised' group (relative risk (RR) 0.79; 99% CI, 0.65–0.96), whereas manual removal of placenta was more common among women in the 'hands-poised' group (RR, 1.6; 99% CI, 1.02–2.78).

A specially designed results brochure (McCandlish et al., 1998b) was sent to women who took part in the study and, during the process of writing the results for publication, a series of 'roadshows' were held in the collaborating centers to discuss the results with midwife collaborators. Nine months after the primary results were first submitted, the main results article was published in the *British Journal of Obstetrics and Gynaecology* (McCandlish et al., 1998a). Secondary dissemination took place in a range of midwifery and consumer publications (McCandlish, 1999a, b), and the members of the original research team made presentations at national and international conferences (McCandlish, 1999c, d) and midwifery study days.

The primary conclusions of the trial were reported as follows (McCandlish et al., 1998a):

The reduction in pain in the 'hands-on' group was statistically significant and the difference detected potentially affects a substantial number of women. The difference related mainly to mild pain at 10 days. At three months [after birth], pain and other outcomes were not found to differ between the groups. Nevertheless, it is hard to recommend that units move to a policy of 'hands poised'. If 'hands-poised' care is used, audit, particularly of third stage care, should be maintained, and midwifery education should prepare practitioners to use either technique. Midwives who are currently in practice and who are requested to offer 'hands-poised' care should have access to clinical support to enable them to develop appropriate skills. Overall the results provide evidence to enable individual women and health professionals to make informed decisions about which of these perineal managements is preferable for them.

There has been no formal evaluation of whether, or how, the HOOP study results have been used in practice, but there has been some debate about the worth of the study and the conclusions drawn in the primary article. For example, the study was criticized for researching aspects of care that were themselves iatrogenic, because the question of what the attendant does with her hands can be considered the result of women being obliged to adopt positions for birth that suit the attendant and facilitate manual interference with the birthing process (Wickham, 2000). The appropriateness of trying to measure something as 'individual and intangible' (Wickham, 2000) as the primary outcome of pain 10 days after birth has also been questioned, and the reported difference in perineal pain may be insufficient to convince practitioners of the value of using one rather than the other technique. In addition, in some practice settings 'midwives are not accustomed to using either of these techniques, and use a mixture of both. The value of this trial to our clinical practice is therefore questionable' (Munro & Spiby, 2000). The issues raised by these critics are important. No matter how well conducted a clinical research study is, it is of little relevance if the results are not meaningful and useful to women accessing care and practitioners offering that care.

The HOOP Study was the largest RCT ever to evaluate a common midwifery practice, and it still provides the best evidence available comparing hands-on and hands-poised management in the context of midwifery care in the United Kingdom. Despite the contention that pain cannot be measured, it is possible (because of the large number of women who contributed information to the study) to estimate the impact of interventions on experiences such as pain. The measurement analyzed and reported was not of each individual's pain but that of the group of women allocated to one method of perineal management compared with those who were allocated to the other. HOOP set out to evaluate the effect of exposing a population of women who were giving birth to a policy of 'hands-on' or 'hands-poised' care and therefore did not estimate the risk of a particular outcome for an individual.

One of the greatest challenges in reviewing research results and thinking through their applicability in particular practice settings is to consider how the midwife's own biases might influence interpretation and application of information. The HOOP Study results did not clearly favor hands on or hands poised, and therefore it is beholden on practitioners to review and critique them carefully and use the information judiciously.

Many aspects of maternity care have been evaluated and classified as having '... effectiveness demonstrated by clear evidence from controlled trials' (for example, absorbable instead of nonabsorbable sutures for skin repair of perineal trauma) and others have been termed 'forms of care likely to be ineffective or harmful' (for example, routine or liberal episiotomy for birth) (Enkin et al., 2000).

'Hands-on' versus 'hands-poised' care cannot be labeled so neatly, and the results have been classified under the category ... evidence in favor of these forms of care [i.e. hands on] is strong, although not established by randomized trials.
(Enkin et al., 2000)

Other strategies to decrease perineal trauma

'Do the right things right (at the right time) to the right people' (Gray, 1997) is an invaluable guide when thinking about whether evidence can be used to inform effective, creative, thoughtful practice. For example, research about using perineal massage in second stage of labor (Stamp et al., 2001) has demonstrated no clear benefit to the practice, although a trend toward a reduction in trauma involving the anal sphincter was observed that did not reach statistical significance. Promising results from other trials that evaluated antenatal perineal massage and its effect on perineal trauma (Shipman et al., 1997; Labrecqe et al., 1999) mean that this kind of care deserves further well-designed, large-scale research.

The considerable research agenda about care that might prevent perineal trauma (and, thereby, reduce important associated morbidity such as perineal pain) is being addressed. For example, a large midwife-led RCT funded by the National Institute of Health and based in New Mexico will begin recruitment in 2001 with the aim of comparing strategies intended to minimize trauma used by midwives during the second stage of labor (Leah Albers, personal communication, 2001).

If we believe that midwifery care does make a difference, then we must be prepared to ask ourselves: how much difference does it make? The paradigm of noninterventionist, expectant, watchful care is often cited as being fundamental to midwifery practice. If this has enduring relevance in contemporary practice, then it is essential to acknowledge that 'doing nothing' or nonintervention, as much as intervention, has the potential to be helpful, harmful, or make no difference at all.

To suture or not to suture: dogma replaced by dogma?

In the developed world during the 20th century, childbearing moved from the home into hospitals staffed by skilled health professionals. Initially, repair of perineal trauma was low priority, unless it included the anal sphincter; however, as early as 1897, MacNaughton-Jones vividly described the dangers of an unsutured perineum by asserting that:

... the negligence of postponing the closure [suturing] of the rent, have cost many a woman an infinity of misery, and, through a septicemia, induced by perineal wounds made in operating and during the puerperal period, have caused, occasionally, peritonitis and death.

Although infection continued to play an important part in the rationale for perineal suturing, the need to restore the integrity and function of the tissue became prominent (Munro-Kerr et al., 1944). Repair became the norm, and the prevailing advice was that 'perineal tears should always be looked for ... The best rule to follow is that every tear, even the smallest, should be sewn up' (Johnstone, 1947).

MacNaughton-Jones (1900) further asserted that:

If surgeons only recognize the ills, immediate and remote, which follow lacerated perineum, we should less frequently hear of 'secondary operations'. The sensible obstetrician stitches the perineum at once when he recognizes the laceration after parturition. The futile plan of binding the knees together were better never conceived, unless, indeed, to be adopted after the immediate operation. It encourages procrastination, and is almost certain to end in failure.

Margaret Myles, a Scottish midwife teacher, wrote in the first edition of her influential *Textbook for Midwives*, published in 1953:

Midwives in the past used to take a pride in delivering the baby without perineal laceration, but in doing so the perineal phase was sometimes unduly prolonged and the infant subject to intracranial injury and asphyxia. The outlook is now more rational. Obstetricians consider it is better for the woman to sustain a laceration of her perineum, which is subsequently repaired in an efficient manner, than to have an over-stretched, although intact, perineum which is too lax to provide adequate support to the pelvic organs.

Universal repair was the standard (and commonly assumed) practice until journals aimed at a midwifery readership began to publish reports of observational studies highlighting the benefits for mothers of not suturing perineal trauma that did not involve the anal sphincter (Head, 1993; Clement & Reed, 1999).

In addition to these reports, an important large RCT designed and conducted by midwives in England compared a policy of two-stage perineal repair in which the skin was left unsutured and a policy of three-stage repair in which the skin was sutured using interrupted or subcuticular stitching among 1780 women who had experienced first- or second-degree trauma (Gordon et al., 1998). The main outcome measures were pain and healing at 24–48 hours postpartum; pain, healing, and need to remove sutures at 10 days after birth; and pain, need for suture removal or resuturing, dyspareunia, and failure to resume pain-free intercourse three months after birth. Data were collected for 99% of women at 24–48 hours and 10 days after birth and 93% at three months. There were no differences in pain at 24–48 hours (62% vs 64%; RR, 0.96; 95% CI, 0.90–1.03) and 10 days (25% vs 28%; RR, 0.90; 95% CI, 0.77–1.06). At three months after birth, among women who had resumed intercourse, there was a significant difference in reports of dyspareunia, with fewer women in the two-stage repair group reporting this outcome (15% vs 19%; RR, 0.80; 95% CI, 0.65–0.99). Of special note, 793 women who had taken part in the trial also were followed up at one year after birth (Grant et al., 2001). The results of the follow-up demonstrated that fewer women allocated to the two-stage repair reported that the perineum felt different from before birth (30% vs 40%; RR, 0.75; 95% CI,

0.61–0.91). There were no other clear differences reported.

Most recently a small RCT was conducted in Sweden comparing 40 women who had undergone suturing of 'grade 1 or 2 lacerations' with 40 who had not (Lundquist et al., 2000).

Women were followed up two to three days, eight days, and six months after birth, and data were collected about participant's experience of pain and discomfort, breastfeeding, and sexual intercourse. The researchers concluded that their study indicated that nonsuturing was appropriate for minor lacerations and concluded that 'minor lacerations can be left to heal spontaneously'. However, the interpretation of the results of this study should be treated with great caution. It has been calculated that to be able to detect a clinically important relative difference of 20% in an outcome such as pain at 12 weeks after birth, almost 14,000 women would need to be randomized. If dyspareunia reported at 12 weeks after birth were taken as the primary outcome of interest, the trial would need to include more than 3000 women to identify such a difference between the groups (McCandlish et al., 2000).

There is reliable evidence that it may be appropriate to offer some women restricted suturing of perineal skin (Gordon et al., 1998), but no such evidence exists to support not repairing trauma involving perineal muscle. The assumed benefits of nonrepair have not been established, and there is insufficient evidence to justify change from conventional care. Therefore, there is an urgent need to systematically question the effectiveness of not suturing compared with suturing. Research about the topic must also include important long-term outcomes such as incontinence and sexual function.

Perineal trauma: prevention and treatment – beyond dogma and into creative uncertainty?

A previous article in the *Journal of Midwifery and Women's Health* provided information and guidance about identifying and reviewing research evidence and information sources for midwifery care (Albers, 2001). There are key issues to consider while one reviews relevant articles to assess whether they hold credible and useful information about perineal trauma care for clinical practice (Dawes, 1999). These include:

- What are the results?
- Are the results valid?
- Are the results relevant?

A structured approach to evaluating the quality of a report is essential to help ascertain whether the evidence is meaningful and applicable in a particular practice context. Using prespecified quality criteria may be particularly efficient (Guyatt et al., 1993).

If you determine that there is robust, relevant, usable evidence on which to base change in practice, then a written guideline should be developed to map this change. Auditing the impact of altering care is the next step in effective evidence-based practice and should involve all participating in provision and implementation of care (including women accessing care) and make up the processes and outcomes associated with care (Wray & Benbow, 2000).

There are important, basic questions to ask about the routine perineal care to which women are exposed. In addressing these questions, high-quality, sufficiently large evaluations of alternative approaches to prevent and treat perineal trauma must ask about outcomes of value and interest to women during pregnancy, labor, birth, and in their lives after childbirth.

Women deserve midwives working *with and for* them (Keirse, 2000) who are prepared to move beyond dogmatic certainty and fixed paradigms of care to bring creative uncertainty into daily practice. In this way, women and midwives can together ask and answer questions about routine care – whether active intervention or nonintervention is likely to provide women with better experiences of birth and lifelong postnatal health.

REFERENCES

Albers L. 2001. Evidence and midwifery practice. J Midwif Women's Health, 46: 130–136

Albers L, Garcia J, Renfrew M, McCandlish R, Elbourne D. 1999. Distribution of genital tract trauma in childbirth and related postnatal pain. Birth, 26: 11–15

Barrett G, Pendry E, Peacock J, Victor C, Thaker R, Mayonda I. 2000. Women's sexual health after childbirth. Br J Obstet Gynaecol, 107: 186–195

Carroli G, Belizan J. 2001. Episiotomy for Vaginal Birth, Cochrane Collaboration Library Issue 2. Update Software, Oxford

Clarke E. 2000. Historical context of research in midwifery. In: Proctor S, Renfrew M (eds), Linking Research and Practice in Midwifery: A Guide to Evidence-based Practice, pp. 38–41. Balliere Tindall, London

Clement S, Reed B. 1999. To stitch or not to stitch? Practising Midwife, 2: 20–28

Dawes M. 1999. Introduction to critical appraisal. In: Dawes M, Davies P, Gray A, Mant J, Seers K, Snowball R (eds), Evidence-based Practice: A Primer for Health Care Professionals. Churchill Livingstone, London

Eason E, Feldman P. 2000. Much ado about a little cut: is episiotomy worthwhile? Obstet Gynecol, 95: 616

Enkin M, Keirse M, Neilson J, Crowther C, Duley L, Hodnett E et al. (eds). 2000. Evaluating care in pregnancy and childbirth. In: Guide to Effective Care in Pregnancy and Childbirth, 3rd edn. Oxford University Press, Oxford

Floud E. 1994a. Protecting the perineum in childbirth. 1. A retrospective view. Br J Midwif, 2: 258–263

Floud E. 1994b. Protecting the perineum in childbirth. 2. Risk of laceration. Br J Midwif, 2: 306–310

Floud E. 1994c. Protecting the perineum in childbirth. 3. Perineal care today. Br J Midwif, 2: 356–361

Garcia J, Redshaw M, Fizsimons B, Keene J. 1998. First Class Delivery. A National Survey of Women's Views of Maternity Care. Audit Commission, London

Glazener CMA, Abdalla M, Stroud P, Naji S, Templeton A, Russell AT. 1995. Postnatal morbidity: extent, causes, prevention and treatment. Br J Obstet Gynaecol, 102: 282–287

Gordon B, Mackrodt C, Fern E, Truesdale A, Ayers S, Grant A. 1998. The Ipswich Childbirth Study: a randomised evaluation of leaving the skin unsutured during postpartum perineal repair. Br J Obstet Gynaecol, 105: 435–440

Government Statistical Service. 2001. NHS Maternity Statistics, England: 1995–96 to 1997–98 (www.doh.gov.uk/public/sb0114.htm)

Grant A, Gordon B, Mackrodt C, Fern E, Truesdale A, Ayers S. 2001. The Ipswich childbirth study: one year follow up of alternative methods used in perineal repair. Br J Obstet Gynaecol, 108: 34–40

Gray JAM. 1997. Evidence-based Healthcare: How to Make Health Policy and Management Decisions, pp. 17–27. Churchill Livingstone, New York

Guyatt GH, Sackett DL, Cook DJ. 1993. Users' guides to the medical literature. II. How to use an article about therapy or prevention. A. Are the results of the study valid? JAMA, 270: 2598–2601

Hall MJ, Popovic JR. 2000. 1998 Summary: National Hospital Discharge Survey. Advance Data from Vital and Health Statistics, No. 316. National Center for Health Statistics, Hyattsville, MD

Head M. 1993. Dropping stitches. Nursing Times, 33: 64–65

Johnstone RW. 1947. A Textbook of Midwifery, 12th edn, p. 393. A&C Black, London

Keirse M. 2000. Foreword. In: Proctor S, Renfrew M (eds), Linking Research and Practice in Midwifery. Balliere Tindall, London.

Labrecque M, Eason E, Marcoux S et al. 1999. Randomized controlled trial of prevention of perineal trauma by perineal massage during pregnancy. Am J Obstet Gynecol, 180: 593–600

Lundquist M, Olsson A, Nissen E, Norman M. 2000. Is it necessary to suture all lacerations after a vaginal delivery? Birth, 27: 79–85

MacNaughton-Jones H. 1897. Practical Manual of Diseases of Women and Uterine Therapeutics. Balliere Tindall & Cox, London

MacNaughton-Jones H. 1900. Practical Manual of Diseases of Women and Uterine Therapeutics. Balliere Tindall & Cox, London

McCandlish R. 1999a. The HOOP Study: a personal view. MIDIRS Digest, 9: 77–78

McCandlish R. 1999b. HOOP study: Hands on or hands poised? A summary of the HOOP Study results. National Childbirth Trust New Digest, 22 June

McCandlish R. 1999c. Care of the perineum at delivery: the HOOP Study. Congress Proceedings of the Perinatal Society of Australia & New Zealand (PSANZ) 3rd Annual Congress, p. A44. PSANZ, Melbourne

McCandlish R. 1999d. Protecting the perineum at delivery; hands on or poised? Conference Proceedings of Common Intrapartum Problems – What Helps?, p. 7. University of Toronto

McCandlish R, Bowler U, van Asten H, Berridge G, Winter C, Sames I et al. 1998a. A randomised controlled trial of care of the perineum during the second stage of normal labour. Br J Obstet Gynaecol, 105: 1262–1272

McCandlish R, Bowler U, van Asten H, Berridge G, Winter C, Sames L et al. 1998b. Hoop Study – The Results: Brochure for Women who took Part in the HOOP Study. NPEU, Oxford

McCandlish R, Albers L, Sandland D, Brocklehurst P, Kettle C, King V. 2000. Suturing versus non-suturing of perineal lacerations [letter]. Birth, 28: 73–74

Munro J, Spiby H. 2000. Evidence based midwifery. Guidelines for Midwifery-led Care in Labour. November, p. 52. Accessed at www.fons.org/networks/ebm/guide.htm

Munro-Kerr JM, Johnstone RW, Young J, Hendry J, McIntrye D, Baird D et al. 1944. Combined Textbook of Obstetrics and Gynaecology, 4th edn, p. 593. E&S Livingstone, Edinburgh

Myles M. 1953. Textbook for Midwives, 1st edn. E&S Livingstone, Edinburgh

Reading A, Sledmere C, Cox D, Campbell S. 1982. How women view post episiotomy pain. BMJ, 284: 243–246

Renfrew M, Hannah M, Albers L, Floyd E. 1998. Practices that minimise trauma to the genital tract in childbirth: a systematic review of the literature. Birth, 25: 143–160

Sackett D. 2000. Introduction. In: Sackett D, Straus S, Richardson W, Rosenberg W, Haynes R (eds), Evidence-based Medicine, 2nd edn, p. 1. Churchill Livingstone, London

Shipman MK, Boniface DR, Teffr ME, McCloghry F. 1997. Antenatal perineal massage and subsequent perineal outcomes. Br J Obstet Gynaecol, 104: 787–791

Sleep J. 1991. Perineal care: a series of five randomized controlled trials. In: Robinson S, Thomson A (eds), Midwives, Research and Childbirth, Vol. 2, pp. 199–251. Chapman & Hall, London

Sleep JM, Grant A. 1987. West Berkshire perineal management trial: three year follow-up. BMJ, 295: 749–751

Sleep J, Grant A, Garcia J, Elbourne D, Spencer J, Chalmers I. 1984. West Berkshire perineal management trial. BMJ, 289: 587–590

Stamp G, Kruzins G, Crowther C. 2001. Perineal massage in labour and prevention of perineal trauma: randomised controlled trial. BMJ, 322: 1277–1280

Sultan AH. 1999. Obstetrical perineal injury and anal incontinence. Clin Risk, 5: 193–196

Sultan AH, Kamm MA, Bartram CI, Hudson CN. 1994. Perineal damage at delivery. Contemp Rev Obstet Gynaecol, 6: 18–24

Wickham S. 2000. 'Perineal pampering' – before, during and after birth. MIDIRS Midwifery Digest, 11: S23–S27

Wray J, Benbow A. 2000. Developing standards for practice. In: Proctor S, Renfrew M (eds), Linking Research and Practice in Midwifery: A Guide to Evidence-based Practice. Balliere Tindall, London

Journal of Midwifery and Women's Health 2001; 46(6): 396–401

A disappearing art: vaginal breech birth

Becky Reed

Following the Term Breech Trial (TBT) (Hannah et al., 2000), it seems that women carrying a diagnosed breech baby at term often no longer have fully informed choice about how their baby may be born. In an article in *Midwifery Matters*, Karen Beckett (2003) states that 'policies, protocols and guidelines continue to be based on the TBT which considers caesarean section to be the only safe option'. However, she also comments that 'undiagnosed breech presentations continue to occur and often lead to safe vaginal breech deliveries'. In a favourite midwifery textbook of mine, Elizabeth Davis (1987) warns all midwives practising home births:

There may come a day when firm abdominal tone, extra belly fat, or excess amniotic fluid confuses your evaluation of position, and suddenly you have a surprise breech on your hands! Be ready for it.

In the group practice in which I work we aim to visit all women at home in labour. This is not only in an attempt to reduce that labour ward 'category X' syndrome, but also and more importantly to keep open the choice of place of birth for all women for whom home birth would be a safe option. The women we look after know that they can choose to stay at home to give birth if all goes well.

As it happened, Rebecca had been planning a home water birth. She was a fit and healthy 36-year-old, was expecting her first baby and did indeed have firm abdominal tone! I booked Rebecca at 14 weeks, and Claire (her second midwife) and I saw her throughout her pregnancy. Although there was a query about the baby's position at 35 weeks, by 38 weeks we were sure that the presentation was cephalic, with the head deeply engaged. The pool was organised and labour awaited.

Rebecca went into spontaneous labour at 39 + 3 weeks. She bleeped me at 9 a.m. to let me know that her waters had broken at 1.30 a.m., with clear liquor draining since. The baby was active, and Rebecca was starting to have some period-type pains; I arranged to visit her later for a check and to do a low vaginal swab. Rebecca felt fine with this arrangement and we agreed that she would call me if things changed or if she had any concerns.

At 2.30 p.m., having heard nothing from Rebecca, I phoned and spoke to her husband, Pete. He told me that she was now contracting well every three minutes or so. We agreed that I would visit her within the hour unless they called me sooner. I completed a postnatal discharge at the hospital and collected Michelle, a student midwife on placement with us. We arrived at the house at 3.20 p.m. Rebecca was on all fours at the top of the stairs, and told me she was feeling like pushing. I observed the next contraction: obvious rectal pressure. I suggested she come downstairs where the pool was ready and waiting.

Rebecca flopped forward over the sofa and I asked her if I could examine her before calling Claire; this was fine. There was a soft anterior lip, easily pushed away, and a confusing presentation… something soft with bone behind – either head with soft caput, or maybe a breech? Whatever it was was at the spines and descending well, so I realised I would know soon enough. I called Claire and warned her that Rebecca's baby might be breech, and asked her to come quickly. Less than five minutes later there was frank meconium at the introitus and my diagnosis was confirmed.

I have attended many breech births, and I felt confident about supporting Rebecca in giving birth vaginally; besides, it seemed there may be no choice as this little baby was apparently hurrying into the world. However, we had not planned for a breech birth at home, and I work as an NHS midwife with clear policies and guidelines to consider. I decided to call an ambulance, with the aim of transferring to hospital if there was time. Rebecca was contracting very strongly every two minutes, with strong expulsive urges and obvious descent occurring.

Between contractions I explained what was happening to Rebecca and Pete, and prepared my equipment for birth at home. Resuscitation equipment was checked, and I asked Pete to prepare warm towels for his baby. Rebecca was feeling scared, not surprisingly, but was coping beautifully with Pete supporting her. Michelle was excited, and ready with her digital camera to photograph the birth! Claire arrived and took over, writing contemporaneous notes. The breech was visible at 3.40 p.m., advancing with each contraction. Claire telephoned the labour ward (as advised in the protocol) and asked to speak to a Senior Registrar; his advice was to transfer immediately to hospital. Two ambulances with four crew arrived at 3.53, by which time the first buttock was beginning to stretch the perineum. I spoke to the ambulance crew and told them that I was making a clinical decision to stay at home for the birth, as I felt that it would be riskier to transfer at this stage. They agreed with me; however, I asked them to stay in case there were any problems with the baby.

By 4.04 p.m. Pete was able to see that he had a daughter, as her bottom began to deliver. By 4.09 her legs and body were born, and I wrapped them gently in a warm towel.

We could clearly see her heart beating at between 60 and 80 b.p.m.; I asked Rebecca to push well with the next contraction as I felt her baby needed to be born soon. At 4.12 p.m. Rebecca pushed out her baby's head. I caught her in a warm towel, and laid her gently on a heating pad in front of her mum. Little Marieta was shocked and floppy at first, but responded well to drying with a towel and some gentle massage; Apgars were seven at one minute, 10 at five minutes. Marieta's mum and dad were shocked, too, but delighted with their beautiful baby girl.

I telephoned the labour ward to let them know of the baby's safe arrival, and at 4.20 the ambulance crew left, delighted that we hadn't needed their services after all. Rebecca pushed her placenta out at 4.33, and we then made her comfortable on the sofa while Pete had a cuddle with his daughter – feet up by her head and sucking her big toe! Clearly, she had been breech all along …

Later, Pete, Marieta and Rebecca all got in the pool and had a 'swim' together, Rebecca feeling a bit sad that she had missed out on her planned water birth. However, I think we were able to convince her that she had done something very special that day – something of which she would always be proud.

With risk management in mind, I phoned the supervisor of midwives on call and discussed Rebecca's birth with her. She warned me that an NCE (Notifiable Clinical Event) form would need to be completed, but reassured me that she felt I had acted appropriately, and congratulated me on the happy outcome.

Following Rebecca's birth, I felt grateful to all those women whose previous breech births had taught me so much. I felt happy for Rebecca and Pete that they had achieved the home birth that they had hoped for. I felt re-confirmed in my belief (and that of others) that with an undiagnosed breech and strong, advancing labour it is safe to aim for a vaginal birth. But most of all I felt sad for all those midwives who will no longer have the opportunity to gain the skills needed to help women deliver their breech babies vaginally, but who may even so come across a situation just like this one. With the new belief that caesareans are the only safe option for diagnosed breeches, are we not doing women like Rebecca, and babies like Marieta, a terrible disservice?

An afterthought: although I felt calm throughout the birth, it's clear that there was just one thing too many to think about. When I look at the wonderful photos, I realise that I forgot to put on my gloves!

Acknowledgements

Thank you to Rebecca, Pete and Marieta for letting me tell their birth story.

REFERENCES

Beckett K. 2003. Breech! Birth or delivery? Whose choice is it? Midwifery Matters, 98: 3–5

Davis E. 1987. Heart and Hands, 2nd edn. Celestial Arts

Hannah ME, Hannah WJ, Hewson SA, Hodnett ED, Saigal S, Willan AR et al. 2000. Planned caesarean section versus planned vaginal birth for breech presentation at term: a randomised multi-centre trial (Term Breech Trial). Lancet, 356: 1375–1382

The Practising Midwife 2003; 6(9): 16–18

Home breech birth

After three traumatic births, a peaceful and caring home birth, even with a breech presentation, was a welcome change

Esther Culpin, with Michel Odent

At a time when breech presentation is almost synonymous with caesarean section, I find it useful to write up the story of the easiest of my four deliveries. In this case, changing the birth environment absolutely transformed the way I gave birth.

Arrangements beforehand

I set out to create a new birthing environment this time around, as my previous births, although loosely defined as 'normal', were definitely not. The births of my three sons followed long and traumatic labours and I experienced excessive blood loss immediately afterwards. Overall, birth appeared to be extremely risky and to contemplate it all over again did not seem like a good idea. The solution to my difficult birth experiences could have been an elective caesarean section. Instead I had the opportunity to look more closely at important issues that might have affected the way my first three births had turned out.

Giving birth at home was a really important factor for me because of the absolute freedom to do as I wished in labour; I needed to arrange for a midwife to be in attendance who would respect my need for a calm and undisturbed environment. Michel Odent was happy to assume this role and was noticeably unperturbed by my traumatic labour and delivery record!

Breech presentation

When, after 30 weeks of pregnancy, my daughter was persistently a breech presentation, I made no change of plan. I was still happy, confident and looking forward to an easier birth in the privacy of my home. At this point technology could have taken over, but all the required information seemed to be available, literally through the midwife's hands. There was never a suggestion that I should undergo an external cephalic version (ECV) and,

having experienced that procedure 14 years previously, I did not feel I wished to undergo it again. Although I was still aiming for the birth to be at home, I booked in at the maternity hospital just a mile away, in case admission to hospital and emergency treatment should be required. Local midwives, although acquainted with home birth, indicated their preference not to be involved with a breech birth if it was to be at home.

Labour

I went into labour a week after my due date. This time around, as part of a strategy for giving birth easily, I aimed to keep myself rested. This was achieved by not doing too many things in a day so that I would be able to cope with the rigours of labour whenever it started. As the process got underway, I found that being at home had a direct effect on the way I coped and on the optimism I felt. (Remember, the baby was breech, I had never experienced an easy birth before and I was at home!)

On the domestic front I was assisted by my husband. Again, considering my history of traumas associated with giving birth, he was superb. His responsibilities were wide-ranging, but his priority was to maintain a safe, dark and secure environment for me, so that I should experience no disturbances.

A birthing pool in the sitting room was filled with warm water, in case it should be needed for pain relief. The children went out to breakfast with their grandparents. For this birth, because I badly wanted things to progress easily, I did not wish to have any distractions at all.

For me, labour in any circumstances remains hard, but given that this time I would be able to adopt any position, and there were no outsiders coming in and out of the room (as there could easily be in the hospital setting), I felt that I was on the way to giving birth quickly and easily.

Breech birth

In fact, for the first time in my experience, labour progressed extremely quickly and I found myself trying to slow things down so that I would not give birth before assistance arrived! What was noticeable at this point was the lack of instructions I was given: Michel gathered silently all the information he needed to assess the situation. I was obviously ready to deliver and, because I was not directed in any way, I decided to get into the pool! At the next contraction and whilst standing upright, my baby's body was born.

I was assisted out of the pool and supported from behind so I could maintain a standing position. Now there was a long pause while the cord, which was wrapped tightly three times around her neck, was unwound. Her head was deflected by inserting a finger into her mouth before her head was delivered. During these few critical minutes there was no discussion about whether I had a girl or a boy.

My daughter lay on the carpet, motionless at first. But, in that situation, I was her life support, just as I had been all along. The fact that I was personally and actively involved in those early moments was of prime importance, whatever the outcome would be.

The position that I adopted at this point, immediately after her birth, was also extremely advantageous. I was leaning over my daughter, who was lying on the ground. This was the optimal position in the early moments of her life: it aided the natural compression of the uterus, and meant that the baby could be readily gathered up as soon as this became appropriate. There was no cutting of the cord, no touching of my abdomen and no administration of artificial hormones.

A physiological third stage of labour

A truly physiological third stage of labour is extremely rare but, for this birth, I had experienced exactly that. After a little while I moved on to a nearby couch and instinctively lay on my side with the baby. The move from floor to couch was easily undertaken, the cord remaining slack in the process. I was now in that wonderful time following birth but had not experienced any preceding trauma.

Probably within the hour the placenta separated, and by that time the cord was lifeless and could be cut and tied. I really preferred the idea that the cord would not be cut in the early moments following birth, since this would maximise all the benefits to the baby. Blood loss was minimal.

Conclusion

This is the story of my birth, which turned out to be easy and untraumatic. Very simple measures were taken to change the factors surrounding birth and these appeared to make a huge difference: I was at home, I had freedom to move around as I wished, I was not watched by anybody (including my husband) and I had faith in 'the midwife'. From my perspective, as the mother, the fact that my baby was in a breech position proved to be a secondary consideration.

Commentary: by Michel Odent

Esther's daughter was born several years before the publication in the *Lancet* of the huge randomised multicentre trial that is considered a landmark in the history of breech births (Hannah et al., 2000). It is easy to summarise what we learnt from this study: we learnt that a breech birth in a conventional hospital and in the presence of an obstetrician is dangerous. The case of Esther's delivery does not belong to this framework. It occurred outside the conventional hospital environment and, in the mind of Esther, I was probably an old friend of the family with an experience of home births and breech births, rather than an obstetrician.

What can we say today to women who want to avoid a caesarean section in spite of a breech presentation at term? I find it useful to transmit some simple rules that I gradually adopted after having the experience of about 300 breech births by the vaginal route:

- The best possible environment is usually a place with nobody else around other than an experienced, motherly and low-profile midwife who is not scared by a breech birth.
- The first stage of labour is a trial. If it is straightforward, easy and fast, the vaginal route is possible. If the first stage is long and difficult, a caesarean section should be decided without any delay, before a point of no return is reached.
- Because the first stage is a trial, it is important not to make it artificially too easy, either with drugs or even with water immersion.
- After the point of no return, privacy remains the key word.
- It is permissible to be more audacious with a frank breech than with a footling breech. A cord prolapse outside the hospital environment can be a disaster.

REFERENCES

Hannah ME, Hannah WJ et al. 2000. Planned caesarean section versus planned vaginal birth for breech presentation at term: a randomised multicentre trial. Lancet, 356: 1375–1383

The Practising Midwife 2003; 6(1): 10–11

To drip or not to drip? A literature review

Myra Parsons

The unnecessary use of intravenous infusions during normal labour is an issue that has been raised time and again, yet the practice continues. Although good intentions accompanied their introduction in the late 1940s, it has since been discovered that they are deleterious to mother, fetus and the progress of labour.

This article gives a historical overview of the use of intravenous fluids during the past 50 years, and questions whether physiologically and psychologically these fluids should ever be used for normal labour.

Introduction

Intravenous therapy as a treatment for labour was first introduced in the late 1940s in response to Mendelson's (1946) research, which recommended that all labouring women should fast as one aspiration prevention strategy for general anaesthesia.

Although originally recommended for women who were considered to have a high-risk pregnancy, it became widespread over time and eventually became routine. No research was ever conducted prior to the introduction of intravenous infusions to substantiate their safety or efficacy during labour (Pengelley & Gyte, 1998).

Today, a policy of fasting labouring women is still widely practised and has led to the continuance of the routine use of intravenous fluids during normal labour in most hospitals in the United States (Sommer et al., 2000; Carr & Schott, 2002) and, anecdotally, in some Australian hospitals. The reason behind the continuation of this practice has been the need to provide fluids, calories and electrolytes during labour in lieu of oral intake (Keppler, 1988; Tourangeau et al., 1999). Yet 'intravenous hydration, however profuse, does not quench thirst' (Simini, 1999, p. 862). This paper examines the use of intravenous fluids for these reasons, along with the consequences for their use, or overuse, during labour.

Intravenous therapy for hydration

The physiological changes associated with pregnancy have a marked effect on fluid balance and prepare the woman's body for the demands of labour. Plasma volume increases by some 40% by the end of pregnancy (Millns, 1991). The total body fluid increases by 6–10 litres, with 3–6 litres being extracellular, depending on the degree of oedema (Grant, 1992).

Renal plasma flow and glomerular filtration rate increase, and are matched by an increase in tubular reabsorption (Millns, 1991). Due to the pregnancy-induced increase in total body fluids and the high level of pituitary antidiuretic hormone, the pregnant woman enters labour fairly 'waterlogged' and well adapted to withstand periods of water deprivation, but her ability to cope with a water load is impaired (Morton, 1993; Odent, 1994; World Health Organisation, 1996).

During labour, water excretion is delayed due to the increased level of plasma antidiuretic hormone (O'Sullivan, 1994). Furthermore, the normal fluid loss caused by respiration and perspiration is reduced due to the relative inactivity of the woman during labour (Odent, 1994).

Intravenous therapy for nutrition

The logic behind administering intravenous fluids for nutrition is based on the body's production of ketones during labour and the belief that they have a detrimental effect on labour. Sabata et al. (1968) theorised that the rise in blood ketones, which occurs during labour, is due to the increasing energy demands which can no longer be met by endogenous glucose only, hence the introduction of intravenous glucose infusions to prevent and treat ketosis and dehydration in labouring women following long periods of fasting (Dumoulin & Foulkes, 1984).

It was not until many years later that scientists studied the effects of intravenous fluids used for healthy labouring women and uncovered the negative consequences, which will be discussed below (Sleutel & Golden, 1999). Interestingly, the rise in ketone bodies at the end of the first stage was found to be significantly smaller in mothers who had eaten during labour than those women treated with intravenous infusions (Sabata et al., 1968; Tourangeau et al., 1999). Whether intravenous therapies are instituted for hydration or nutritional requirements, they have both physiological and psychological implications for the mother, her fetus and the labour.

Physiological implications

Fasting causes an increase in the incidence of dehydration and ketosis, and it was believed that intravenous therapy would meet the fluid and nutrient requirements of the fasting labouring woman. It was not until the mid-1970s that research began to demonstrate the adverse effects to the mother and fetus caused by intravenous infusions (e.g. Ames et al., 1975; Lawrence et al., 1982). These adverse effects are both physiological and psychological.

Physiologically, the first problem is water intoxication. The 'waterlogged' condition of the woman at the start of labour is further increased when oxytocin and/or opiates, which have an antidiuretic effect, are used for augmentation or pain relief during labour (Schwartz & Jones, 1978; MacLennan, 1986). Add to this a preload for an epidural anaesthesia, which is a common form of labour pain management these days (NSW Health Department, 2001), and the labouring woman may be compromised severely (Keppler, 1988).

Concerns have been raised that fluid overload may contribute to the development of pulmonary oedema, causing and aggravating the effect of pulmonary aspiration if it occurred (McKay & Mahan, 1988). Therefore, intravenous fluids are seldom required, even with a 24-hour labour (Lind, 1983), especially if healthy labouring women have access to unlimited oral fluids (O'Sullivan, 1994).

Fluid overload can also lead to postpartum cerebral oedema, convulsions, severe brain damage, severe visual deficit, dysphasia and maternal death (Gupta & Cohen, 1972; Paech, 1998). It has been recommended that a maximum daily intravenous intake should be 1200 ml during labour due to the woman's impaired water excretion (Tarnow-Mordi et al., 1981).

Not only does intravenous infusion increase the workload for midwives and doctors, but it is a potential source of infection and phlebitis (Swift, 1991). Other adverse physiological effects of intravenous therapies depend on the type of infusion used. Three types have been used in labour over the past 50 years: dextrose, normal saline and Hartmann's. The effect of these intravenous fluids is further discussed below.

1. Dextrose infusion

Dextrose (glucose) infusions were the first intravenous fluids to be used, as it was believed that they would eradicate ketosis during labour (Sabata et al., 1968). Although high-dose glucose infusions in labour rapidly reverse maternal ketosis (i.e. the concentration of D-3-hydroxybutyrate in the blood), they cause a significant rise in lactate concentrations, leading to hyperglycaemia.

It was not until some 20–30 years after their introduction for labour that research found dextrose infusions caused hyperglycaemia and hyperinsulinaemia in the mother (Morton et al., 1985), and hyperinsulinaemia (Mendiola et al., 1982) and lactic acidosis in the fetus (Singhi et al., 1982).

Large volumes of glucose solutions are also believed to increase maternal blood volume, resulting in an increased cardiac output (Enkin et al., 1995). When given as a 10% dextrose infusion, it was associated with a significant increase in osmotic diuresis in the labouring woman. When given for hydration purposes, it makes this form of intravenous fluid illogical (Morton et al., 1985).

Other findings associated with high-dose glucose infusion during labour were a lowering of the labouring woman's pain threshold (Odent, 1994), a slowing down of labour (Anderson et al., 1982), an increased incidence of neonatal jaundice (Gabbe, 1988) and an increased weight loss in the newborn in the first two days of life (Keppler, 1988). It has been suggested that the potential hazards caused by glucose infusions may be obviated by using a more physiological approach – that is, allowing oral intake of both food and fluids during labour to supply the calories and fluid requirements (Johnson et al., 1989).

Glucose infusions, being salt free, can lead to both maternal and fetal hyponatraemia (Stratton et al., 1994), as glucose draws water from the cells, diluting the concentration of sodium in the plasma (Tarnow-Mordi et al., 1981). Maternal hyponatraemia has been known to result in vomiting, cerebral oedema, pulmonary oedema, oliguria, coma and convulsions (Gupta & Cohen, 1972; Keppler, 1988).

Fetal hyponatraemia can produce convulsions, apnoea, cyanosis, respiratory distress, feeding difficulties (Dahlenburg et al., 1980) and transient tachypnoea (Sleutel & Golden, 1999).

Due to the substantial body of evidence that glucose administration can be harmful in labour, there has been a dramatic change away from routine intravenous therapy, particularly with dextrose and especially for low-risk labouring women (Morton, 1993).

2. Normal saline infusion

For a time, normal saline solutions were used to replace glucose solutions. Their sole or excessive use, however, was found to lead to fluid overload, thus contributing to pulmonary oedema and hypernatraemia (Gabbe, 1988; Enkin et al., 1995). In pregnancy, and especially during labour, common obstetric and anaesthetic procedures may interfere with the mechanisms that protect against pulmonary oedema (MacLennan, 1986), adding to the risk of pulmonary oedema.

Ramanathan et al. (1984) compared the infusion of solutions containing glucose, saline, lactate or acetate administered to labouring women and concluded that, although high plasma lactate concentrations were observed following all fluids, fetal-neonatal outcomes were similar. These authors recommended Hartmann's solution, as opposed to normal saline, for use during labour due to the higher lactate concentration found in saline.

3. Hartmann's infusion

Hartmann's (Lactated Ringer's) solution containing 5% glucose is in common use today as an intravenous therapy for labouring women based on the accelerated starvation theory of pregnancy, and the assumed intrapartum metabolic demands and increased caloric needs of the mother. This low-dose infusion of glucose via Hartmann's solution is believed to have a beneficial affect for both the mother and her fetus (Fisher & Huddleston, 1997). Morton (1993) advocated a more detailed look at intravenous therapy used for epidural preloading and maintenance, and believes that the amount infused and the consequences for the mother and fetus have not been considered.

Many articles over the past decade have debated the type of intravenous fluids to use (e.g. Keppler, 1988; Morton, 1993; Fisher and Huddleston, 1997). Studies have investigated the feasibility of dextrose-containing solutions administered at very low concentrations during labour. Evans et al. (1986) found that a modest glucose infusion rate (6 g of glucose per hour) was sufficient to prevent severe ketosis without compromising mother or baby.

A more recent study comparing normal saline with a 5% dextrose solution infused at 180 ml/hour (i.e. 9 g of glucose per hour) found that this rate of dextrose was also safe from complications incurred with higher doses administered more quickly (Nordstrom et al., 1995). These researchers have recommended the use of 5% dextrose if a labouring woman develops ketonuria.

Psychological implications

The psychological effects of intravenous therapies have also been investigated (Newton et al., 1988). The attitude of some health professionals caring for labouring women is that intravenous therapy is a benign intervention (Davis & Riedmann, 1991). However, the intravenous apparatus causes pain and restriction of movement.

The body's release of catecholamines in response to pain and fear, along with the woman's immobilisation, has been associated with reduced uterine efficiency and slow progress of labour (Broach & Newton, 1988; Davis & Riedmann, 1991), resulting in the 'medical intervention cascade' (Mold & Stein, 1986). It has also been argued that it is just as stressful for a labouring woman to be virtually immobilised by an intravenous apparatus as it is to have oral fluids withheld (O'Sullivan, 1994).

Are intravenous fluids necessary?

The growing realisation of the deleterious effects of intravenous fluids for the mother and her fetus during labour has led to recommendations for careful control of these fluids (Gabbe, 1988). The practice of instituting intravenous fluids in labour should be weighed carefully against the alternative approach of allowing women unrestricted oral food and fluids (Pengelley & Gyte, 1998). It was concluded by Enkin et al. (1995), after reviewing current literature on this subject, that there is no compelling evidence to support the routine administration of intravenous fluids and that they do not provide any benefit in the care of low-risk labouring women.

But are oral fluids the answer?

With the complications attributed to intravenous fluids in mind, the hydration saga pursued a new direction. To prevent the risk of overloading the woman with intravenous fluids, a push with oral fluid has erupted. Odent (1994) believes the need for oral fluids during labour is also overestimated and can lead to water intoxication and hyponatraemia. The woman's nutritional needs during labour are too complex; women therefore should rely on what they feel they need (Odent, 1994).

Conclusion

The articles reviewed regarding the use of intravenous fluids during labour present well-founded, scientific and clinical arguments against their routine and often unnecessary use as a compensation for the restriction of oral intake. There is no current research which supports the use of intravenous therapy during labour, nor is there any evidence purporting any beneficial effects of this practice for the woman, her fetus or her labour.

Scientific knowledge demonstrates that the pregnancy-induced changes to a woman's body adequately prepare her to cope with the ordeal of labour. There may be labouring women who do require intravenous therapy, but the needs of a few should not be interpreted as beneficial to all.

REFERENCES

Ames AC, Cobbold S, Maddock J. 1975. Lactic acidosis complicating treatment of ketosis of labour. Br Med J, iv: 610–613

Anderson GG, Cordero L, Hon EH. 1982. Hypotonic glucose infusion during labour. Obstet Gynecol, 36: 405–414

Broach J, Newton N. 1988. Food and beverages in labour. Part I: cross-cultural and historical practices. Birth, 15: 81–85

Carr CA, Schott A. 2002. Difference in evidence-based care in midwifery practice and education. J Nurs Schol, 34(2): 153–158

Dahlenburg GW, Burnell RH, Braybrook R. 1980. The relation between cord serum sodium levels in newborn infants and maternal intravenous therapy during labour. Br J Obstet Gynaecol, 87: 519–522

Davis L, Riedmann G. 1991. Recommendations for the management of low-risk obstetric patients. Int J Gynecol Obstet, 35: 107–115

Dumoulin JG, Foulkes JE. 1984. Ketonuria during labour. Br J Obstet Gynaecol, 91: 97–98

Enkin M, Keirse MJ, Renfrew M et al. 1995. A Guide to Effective Care in Pregnancy and Childbirth. Oxford University Press, Oxford

Evans SE, Crawford JS, Stevens ID et al. 1986. Fluid therapy for induced labour under epidural analgesia: biochemical consequences for mother and infant. Br J Obstet Gynaecol, 93: 329–333

Fisher AJ, Huddleston JF. 1997. Intrapartum maternal glucose infusion reduces umbilical cord acidemia. Am J Obstet Gynecol, 177: 765–769

Gabbe S. 1988. Commentary: current practices of intravenous fluid administration may cause more harm the good. Birth, 15: 73–74

Grant J. 1992. Nutrition and hydration in labour. In: Alexander J, Levy V, Roch S (eds), Midwifery Practice: Intrapartum Care: A Research-based Approach. MacMillan Press, London

Gupta DR, Cohen NH. 1972. Oxytocin, "salting out" and water intoxication. JAMA, 220: 681–683

Johnson C, Keirse MJ, Enkin M et al. 1989. Nutrition and hydration in labour. In: Chalmers I, Enkin M, Keirse MJ (eds), Effective Care in Pregnancy and Childbirth, Vol. 2, pp. 827–832. Oxford University Press, Oxford

Keppler A. 1988. The use of intravenous fluids during labour. Birth, 15: 59–75

Lawrence GF, Brown VA, Parsons RJ et al. 1982. Feto-maternal consequences of high-dose glucose infusion during labour. Br J Obstet Gynaecol, 89: 27

Lind T. 1983. Fluid balance during labour: a review. J Royal Soc Med, 76: 870–875

MacLennan FM. 1986. Maternal mortality from Mendelson's syndrome: an explanation? Lancet, 1: 587–589

McKay S, Mahan C. 1988. How can aspiration of stomach contents in obstetrics best be prevented? Birth, 15: 222–229

Mendelson CL. 1946. The aspiration of stomach contents. Am J Obstet Anesth, 52: 191–205

Mendiola J, Grylack LJ, Scanlon JW. 1982. Effects of intrapartum maternal glucose infusion on the normal fetus and newborn. Anesth Analg, 61: 32–35

Millns JP. 1991. Fluid balance in labour. Obstet Gynaecol, 1: 35–40

Mold JW, Stein HF. 1986. The cascade effect in the clinical care of patients. New Engl J Med, 314: 512–514

Morton KE. 1993. Fluid management during labour: a British view. Int J Obstet Anesth, 2: 147–151

Morton KE, Jackson MC, Gillmer MD. 1985. A comparison of the effects of four intravenous solutions for the treatment of ketonuria during labour. Br J Obstet Gynaecol, 92: 473–479

Newton N, Newton M, Broach B. 1988. Psychological, physical, nutritional and technologic aspects of intravenous infusion during labour. Birth, 15: 67–72

Nordstrom L, Arulkumarin S, Chua S et al. 1995. Continuous maternal glucose infusion during labour: effects on maternal and fetal glucose and lactate levels. Am J Perinatol, 12: 357–362

NSW Health Department. 2001. New South Wales Mothers and Babies 1999. NSW Health Department, Sydney

Odent M. 1994. Labouring women are not marathon runners. Midwif Today, 31: 23–24, 43, 51

O'Sullivan G. 1994. The stomach – fact or fantasy: eating and drinking during labour. Int Anesth Clinic, 32: 31–44

Paech MJ. 1998. Convulsions in a healthy parturient due to intrapartum water intoxication. Int J Obstet Anesth, 7: 59–61

Pengelley L, Gyte G. 1998. Eating and drinking in labour (1). A summary of medical research to facilitate informed choice about the care of mother and baby. Pract Midwif, 1: 34–37

Ramanathan S, Masih AK, Ashok U et al. 1984. Concentrations of lactate and pyruvate in maternal and neonatal blood with different intravenous fluids used for prehydration before epidural anesthesia. Anesth Analg, 63: 69–74

Sabata V, Wolf H, Lausmann S. 1968. The role of free fatty acids, glycerol, ketone bodies and glucose in the energy metabolism of the mother and fetus during delivery. Biol Neonatol, 13: 7–17

Schwartz RH, Jones RW. 1978. Transplacental hypronatraemia due to oxytocin. Br Med J, 1: 152–153

Simini B. 1999. Preoperative fasting. Lancet, 353: 862–863

Singhi S, Kang EC, Hall J. 1982. Hazards of maternal hydration with 5 per cent dextrose. Lancet, ii: 335

Sleutel M, Golden SS. 1999. Fasting in labour: relic or requirement. J Obstet Gynecol Neo Nurs, 28: 507–512

Sommer PA, Norr K, Roberts J. 2000. Clinical decision-making regarding intravenous hydration in normal labour in a birth centre setting. J Midwif Women's Health, 45: 114–121

Stratton JF, Stronge PC, Boylan PC. 1994. Hyponatraemia and non-electrolyte solutions in labouring primigravida. Eur J Obstet Gynecol Reprod Biol, 59: 149–151

Swift L. 1991. Labour and fasting. Nurs Times, 87: 64–65

Tarnow-Mordi WO, Shaw JG, Lin D et al. 1981. Iatrogenic hyponatraemia of the newborn due to maternal fluid overload: a prospective study. Br Med J, 283: 629

Tourangeau A, Carter N, Tansil N et al. 1999. Intravenous therapy for women in labor: implementation of a practice change. Birth, 26(1): 31–36

World Health Organisation. 1996. Care in Normal Birth: A Practical Guide. World Health Organisation, Geneva

The Practising Midwife 2003; 6(9): 25–27

Blood gases and babies

Penny Champion

Taking blood from babies and from their cords around the time of birth has become a common practice in many obstetric units. I have found that both the student midwives and midwives I meet in my work as a midwife teacher find it difficult to understand and explain the physiology and interpret the results of this investigation. In my quest to find adequate information I have never found an article or reference book that explains the physiology and interpretation to my satisfaction. I feel that it is important as a midwife to be able to explain any investigation performed on a baby, to the parents and to student practitioners, and I hope that this article will help midwives to do just that.

Background

This article focuses on cord blood analysis, but the physiology and interpretation is also relevant to fetal blood samples taken from the scalp during labour. In 2001 the National Institute for Clinical Excellence (NICE) produced a guideline about electronic fetal monitoring. The recommendations in that document have been widely implemented in obstetric units throughout the UK and include the following:

'Intermediate fetal/neonatal measures of fetal hypoxia to be collected should be:
- *umbilical artery acid–base status*
- *Apgar score at five minutes*
- *neonatal encephalopathy.*
  These should be collected on a local (hospital/trust) level.

Umbilical artery acid–base status should be assessed by collection of paired samples from the umbilical artery and umbilical vein.

Umbilical artery acid–base status should be performed as a minimum after:

- *emergency caesarean section is performed*
- *instrumental vaginal delivery is performed*
- *a fetal blood sample has been taken in labour*
- *birth, if the baby's condition is poor.'*

(NICE, 2001, p. 8)

This means that cord blood analysis is becoming a routine investigation following any kind of complicated birth and in some units after every birth (Shallow, 2003, p. 28).

The measurement of the acid–base status of a baby around the time of birth is considered to be an objective observation of the fetal response to labour. In other words, we can tell by interpreting a set of numerical results how a baby has coped with the relatively hypoxic environment which prevails during labour (cord blood sampling) or how a baby is coping during labour (fetal blood sampling). We can also use this information to predict what may happen to a baby in the future.

Prior to the availability of this test, the Apgar score has been the only scoring system used. It is based on observation of the newborn baby and is felt to be both subjective and prone to inter-observer variation (Clark & Hakanson, 1998, p. 203).

The Apgar score will continue to be used because it has become so ingrained in our practice, and certain elements of it are crucial in our assessment of a baby's need for resuscitation. However, cord blood analysis adds another dimension to our knowledge: numerical data.

The results of cord blood analysis are particularly significant in litigation cases because they are felt to be more objective.

It provides objective information which is a useful adjunct to subjective methods of assessment of newborn babies and enables a group of neonates at risk of morbidity to be identified.
(Harris et al., 1996, p. 149)

Physiology

OK, back to chemistry lessons now!

- The more hydrogen ions (H^+) there are in a solution, the more acidic it is.
- On the pH scale, 7 is neutral and is the pH of water.
- In the human body the normal pH is 7.35–7.45 (a slightly alkaline environment).
- If the pH of the blood is below 7.35, the person is considered to be acidemic.
- If it is above 7.45, the person is alkalemic.

Now on to the baby:

Respiration. In the uterine world the baby uses the placenta rather than its lungs for receiving oxygen and getting rid of carbon dioxide. Blood that is rich in oxygen travels along the umbilical vein from the placenta to the baby. Blood with a higher carbon dioxide content travels from the baby to the placenta via the two umbilical arteries. Carbon dioxide is an acidic substance so the blood in the umbilical arteries will have a lower pH than that in the umbilical vein.

Energy production. The other basic process that is going on is the production of energy. This is achieved by a process called aerobic metabolism. This requires adequate supplies of oxygen and glucose, and the waste product of the process is carbon dioxide. (Think of 'air-obic' to help you remember the normal process!)

Homeostasis. The final physiological process that is relevant here is homeostasis or keeping a balance. Both the respiratory process and the metabolic process produce acid waste that will cause the pH of the blood to fall and become more acidic. The body has a number of ways of keeping the blood pH stable. One of the substances which helps to 'buffer' or neutralize this acid is bicarbonate. Buffering substances are also known as 'bases' and the normal ratio of base to acid is 20:1 (Simpson & Popat, 2002, p. 31). This means that there are plenty of reserves within the body to cope with excess acid. Other bodily systems such as excretion by the kidneys and normal respiration also help to maintain the balance. (For a more detailed explanation of the physiology, please refer to Askin, 1997.)

From these three basic processes we gather information, which forms the results of a cord blood analysis (Table 5.6.1).

During labour we understand that the contraction of the uterine muscle reduces the flow of blood to and from the placenta. This means that the flow of oxygen and glucose from mother to baby is reduced and that waste products such as carbon dioxide cannot escape. This reduction in blood flow occurs for about 50–70 seconds (Harris et al., 1996, p. 147) and then, as the muscle relaxes, the normal chemical balance is restored. This

Table 5.6.1

pH	How acid/alkali the blood is
pCO_2	How much carbon dioxide is in the blood
pO_2	How much oxygen is in the blood
Standard bicarbonate, HCO_3	How much bicarbonate or base is in the blood
Base deficit/base excess	The buffering ability of the blood (explained in more detail later)

means that the gaps between contractions are very important to the baby's well-being and homeostasis. A healthy, well-grown baby is able to cope with increasing length and strength of contractions.

There are other events, which sometimes occur due to intervention or spontaneously, which can further reduce the amount of oxygen reaching the baby. These are things like hypercontractility of the uterus when using syntocinon, maternal hypotension secondary to epidural analgesia, cord prolapse, placental abruption, bleeding placenta praevia, cord occlusion, and also a baby who has intrauterine growth retardation, who will not have the same resources to cope with even normal labour stresses.

The baby in these circumstances will work hard to compensate for the lack of oxygen and glucose coming in and the increasing amounts of carbon dioxide that cannot escape.

- Its condition will gradually deteriorate if oxygen supply is not restored.
- The baby retains carbon dioxide, which will make the blood more acidic and lower the pH.
- This initial response is called *respiratory acidosis*, because it is primarily caused by failure of respiration.

If the oxygen supply to the baby is not restored then it will become increasingly acidotic as carbon dioxide is retained. (Remember the oxygen supply can be restored by delivering the baby and assisting with respiration if necessary or by restoring the placental perfusion.)

- The baby will also begin to use *anaerobic metabolism* to provide energy. This is a way of producing energy without oxygen.
- The baby will use stores of glycogen from the heart muscle, liver and other muscles to produce energy.
- The waste product of this process is lactic acid.
- The accumulation of this acid will produce a *metabolic acidosis*.

So, acidosis can have a respiratory part caused by excess carbon dioxide and a metabolic part caused by the accumulation of lactic acid. Measuring pH alone can tell us that a baby is acidotic and struggling to maintain optimal blood chemistry. But what we need to know in addition is how much of the acid is being produced by respiratory acidosis and how much by metabolic acidosis, because this will give us some idea of how long the baby has been lacking oxygen.

This is where we have to look at the phrases 'base deficit' and 'base excess'.

We know that base also means alkali and that it is present in the blood at a ratio of 20 (base):1 (acid); in other words, there is plenty of it to mop up any excess acid. Think of base as a receptor for hydrogen ions and acid as a donator of hydrogen ions. As the base receptors become full there is less base available to mop up excess hydrogen ions. Bicarbonate is an important base substance and it is measured as part of cord blood analysis.

A final calculation that is made as part of the analysis is that of base deficit of the extracellular fluid (BDecf). The calculation is made using the pH level and the accumulated CO_2 level. It is important to note that the deficit is calculated using fetal/neonatal values and taking the larger extravascular fluid compartment into account, otherwise there will be an overestimation of the metabolic component of the acidaemia (Harris et al., 1996, p. 147). The BDecf value tells us how much base it would take to get the blood back to a normal pH when respiratory factors are taken out of the equation (Barrett, 2003, p. 5). So, the higher the result the more base is required, which means that the baby has used up lots of base to correct any acidosis.

BDecf values of greater than 12mmol/l with a pH of 7.05 or lower are currently felt to be suggestive of adverse outcomes for the neonate.
(NICE, 2001, p. 79)

In order to understand why the base excess/deficit result can tell us about the metabolic component of acidosis, we have to note that during the calculation the respiratory factors are removed, which leaves only the metabolic component of the acidosis. As the BDecf level rises, it indicates that the baby is using anaerobic metabolism more, which really means there is less and less oxygen around in the baby's system.

Some blood gas analysers give the result of this calculation as base excess (BE), and you can see from the normal values given below that there generally isn't much excess; in fact, the BE levels are minus values. If the result is given as a BE then the greater the number behind the minus sign the more acidotic the baby is.

Now we need to look at how to interpret the results we see in practice.

A normal healthy baby's results are given in Tables 5.6.2 and 5.6.3.

From this we can see that the pH is lower in the artery measurement and the pCO_2 is higher, which we would expect in blood returning from the baby to the placenta. We can also see that the base deficit value is low in both samples, which means that not much base is required to balance the biochemical picture.

It is worth noting here that it is difficult to find any consensual statement in the literature about normal or abnormal values. Loh et al. (1998, p. 150), Wallman (1997, p. 73) and Westgate et al. (1994, p. 1054) all acknowledge the lack of consensus, and Shallow (2003, p. 31) uses this inconsistency to argue against this test becoming routine.

Having looked at the physiology and the normal picture, we can now look at some abnormal results and interpret what they might mean.

A set from fetal blood sampling performed because of reduced variability, shallow early decelerations and a raise in baseline rate is shown in Table 5.6.4.

We have to assume that if the sample is taken from the baby's scalp it is venous blood. We can see that in the 35 minutes between samples the biochemical picture has improved. Whilst the pH has remained stable, indicating no deterioration in the acid status, the oxygen

Table 5.6.2 Arterial cord blood sample

pH	7.27–7.28
pCO_2 (mmHg)	49.2–50.3 (6.56–6.71 kPa)
BE (mmol/l)	–2.7 to –3.6
BDecf (mmol/l)	2.4 (Westgate et al., 1994, p. 1059)
Standard bicarbonate (mmol/l)	22.0–23.1

Table 5.6.3 Venous cord blood sample

pH	7.34–7.35
pCO_2 (mmHg)	38.2–40.7 (5.09–5.43 kPa)
Base excess (mmol/l)	–2.4
BDecf (mmol/l)	3.0 (Westgate et al., 1994, p. 1059)
Standard bicarbonate (mmol/l)	20.4–21.4

Source: Wallman (1997, p. 74).

Table 5.6.4

	Time	
	15:25	16:00
pH	7.2	7.2
pCO_2 (kPa)	7.23	6.8
pO_2 (kPa)	1.7	1.85
Base excess (mmol/l)	–8.8	–8.51

level has increased, the CO_2 level has decreased and the base excess has increased by 0.3, which means there must be less acid around in the blood.

This is a reassuring finding, and this is reflected in the outcome; an emergency section was considered before the first sample, and after the second sample the woman had a vaginal birth of a baby who had a cord pH of 7.23 and a base excess of –9.3 mmol/l.

We now need to look at some more serious results, which indicate respiratory and metabolic acidosis (Table 5.6.5):

- In respiratory acidosis there is a low pH, high pCO_2, normal BDecf.
- In metabolic acidosis there is low pH, normal to high pCO_2, high BDecf.

These results show a pH value which indicates acidosis at a concerning level. The pCO_2 levels are high, indicating an element of respiratory acidosis. The base deficit is raised, but not as high as the adverse outcome level previously suggested. Westgate et al. (1994, p. 1059) suggest that a BDecf of less than 10 mmol/l is generally associated with respiratory acidosis and anything higher indicates a metabolic component. So, there is some respiratory but probably no metabolic element.

This baby was born by emergency lower segment caesarean section because of placental abruption; the CTG showed a bradycardia and poor baseline variability. The baby's Apgar scores were 9 at one and five minutes.

The results in Table 5.6.6 show a pH value which indicates acidosis at a concerning level. The pCO_2 levels are very high, indicating respiratory acidosis. The BDecf levels are much higher than the adverse outcome level previously suggested. There is respiratory and metabolic acidosis at a level that would suggest an adverse outcome.

This baby was delivered by ventouse following an augmented labour in a woman who had had a previous caesarean section. There was a prolonged bradycardia noted on the CTG, which prompted the assisted birth.

The baby's Apgar scores were 0 at one minute and 2 at five minutes. This baby died when it was 99 days old.

The literature that I have looked at has revealed several other important points for practice:

- Both arterial and venous samples must be taken and verified (this means that the minimum difference in pH seen between the two samples should be 0.02, but there is no consensus on this). This is because arterial cord blood reflects fetal acid–base status and venous cord blood reflects a combination of maternal acid–base status and placental function. On its own, either result could give us a false impression of the baby's well-being (for a good example, see Westgate et al., 1994, p. 1059).
- A large arterial-venous BDecf difference is usually the result of cord entanglement or stasis of umbilical cord flow (Westgate et al., 1994, p. 1059).
- A pH fall from 7.1 to 7.0 is much more significant than a fall from 7.3 to 7.2. This is because the relationship between pH and hydrogen ions is logarithmic, not linear. A 0.1 unit decrease in pH from 7.3 to 7.2 is associated with a rise in hydrogen ions of 13 nmol/l, but a similar fall from 7.0 to 6.9 means a rise in hydrogen ions of 26 nmol/l (Westgate et al., 1994, p. 1062).
- There is not a linear relationship between pH and Apgar scores. Because a healthy baby can compensate for hypoxia it is possible to have a low scalp pH and then be awarded a high Apgar score at birth.

At the beginning of this article we talked about cord blood analysis giving us objective information. By looking at the underlying physiology and discussing the interpretation of results, we can see that the numerical data is just one part of the information that we need to provide a complete picture of the baby's condition at birth. The other observations that we make of the mother's well-being and the baby's behaviour during labour and at the time of birth are just as important in helping us to make sense of the results.

Table 5.6.5 Example 1 (taken from Loh et al., 1998, p. 152)

	Arterial result	Venous result
pH	6.983	7.034
pCO_2	94.5	81.5
BDecf	7.7	6.6

Table 5.6.6 Example 2 (taken from Loh et al., 1998, p. 152)

	Arterial result	Venous result
pH	6.688	6.71
pCO_2	121.6	116.2
BDecf	24.6	24.0

REFERENCES

Askin DF. 1997. Interpretation of neonatal blood gases, Part 1: Physiology and acid–base homeostasis. Neonatal Network, 16(5): 17–21

Barrett DH. 2003. Acid–base balance and interpretation of blood gas results. World Anaesthesia, Issue 16; www.nda.ox.ac.uk/wfsa/html/u16/u1602_01.htm accessed 25 September 2005

Clark DA, Hakanson DO. 1998. The inaccuracy of Apgar scoring. Journal of Perinatology, 8: 203–205

Harris M, Beckley SL, Garibaldi JM, Keith RDF, Greene KR. 1996. Umbilical cord blood gas analysis at the time of delivery. Midwifery, 12: 146–150

Loh SF, Woodworth A, Yeo GSH. 1998. Umbilical cord blood gas analysis at delivery. Singapore Medical Journal, 39(4): 151–155; www.sma.org.sg accessed 22 September 2005

NICE. 2001. The Use of Electronic Fetal Monitoring, p. 8. RCOG, London

Shallow H. 2003. Should cord pH be performed routinely after normal birth? Midwives, 6(1): 28–31

Simpson PJ, Popat M. 2002. Understanding Anesthesia, 4th edn, p. 31. Butterworth-Heinemann, Oxford

Wallman CM. 1997. Interpretation of fetal cord blood gases. Neonatal Network, 16(1): 72–75

Westgate JA, Garibaldi JM, Greene KR. 1994. Umbilical cord blood gas analysis at delivery: a time for quality data. British Journal of Obstetrics and Gynaecology, 101: 1054–1063

5.7

Don't take it lying down!
The NCT calls on UK midwives to help mums get active

Gillian Fletcher

As President of the NCT I have recently attended numerous childbirth conferences and also a number of different committee or working group meetings based at the RCM or RCOG. I have been struck by one strong, common theme coming through them all. Real concern is being expressed about the continued erosion of normality in childbirth. There is concern about the barriers many midwives face in supporting and empowering women in units where a mechanised and medical approach to labour predominates. Debate often centres on what we mean by the term 'normal'. The goalposts seem to have shifted over recent years so that normal now seems to mean what is 'usual' or common practice, and is likely to include different interventions such as ARM and augmentation rather than what is physiological and without intervention.

In their article 'Has the medicalisation of childbirth gone too far', Johanson et al. (2002) explore many of the factors that influence midwives' practice and those that are more likely to enhance a woman's ability to achieve a straightforward vaginal delivery. They highlight research which shows the importance of health professionals' attitudes. It seems that units which develop a culture of pride in low intervention rates and birth as a normal physiological process have more normal births. Other factors like good midwifery and medical leadership and teamwork also seem to be key.

In September 2002 the NCT launched a 'Don't take it lying down' campaign, providing information through the press about the value of keeping mobile in labour and finding upright positions. We invited maternity units to display the new NCT labour positions posters as a way of encouraging more women to be active in the first and second stages of labour. The posters aim to encourage positions for the actual birth that work with the body's own mechanisms for ensuring a straightforward birth. In a poll of NCT members we asked women to tell us what position they had given

birth in. We found that more than one-third (40%) had not been encouraged to have an active birth and had found themselves propped up on the bed in a semi-reclining position.

These findings reflect those of the Audit Commission (1997), in which many women remarked that they were unable to move around and choose the position that made them feel most comfortable.

Of course, many thousands of babies have been born successfully in this semi-recumbent position over the years and, yet, with what consequences?

We know that with the mother in a semi-sitting position, the coccyx will be compressed. This reduces the helpful effects of relaxin on the ligaments that enable the pelvis to move and open to accommodate the baby as he/she descends. The MIDIRS Informed Choice leaflet (1999) documents the many advantages of upright postures in labour and reflects women's feelings about positions for birth. Most women who gave birth lying down preferred a different position for their next birth, while those who had been upright wished to remain so next time.

In antenatal classes, when exploring the stages of labour with expectant parents, I often ask them to draw a diagram of the position they think they might be in at the actual moment of birth. I suggest that they use stick figures to depict the woman, her partner, the midwife and anyone else they expect to be in the room. We then discuss their suggested positions and where these perceptions of birthing positions come from. The influence of TV, books and magazines is very strong and many people will draw the woman in the 'traditional', semi-recumbent, propped up on the bed position, although an equal number will usually suggest that they would like to try a more upright position, such as kneeling over the back of the bed.

Using these diagrams as a trigger for discussion we can then explore the pros and cons of each position in terms of comfort, the effort required to adopt and maintain the position, and the potential effect on the pelvis and progress of labour. We also discuss the likelihood of being able to implement your choice when in labour. What impact might feeling stressed in a strange, uncomfortable and unfamiliar environment have on your behaviour? What additional effect might be added if you are with people you don't know? In practice, it seems that many women giving birth in a hospital maternity unit do not feel able to adopt positions that are not the norm within the unit's culture and environment.

At a recent meeting of the steering group for the RCM's Virtual Institute for Normal Birth, a lecturer in midwifery talked about how difficult it is for some student midwives to implement practices that promote normality, as taught in the classroom, when they arrive on a 'high-tech' maternity unit. How easy it is to feel disempowered when faced with an NHS culture of fear and blame, and one that is dominated by risk management. I was very struck by the similarity to the barriers that face couples trying to make choices in an environment where they feel disempowered.

So what could midwives do to bring about a change?

The NCT would like to see positions posters displayed in all labour and delivery rooms, so that on arrival in the room expectant parents get the positive message that active positions are understood and valued here. Even if the room seems alien and they do not know the midwife caring for them, we hope this will enable more women to avoid falling into 'passive hospital patient mode', labouring on the bed with their mobility restricted by an electronic fetal monitor. Thankfully, implementation of the NICE guidelines on electronic fetal monitoring means that routine admission traces are being used much less frequently. Intermittent auscultation should be offered and recommended to healthy women with a normal pregnancy.

We would like to see expectant couples encouraged in antenatal classes to try out the different positions and weigh up the pros and cons of each for themselves. The NCT has produced laminated cards of each position and in my classes I use post-it notes on the back of each card so that couples can jot down the advantages and disadvantages of each position they try and then discuss them with other couples when swapping cards to try out a different position.

By actively engaging them in this way the woman is far more likely to adopt different positions during labour, especially if reinforced by the policy, practice and supportive attitudes of the midwives they encounter on the labour ward.

The way midwives talk to women can either convey the message that moving the bed and using beanbags or a birth ball to make the space more comfortable for them is expected. Or it can suggest that it would be unusual, awkward or difficult to do these things in this unit.

At the recent Antenatal Education Conference, a midwife from the Birmingham Women's Hospital outlined the format of their innovative Birth Ideas workshops, which replace the traditional labour ward tour. These workshops enable expectant couples to familiarise themselves with the delivery rooms and explore, with the midwife, how they might move the furniture and try out different positions for an active labour in the real setting.

Walsh (1999) demonstrated how combining evidence with audit was successful in bringing about a change in midwifery practice. The project, based in a large consultant unit in Leicester, increased the number of women adopting off-the-bed positions for childbirth from 18% in 1996 to 43% in 1998. They selected four areas of practice where strong evidence about clinical efficacy existed, such as EFM and positions for childbirth, and used a variety of different strategies to encourage changes in practice. Is there regular audit of the positions that women are labouring and giving birth in, in your unit? Has there been a change of practice regarding routine admission traces?

Midwives can increase the number of normal births by empowering women to choose upright positions and mobility in labour. The NCT has produced some tools for you to use and the response from many midwives has been very positive, so now it's over to you.

REFERENCES

Audit Commission. 1997. Improving Maternity Services in England and Wales. Audit Commission, London

Johanson R, Newburn M, Macfarlane A. 2002. Has the medicalisation of childbirth gone too far? BMJ, 324(7342): 892–895

MIDIRS. 1999. Positions in Labour and Delivery. MIDIRS, Bristol

Walsh D. 1999. Changing midwifery birthing practice through audit. British Journal of Midwifery, 7(7): 432–435

The Practising Midwife 2003; 6(2): 14–15

Going backwards: the concept of 'pasmo'

Ina May Gaskin

I learned a new Spanish word while lecturing in New York City on a book promotion tour during the spring of 2003. The Puerto Rican nurse who explained it to me said that in the countryside where she grew up it is used like this:

One woman might say: 'I heard that your sister was in labour. Has she had the baby yet?' She might get this answer: 'She went to the hospital, but when she got there, she went into pasmo and they sent her home.'

'Pasmo' is a word with no English equivalent. It means the reversal of labour once it has already started. It may mean that uterine contractions, once started, come to a stop, and sometimes it is characterised by a significant reduction in cervical dilatation. Assuming that this uterine capability is real, we might be justified in asking why no word for the arrest or reversal of labour exists in everyday English. I don't know that we'll find any answers.

In US English medical language, though, there are some words or phrases that describe this phenomenon, but these aren't in everyday use among women. For instance, we have 'uterine dysfunction' and 'uterine inertia' – both terms that point to a supposed defect in the uterus. Nowadays, once this diagnosis is made after a labour has begun or a woman has been admitted to hospital, several courses of action are common. They include amniotomy, induction or augmentation of labour, or caesarean section. In times past, women whose labours stopped or slowed significantly after admission were sent home or advised to walk the halls of the labour ward in an attempt to stimulate stronger contractions. Now, elective induction is considered acceptable in a majority of US hospitals. Elective caesarean, too, has gained acceptance in a growing number, despite the clear evidence pointing to an elevation of risk in terms of maternal morbidity and mortality.

I was fascinated to know that the concept of pasmo has survived in Puerto Rican culture, even though more than 99% of women there give birth in hospital – approximately the same percentage as in the USA. However, the phenomenon that it describes exists wherever there are childbearing women.

An experience of 'pasmo'

I first became aware of the phenomenon of pasmo in 1973 – my third year of attending births – while attending a friend's first labour. Her cervix dilated to 8 cm in just a few hours. At this point, though, her manner changed noticeably. Whereas before she had been light-hearted, laughing and joking with her partner, my assistant and me, her emotional state changed considerably as she approached transition. No longer did she laugh, and she seemed afraid even to clear her throat in her usual manner. Because her uterine contractions had greatly lessened in their intensity and I was scheduled to leave on a bus trip within a few hours, I asked her if I could do a vaginal exam. She gave her consent. I was astounded to find that her cervical dilation was now only 4 cm. I was certain that I had correctly assessed her dilation at 8 cm only 20 minutes or so earlier, so I guessed that it might be a good idea for her to reactivate her sense of humour during the next few contractions, in hopes that her cervix might reopen. 'Laugh at our jokes like you did before,' I suggested. 'It just might work.' And it did. Her baby was born within two hours.

That experience sent me to the medical library for a deeper search about the (to me) unusual phenomenon I had just observed. Never before had I observed any reduction in cervical dilatation in a particular woman. I had observed stalled labours that were resolved by mere words and described these in my first book, *Spiritual Midwifery*, but I had never before observed someone going backwards in labour.

I hadn't spent very long reading in the medical library before I saw that I was not going to find any mention of pasmo or anything like it in a midwifery or medical textbook in English. And yet I knew that my friend's cervix closed from 8 to 4 cm without her even moving her body in any significant or visible way besides a change in facial expression.

The medical viewpoint

During this same period, I occasionally lectured to groups of US midwives, nurses or physicians, and I asked them if they had ever observed the reversal of cervical dilation in a labouring woman. All of the midwives and nurses had. I soon learned from them that this phenomenon probably took place more often in their hospital-based practices than my partners and I saw in our home birth practice. But I met no physicians who were aware of the capacity to reverse labour. When I asked nurses and midwives about this difference, I was told that whenever they documented a lesser dilation on a woman's chart, they were told they had made a mistake. I realised that physicians and medical students almost never have the chance to observe women's labours from start to finish, so it became obvious to me that they were not in a good position to know about the true physical capacities of women in labour. They were actually far less qualified to comment on the behaviour of women in labour than the lower-ranking professionals, whether midwives or nurses, who spent more time in the labouring woman's presence than they did.

I knew then that the lack of mention of pasmo in labour has much to do with the nature of medical hierarchy. Physicians outrank midwives and nurses in status and in income, and this higher status gives their perceptions of labour phenomena a higher value when it comes to formulating the accepted knowledge of how women's bodies work than the observations made by midwives.

A historical perspective

My documentation of a case of labour reversal in *Spiritual Midwifery* more than 25 years ago has made no difference in this state of medical and midwifery knowledge. As far as the textbooks are concerned, human females lack the capacity to close their cervices during labour. If such a thing happens, the assumption is that the uterus itself is defective, and medical intervention is warranted.

But my research at the medical library did yield some interesting information and evidence having relevance to the pasmo phenomenon. In the library's rare books collection, I found the following excerpts in medical textbooks published between 1837 and 1901:

... it is to be understood, the fact of there being a continuance of regular pains, for it sometimes happens that, *after regular pains have commenced, the agitation of the patient, or the mismanagement of the attendants, occasions a suspension of some hours.*
(Hamilton's Practical Observations, 1837)

As soon as you arrive, let the husband, or some familiar friend, inform the lady, and then you should remain in the ante-chamber till she requests your presence. A sudden surprise, especially if attended with the fear of severe treatment, will greatly retard the process, and, in many cases, cause the foetus to retract. When you enter the room, let your mind be calm and collected, and your feelings kindly sympathize with those of the patient.
(Curtis, Lectures on Midwifery, 1846)

In 1792, I was called to attend a Mrs C, in consequence of her midwife being engaged. As I approached the house, I was most earnestly solicited to hasten in, as not a moment was to be lost. I was suddenly shown into Mrs C's chamber, and my appearance there was explained by stating that her midwife was engaged. As I entered the room, Mrs C was just recovering from a pain – and it was the last she had at that time. After waiting an hour in the expectation of a return of labour, I took my leave, and was not again summoned to her for precisely two weeks. And Dr Lyall says, 'We have been informed by a respectable practitioner of a labour that had nearly arrived at its apparent termination, suspended for more than two days, in consequence of a gentleman having been sent to the patient, against whom she had taken a prejudice.' Every accoucheur has experienced a temporary suspension of pain upon his first appearance in the sick chamber; but so long a period as two weeks is very rare.
(Dewees' System of Midwifery, 1847)

Uterine action, and therefore labour-pains, may be suspended or removed by many causes ... The disappointment occasioned by a stranger entering the room when the patient expected her own attendant has been known to stop a labour, in the midst of its most active operation, and to suspend it for many hours. It is principally on this account that we are careful to prevent a woman in labour becoming suddenly acquainted with any news that is likely to shock her.

... On arriving at the patient's residence it is better not abruptly to obtrude one's-self into her presence, unless there be some immediate necessity for our attendance. Information should be sought from the nurse, on such points as will enable us to judge whether labour has actually commenced. On being ushered into her chamber, we may engage her in some general conversation, which will give us an opportunity of observing the frequency, duration, strength, and character of the pains; and our conduct must be framed accordingly.
(Ramsbotham, The Principles and Practice of Obstetric Medicine and Surgery, 1861)

Cazeaux also had much to say on the subject in his well-known text published in 1884:

I am well aware that books furnish some cases of women who had the power of suspending the contractions at will; but if the facts have even been well observed, they have failed perhaps to receive the most rational interpretation. In the cases related by Baudelocque and Velpeau, in which the labour ceased when the students were summoned to witness it and began again when these numerous observers retired, the will had probably less to do than the imagination and modesty, with the alternations of retardation and acceleration; for though the influence of the will may be reasonably doubled, it cannot be denied that moral disturbances appear to affect the contractility of the uterus; thus, a violent emotion has often sufficed to arouse it long before the ordinary term of gestation, and it is not at all uncommon for the contraction to diminish or disappear for several hours, or even days, under the operation of such causes. [Cazeaux then quotes Betschler, who cited a case 'in which the pains were suddenly suspended by a violent tempest, so that the neck, though widely dilated, closed again, nor did the labour recommence until nineteen days had elapsed.']

Every day, indeed, we witness a suspension of the pains for half an hour, and sometimes even for several hours, upon visiting women whose modesty is shocked by our presence. The exercise of this function is seldom of long duration, lasting for a few seconds only – rarely beyond one or two minutes, and then the organ which was so strongly contracted and hardened gradually regains its primitive state, and remains in repose, until, under the influence of the same stimulus, it is again thrown into action. The organic contractility, like all muscular power, is expended by a prolonged exercise, and hence we can understand why the pains so often become at once more slow and feeble or even cease altogether after a prolonged labour.

Any vivid moral impressions operating during the labour, any unexpected news or sharp discussions, the announcement of a child of an unwished-for sex, and the arrival or presence of persons disagreeable to the lying-in woman, may determine a cessation of the pains; and in these cases the removal of the cause is the only remedy. But, unfortunately, it is not always an easy matter to ascertain what that cause may be.

On arriving at the house the practitioner should have his visit announced to the patient, and he will very often find that the first effect of his presence is to arrest the pains that have been hitherto progressing rapidly, thereby affording a very conclusive proof of the influence of mental impressions on the progress of labour. If the pains be not already propulsive, it is well that he should occupy himself at first in general inquiries from the [female] attendants as to the progress of labour, and in seeing that all the necessary arrangements are satisfactorily carried out, so as to allow the patient time to get accustomed to his presence.

(Playfair's System of Midwifery, 1889)

Just so long as there is no evidence of maternal or foetal exhaustion, and just so long as the clinical course of labor is proceeding after the normal fashion, the physician's policy is a waiting one, and his immediate attendance is not requisite; on the contrary, his presence in the lying-in room simply excites the anxiety of the woman.

(Grandin & Jarman, Pregnancy, Labor, and the Puerperal State, 1895)

On The 'Pains' or Uterine Contractions … Mental emotion of any kind will temporarily diminish their intensity or even absolutely suppress them; the entrance of the physician into the lying-in room may have the same effect.

(Dorland, Modern Obstetrics, 1901)

Taken together, the above excerpts constitute strong evidence that until relatively recently there was an operating consensus that women's labours could be stopped or slowed down by the mere presence of a strange male – the doctor himself (doctors a century ago were virtually always male). In fact, in textbooks published previous to the time when institutionalisation became the norm for childbirth, virtually all texts contained some mention of the sensitivity of labouring women and the need to avoid upsetting them if labour was to continue its normal course.

We know that throughout the world, since time immemorial, when women have given birth they have most often been assisted by other women. While in some societies, husbands traditionally assisted the birth of their children, in most, men have been excluded from participating in birth except in extraordinary circumstances. Up until the beginning of the 20th century, the birth room was still the domain of the labouring mother and her female attendants. These most likely included her mother, her sisters, her cousins or close friends.

'Pasmo' in the animal kingdom

Now, let's consider for a minute the behaviour during labour of mammals other than us humans. Is the phenomenon of pasmo unknown to them? Of course not. One has only to watch film or video of wildlife to know that gazelles, giraffes, antelopes and wildebeest, among others, all have the ability, given the sudden presence of a predator, to discontinue labour and suck the fetus back inside their wombs, even when birth is imminent. Those who raise animals know that various species share something in common: labour at term is most likely to take place when the pregnant female has maximum privacy. Farm animals may be shocked out of labour by the sudden presence of a stranger or predator. Such behaviour is well known to anyone who has any familiarity with the reproductive lives of animals. Considering this, how likely is it that the human female would be the only mammal to lack the capacity to reverse labour once it is well established?

In the USA and the UK, as well as in many other countries around the world, caesarean section rates are rising. Some of this rise can surely be attributed to the fact that maternity ward policy at many hospitals is more likely now than formerly to call for induction or augmentation in case of pasmo than to send a woman home to await the eventual onset of labour. The higher incidence of caesarean section after a failed induction or augmentation of labour is well documented.

How would hospitals and maternity clinics differ if the true physiology of labouring women were understood and taken into account? I believe that they would be organised in much the way that Michel Odent

outlined in his early book *Birth Reborn*. Women would give birth in quiet, dimly lit rooms furnished simply with mats on the floor and a good-sized tub of water. There might be ropes or ladders attached to the wall for the labouring woman to pull on. And if there is a double bed in the room, it is a double bed large enough to accommodate her partner. If a caregiver who has not been in the room needs to check on the woman's progress, she or he would knock on the door and enter quietly enough not to destroy the mood and the atmosphere in the room. What I have described is the best way to reduce the occurrence of pasmo in modern, high-tech hospitals. I am sure that redesigning hospital maternity wards and altering maternity care policies with the goal of preventing pasmo would significantly lower current rates of unnecessary caesarean section for 'failed' labour. How good it would be to see hospitals do this during my lifetime.

REFERENCES

Cazeaux P. 1884. Obstetrics in Theory and Practice: Including the Diseases of Pregnancy and Parturition, Obstetrical Operations, Etc. P Blackiston, Philadelphia

Curtis A. 1846. Lectures on Midwifery and the Forms of Disease Peculiar to Women and Children Delivered to the Members of the Botanico-Medical College of the State of Ohio. C. Nagle Cincinnati, OH

Dewees WP. 1847. A Compendious System of Midwifery. Lea & Blanchard, Philadelphia

Dorland WAN. 1901. Modern Obstetrics: General and Operative. WB Saunders, Philadelphia

Gaskin IM. 2002. Spiritual Midwifery, 4th edn. The Book Publishing Company, Summertown, TN

Grandin E, Jarman G. 1895. Pregnancy, Labor, and the Puerperal State. FA Davis, Philadelphia

Hamilton J. 1837. Hamilton's Practical Observations on Various Subjects Relating to Midwifery. A Waldie The Dunglison's American Medical Library, Philadelphia

Odent M. 1984. Birth Reborn. Pantheon Books, New York

Playfair WS. 1889. A Treatise on the Science and Practice of Midwifery. Lea Brothers & Co, Philadelphia

Ramsbotham, FH. 1861. The Principles and Practice of Obstetric Medicine and Surgery in Reference to the Process of Parturition, 3rd edn. Lea & Blanchard, Philadelphia

The Practising Midwife 2003; 6(8): 34–37

Where might we go from here?

Although little has been written about the concept of 'pasmo', it is something that I suspect a significant number of midwives will have experience of – which is precisely why this was chosen as the question to which we are inviting responses. The questions to which we are inviting responses include:

- Is this something you have seen or experienced, either personally or through hearing about the experience of another midwife?
- If so, what was the situation, and what happened?
- Have you noticed anything which has led you to think about why this might happen, or what might be going on?
- Is there anything else that you could say about this phenomenon which has not been discussed in the article from your own experience (either as a midwife or a birthing woman)?

We look forward to hearing from you! Please feel free to add anything else that seems relevant but which hasn't been asked here!

Focus on...
Birth Centres

SECTION CONTENTS

A 'cycle of empowerment': the enabling culture of birth centres

Mavis Kirkham

Birth centres are important for midwives because they can provide a focus for a social rather than medical model of maternity care. Home births also use this model but they are, by their very nature, private. Birth centres, on the other hand, are clearly identified as places where the complex skills and supportive relationships underpinning normal birth can be developed, nurtured and learned. Their importance as centres offering an alternative to the mainstream medical model explains both why they matter and why they are often threatened.

Birth centres vary greatly, and some call themselves by different titles. Yet underlying beliefs recur: women as active in birth; care adapted to women and families; and the importance of relationships, trust and a nurturing environment, all on a scale where individuals matter and relationships can be developed. The small scale and separate identity of birth centres are important. It is probably true to say that, where separation from a consultant unit is chosen rather than determined by geography, this is to protect the small, safe space within which a philosophy – very different from that of a consultant unit – is held in common by staff and clients.

Effective care

Clinical effectiveness

A number of studies have demonstrated that, when evaluated against obstetric outcomes of safety, births for low-risk women are as safe in small, low-risk maternity units as in hospitals.

Economic effectiveness

There is no economic evidence to support the centralisation of maternity services. Surveying the economic evidence, Campbell and Macfarlane (1994, pp. 113–114) concluded:

The continuing closure of small units and centralisation of maternity care are not based on good evidence ... [and] may simply represent a transfer of costs between sectors of the economy, in particular from NHS to individual families or to social services and social security. Districts may lose unmeasured resources, as voluntary support for community hospitals may not be transferred to the district hospital on closure of the small units.

Satisfaction

Birth centre care is linked with high satisfaction. This was evident with regard to maternal satisfaction in Edgware and Stockholm birth centres (Boulton et al., 2003; Waldenström, 2003). It is noteworthy that satisfaction is also reported by socially marginalised women from several cultures (Esposito, 1999). Fathers expressed satisfaction with the support and respect which they received in the Stockholm birth centre (Waldenström, 1999, 2003), reflecting the focus of birth centre care on the family rather than only the birth.

Being treated with respect is a theme that recurs in evaluations of birth centre care, particularly with regard to groups who often do not report such treatment. Such respectful care is intended to be a powerful educational experience for women:

When all women are treated with this degree of care, their confidence in every aspect of their lives will grow, and they in turn will treat others, including their babies, with equal care.
Midwife owner of a Japanese birth centre (Turner, 2002, p. 35)

Midwives too report satisfaction with working in birth centres (e.g. Saunders et al., 2000) despite, or perhaps because of, the difference from working in a hospital and the greater responsibility.

When new birth centres are opened, users of the service are likely to be a special group. Such women were described in the Edgware evaluation as 'clinically and self-selected for non-intervention in pregnancy' and in the birth centre 'their own aspirations for natural childbirth were supported by the midwives' (Boulton et al., 2003).

Over time, the availability of birth centre care changes local expectations. Once women have friends or neighbours who have delivered in a birth centre and are satisfied with their care, more women consider this option. Established birth centres are accepted as a local option for childbirth (Esposito, 1999), or the only option for those who wish to give birth locally in some rural areas.

New birth centres similarly attract a special group of midwives. In hospital maternity care, midwives are subject to considerable pressures to conform, which are often reinforced by hierarchical disapproval or 'horizontal violence': bullying by one's peers (Kirkham, 1999; Kirkham & Stapleton, 2001). Such a culture can stifle creativity and clinical judgement. It is therefore not surprising that when the Edgware birth centre was set up it was not able to recruit midwives locally, even with the job security of secondment, yet national advertisement brought a flood of applicants willing to relocate for jobs with short-term contracts. The midwives recruited 'share a common philosophy of midwifery care and an enthusiasm for putting it into practice. In their commitment to the birth centre, they have forged a dedicated and cohesive team. It is the philosophy they share and the commitment they have made to it that define the character of the birth centre and evoke the praise and loyalty of their clients' (Saunders et al., 2000, p. 74).

Relationships

The small scale of a birth centre has a real influence on the relationships within it. This is especially true of the relationships between midwives and women. The opportunity to develop relationships with women changes the midwife's professional allegiances (Brodie, 1996a, b; Coyle et al., 2001). It can allow a shift in power from the professional toward the woman.

The philosophy and the small scale of birth centres make it possible to develop relationships between midwives that are supportive and foster growth.

The women and midwives who chose birth centres have common aims and grow in confidence and skill as trust develops between them. As Jones (2000) notes: 'Confident midwives who extend the boundaries of their knowledge and practice assist women in making informed choices about their care'. At the same time, 'women learn to expect choice' and to exercise this choice (Griew, 2003). The 'focus upon childbirth as something normal' led midwives to be 'more guided by the woman's own needs than by established routines' (Waldenström, 2003). This mutual development led Olive

Jones (2000) to speak of 'the cycle of empowerment' and positive feedback for staff and families in birth centres: 'As long as the cycle of empowerment remains unbroken, it is self-perpetuating'.

Thus, expectations are changed and skills are developed. Confident midwives transmit confidence to women and expectations rise, are confirmed and fed back into the local community. Midwives who grow and develop in this way may be less vulnerable to burnout, since they experience less of the alienating work experiences reported by those who leave midwifery (Ball et al., 2002), and are protected by their relative autonomy and relationships of respect with colleagues and clients. Despite the overall shortage of midwives, birth centres have waiting lists with the names of midwives wanting jobs. For midwives, as for women, the birth centre option changes expectations.

Midwifery skills

Midwives in birth centres in many countries speak of the freedom from technology and bureaucracy which enables them to give more attention to women and families. In this situation different skills can develop.

Marion Hunter (2000, p. 143) draws from her research in New Zealand a list of the additional skills required by midwives providing intrapartum care in small units:

- Being confident to provide intrapartum care in a low-technology setting
- Being comfortable to use embodied knowledge and skills to assess a woman and her baby as opposed to using technology
- Being able to let labour 'be' and not interfere unnecessarily
- Being confident to avert or manage problems that might arise
- Being willing to employ other options to manage pain without access to epidurals
- Being solely responsible for outcomes without access to on-site specialist assistance
- Being confident to trust the process of labour and be flexible with respect to time
- Being a midwife who enjoys practising what the participants call 'real midwifery'.

This list is strikingly different from the usual list of midwifery skills or competencies, although it contains within one competency the emergency skills so necessary for isolated practice. The skills on this list are all states of 'being', statements regarding the midwife's self, and her use of self, rather than tightly defined manual or intellectual skills. These are skills for relationships, not for narrowly defined tasks. While it is unusual to see midwifery skills concerned with 'being', I have never before seen a list that contains the word 'enjoy', which is appropriate for midwives who have chosen to work in such settings.

Trust is highly significant. The woman learns to trust her body and the midwife to trust her own judgement (Griew, 2003), as well as to trust each other and the process of labour. Trust is infectious and the midwife's trust is conveyed to the woman. This is different from the self-fulfilling prophesy of intervention 'just in case'.

Being able to 'let labour be' is also in contrast to medicalised practice. Obstetrics is geared toward action. To be seen to have done everything that could be done is widely viewed as good, if defensive, practice. Yet midwives' ability to not act enables women to be active (Leap, 2000).

A threatening model

Birth centre practice deviates from the medicalised birth which is now the norm in Western countries. It demonstrates other ways of doing birth, and this alternative can be perceived as a threat.

In order for women and families to play the key roles in birth, professionals need to acknowledge that their role is a supporting one. This does not fit well with the image of active professionals rescuing needy women from pain or risk, combating emergencies and delivering babies. The birth centre midwife's role is one of prevention and vigilance – states of calmness and readiness, not of activity.

Maternity services sometimes become so rigid as to exhibit a fear of excellence. Where diversity cannot be tolerated, the social model of birth is likely to be seen as a threat to mainstream services. Ironically, this is where birth centres are most needed.

A threatened model

Small units are vulnerable. They can easily be identified as centres of a mode of practice that is different from that of obstetric hospitals and as areas of potential savings.

The pressure to provide the full range of clinical services (which usually comes from those who provide services such as paediatrics or anaesthetics) has led to the closure of units with fewer than 300 births per year in France and 500 births per year in Italy. The belief that such services are needed for all women, 'just in case', is the opposite of the positive outlook of the social model of birth. Yet, like much public policy on birth historically, this medical model of birth is accepted as the one that is obviously right because it is supported by authoritative experts. Like the obvious economics of centralisation, it usually goes unquestioned.

Partnership and cooperation

Working in birth centres on this small scale, midwives come to feel accountable to individuals rather than to the system. This builds confidence, autonomy and generosity, which equip them well to collaborate with other professionals as equals. This is different from the culture of deference and 'passing the buck', which is common in hospitals.

Ironically, midwives and clients, who gain confidence in birth centres, are the groups least likely to develop confidence or autonomy in hospitals, where they are at the bottom of a hierarchy that tends to pass blame downwards.

An enabling culture

Birth centres provide a focus for midwives, a safe haven for the practice of 'real midwifery', a place where like-minded midwives can turn the rhetoric of modern maternity care into reality, without feeling vulnerable and defiant.

Separation from obstetric units is necessary for midwives to be able to attend to families without the fragmentation of their attention which, like fragmented care, results from industrialised obstetrics.

Birth centres develop the transferable skills without which humane care is impossible. They are a positive model for change in the scale of services and for change within neighbouring maternity hospitals.

There is still much resistance to this model of care, yet its existence demonstrates that alternatives to a single, industrialised model of birth are possible.

REFERENCES

Ball L, Curtis P, Kirkham M. 2002. Why Do Midwives Leave? Royal College of Midwives, London

Boulton M, Chapple J, Saunders D. 2003. Evaluating a new service: clinical outcomes and women's assessments of the Edgware Birth Centre. In: Kirkham M (ed.), Birth Centres: A Social Model for Maternity Care. Books for Midwives, Oxford

Brodie P. 1996a. Australian team midwives in transition. International Confederation of Midwives, 24th Triennial Conference, Oslo

Brodie P. 1996b. Being with women: the experience of Australian team midwives. Unpublished MA, University of Technology, Sydney, Australia

Campbell RM, Macfarlane A. 1994. Where to be Born? The Debate and the Evidence. National Perinatal Epidemiology Unit, Oxford

Coyle K, Hauck Y, Percival P, Kristhanson L. 2001. Ongoing relationships with a personal focus: mothers' perceptions of birth centre versus hospital care. Midwifery, 17: 171–181

Esposito NW. 1999. Marginalised women's comparisons of their hospital and free-standing birth centre experiences: a contrast of inner-city birthing systems. Health Care for Women International, 20: 111–126

Griew K. 2003. Birth centre midwifery down under – creating an environment that enables you to truly listen. In: Kirkham M (ed.), Birth Centres: A Social Model for Maternity Care. Books for Midwives, Oxford

Hunter M. 2000. Autonomy, clinical freedom and responsibility: the paradoxes of providing intrapartum midwifery care in a small maternity unit as compared with a large obstetric hospital. Unpublished MA, Massey University, Palmerston North, New Zealand

Jones O. 2000. Supervision in a midwife managed birth centre. In: Kirkham M (ed.), Developments in the Supervision of Midwives. Books for Midwives, Manchester

Kirkham M. 1999. The culture of midwifery in the NHS in England. Journal of Advanced Nursing, 30(3): 732–739

Kirkham M (ed.). 2003. Birth Centres: A Social Model for Maternity Care. Books for Midwives, Oxford

Kirkham M, Stapleton H (eds). 2001. Informed Choice in Maternity Care: An Evaluation of Evidence-Based Leaflets. NHS Centre for Reviews and Dissemination, York

Leap N. 2000. The less we do the more we give. In: Kirkham M (ed.), The Midwife–Mother Relationship. Macmillan, London

Saunders D, Boulton M, Chapple J, Ratcliffe J, Levitan J. 2000. Evaluation of the Edgware Birth Centre. Barnet Health Authority, London

Turner S. 2002. Midwifery in Tokyo. The Practising Midwife, 5(4): 34–35

Waldenström U. 1999. Effects of birth centre care on fathers' satisfaction with care, experience of the birth and adaptation to fatherhood. Journal of Reproductive and Infant Psychology, 17: 357–368

Waldenström U. 2003. The Stockholm Birth Centre. In: Kirkham M (ed.), Birth Centres: A Social Model for Maternity Care. Books for Midwives, Oxford

The Practising Midwife 2003; 6(11): 12–15

'Home from home': the key to success

Morwenna Davies, Shirley McDonald, Denise Austin

Lichfield Victoria Maternity Unit in Staffordshire is a nine-bed, stand-alone unit linked to the local consultant unit. Care is women-centred, provided by a small team of midwives and midwifery assistants who are friendly and highly skilled. Our team's skills, though, aren't confined to midwifery; we are successful fundraisers too. In fact, we could be said to be Lichfield's answer to the Women's Institute's 'Calendar Girls' because of our dedication, with the help of local businesses, to raising money for the unit. With money raised and our combined expertise at sewing and decoration, we have managed to create a wonderful, homely environment within the unit. It has a welcoming, non-clinical feel, with plenty of privacy and space.

Antenatal care

We have a flexible antenatal system which provides an opportunity for more individual care. This includes 24-hour access to midwifery advice for women and their families. Midwives at weekly booking clinics perform ultrasound scans, and it is at this time that the women are able to discuss at length their hopes and fears for their birthing experience. The unit also offers a successful parent education package, which has evolved over the years to reflect changes.

Fantastic facilities

The unit offers individually designed birthing rooms with en-suite facilities, including jacuzzi baths. Our most recent addition is a state-of-the-art pool room, of which we are very proud. We successfully raised over £5000 to provide a brilliant, contemporary design for the birth pool room. Due to the increasing popularity of the 'pool birth' facility with local women, the unit has seen a massive 20% increase in births so far this year, compared with last year. Although our service is predominantly for local women, word is spreading about the unique service we offer and, increasingly, we are attracting women from a wider radius.

A complementary approach

We believe in a holistic approach to care and, as part of this, we offer complementary therapies to most women booked for birth in the unit, with midwives trained in both reflexology and aromatherapy. Reflexology is offered to help minimise the effects of many of the minor disorders of pregnancy. It is provided on an appointment basis at times suitable to both the woman and the staff responsible for the treatment. This allows for flexibility for all concerned. Specific aromatherapy oils are blended by our trained aromatherapist in order for any untrained staff to administer to women both in labour and in the immediate postnatal period. Aromatherapy oils also have an important role in our 'Preparation for labour' package. We also offer post-mature women reflexology at approximately term plus five days. We combine this with a labour blend of aromatherapy oils, designed to relax and so encourage the onset of uterine action.

Working with the consultant unit

Women who are not in labour after 10–14 days are then transferred to the consultant unit for induction of labour, about 10 miles away. They are given priority if they wish to return to us for postnatal care, as are any others who have had to be transferred, for whatever reason, to the consultant unit. This enables them to continue their initial postnatal care in calm, unhurried surroundings, benefiting both mother and baby, and is especially valuable for women with specific postnatal needs.

Training

The care women receive is constantly evolving. Changes often take place after staff attend training workshops and study days. In addition, our midwives keep in regular contact with other birth centres to discuss new ideas and relevant research – even embracing new technology!

In-house, we facilitate monthly 'skill drill' training, attended by midwives, midwifery assistants and community staff. These complement compulsory sessions provided by the consultant unit.

How do we do it?

All of this is achieved by a shared vision: each member of the team is valued for their individual skills. Our philosophy is continuity of care, not carer. The whole team adopting a flexible approach to work patterns, and working as one, achieves this. A midwife and midwifery assistant, usually working one shift out of three over a 24-hour period, cover each shift. Flexibility enables us to call on other colleagues as required, to maintain our standards of care.

The Practising Midwife 2003; 6(11): 16–17

Staff retention has never been an issue for us. In fact, not only is the unit a 'home from home' for the women and their families, but it is also true for its staff. This is clearly illustrated by the dedication the team shows in and out of working hours.

We have found that those who leave, through promotion or for other reasons, have continued to support the team whenever possible, both professionally and socially.

The team also includes invaluable support staff, community midwives and GPs, plus the ongoing professional support of the consultant unit. In essence, we are a dedicated team ready to go the extra mile.

The key to the team's success lies in our willingness to embrace change, dedication, cooperation and interaction with one another, not only professionally but socially too. Last night at the proms, a day at the races – life is never dull for the Victoria Calendar Girls! And finally – behind every good midwife there is a supporting and understanding family and the ever-necessary babysitter, without whose support the unit's unique cohesiveness could not be maintained.

A compromise for change?

Sara Wickham

When I first became involved with birth centres in the USA, they were seen as something of a compromise by many of those involved in setting them up – offering neither the benefits of hospital surgical facilities nor the environmental advantages of being at home (Katz Rothman, 1983). Yet the compromise worked, with birth centres springing up in different states and offering women havens for normal birth experiences amid a rising caesarean rate and proliferation of birth technology. Although some of these birth centres have inevitably fallen along the way, others are now well-established community centres, celebrating significant birthdays with the help of hundreds of the children who were born there.

Some years later, midwives, mothers and supporters of out-of-hospital birth began campaigns in the UK, in an attempt to make the birth centre compromise an option for women over here. We have also lost some of our first birth centres but, again, others have survived and are showing just how effective this model can be for everybody involved in pregnancy and birth. But while compromise has been a useful tool in enabling small groups of women to achieve the birth they envisioned, there is little room for complacency.

Kitty Ernst (1986, p. 32) defined a birth centre as 'a place where women give birth' (as opposed to being 'delivered' by somebody else) and 'a place for the practice of midwifery'. It seemed to me that she was searching for a broad definition which would encompass a wide range of examples, yet also place boundaries between midwifery as an autonomous, woman-centred art and midwifery as an adjunct to obstetric practice. Yet, in this urge to recognise that there are always examples that embody the spirit of the definition if not the letter, I fear we may, in the UK, be in danger of missing the point.

I have heard several people involved in the birth centre movement talk about the fact that a number of places described as birth centres may not actually be birth centres when we analyse what this term really means. If you look at some of the maps depicting the location of UK birth centres, you will see more dots than you might expect. Whether every one of these dots represents a place that is truly centred on the experiences of women and the practice of authentic midwifery in a home-like setting is debatable.

For sure, birth centres are not only about comfy double beds, patchwork quilts and nice paintings on the walls. But all of these things serve to add ambience – and to make the setting more home-like and relaxed. While I totally acknowledge that the atmosphere and philosophy of the birth centre and its staff are far more important than the décor, I would ask whether the term 'birth centre' is appropriate for a setting that more closely resembles a clinical area than somebody's living area or bedroom.

Equally, being 'freestanding' has been a key component of the birth centre philosophy in a number of countries. I don't suppose there is a single midwife who has received babies at home or in a birth centre who hasn't had at least one moment when she wished that she and the woman were in the hospital, but for every one of the scary moments there are thousands of happy ones when everybody was delighted they were not. There is a palpable difference between being in a place that is simply and clearly about normal birth and midwifery, and being somewhere that is a 'holding tank' for the next-door labour ward only as long as your labour remains normal.

I suppose it really depends on whether one sees 'birth centre' as simply another term for a place where babies are born, or as a concept which is intensely political, grounded in the normalcy of birth and autonomous midwifery and needing careful nurturing by those who value this. If we are not careful, we will be turning the compromise on its head.

We could seek to attain a truly useful compromise by having a home-like environment that isn't quite home and skilled, autonomous midwives who have appropriate technology but not a fully staffed operating theatre. Yet, if we don't hold on to what a birth centre really means to women and midwives, we might be offering women so-called birth centres which bear no resemblance to people's homes at all, but have all the staff you could ever need on the other side of a door. Which, when you think about it, comes pretty close to the definition of a hospital...

REFERENCES

Ernst EKM. 1986. Nurse-midwifery in the freestanding birth center. In: Rooks J, Haas JE (eds), Nurse-Midwifery in America. A Report of the American College of Nurse-Midwives. ACNM Foundation, Washington, DC

Katz Rothman B. 1983. Anatomy of a compromise; nurse-midwifery and the rise of the birth center. Journal of Nurse-Midwifery, 28(4): 3–7

The Practising Midwife 2003; 6(11): 23

Birth centres in Wiltshire (1)

Vicky Tinsley

This article discusses why midwifery-led birth centres are important, and introduces the work of the West Wiltshire Primary Care Trust (WWPCT) in developing this service. The concluding article examines education and maintaining competencies and care in emergency situations.

Introduction

The WWPCT delivers approximately 5200 babies a year, with 1800 births (37% of the total) being conducted either in birth centres or at home. The overall normal birth rate trust-wide is 68%. The maternity service managed by the WWPCT operates at seven birth centres and also at a consultant unit, the Princess Anne Wing (PAW) in Bath, where women with more complicated pregnancies give birth.

Birth centres are located at Malmesbury, Chippenham, Devizes, Trowbridge, Frome, Shepton Mallet and Paulton (see Table 6.4.1). The community-based service aims to provide antenatal, intrapartum and postpartum care for low-risk mothers and their babies, as well as antenatal care to women who live in their geographical catchment areas. Each centre has developed and evolved in its own unique way according to local circumstances. Since 1995, all these units have been in various stages of development towards becoming midwifery-led birth centres. Transfer-in-labour time from the birth centres to the consultant unit is approximately an hour.

These birth centres are all stand-alone facilities. They are midwifery managed with no medical input, and are isolated from consultant obstetric services by between 12 and 24 miles. They extend the choice for women who meet the acceptance criteria for birth without active intervention in a home-from-home setting. In practice, this has evolved into a concept of family-centred care as partners, children and grandparents immediately share

in this major life event. The midwives seek to facilitate informed choice and foster a non-intrusive, non-intervention approach to birth. Such a philosophy has evolved to enable women and their families to experience a positive start to parenthood.

The shift towards birth centres

Campbell and Macfarlane (1994) concluded that there was no evidence to support the claim that hospital was the safest place in which to give birth. They also recommended that the closure of small obstetric units on the grounds of safety be stopped. Zander and Chamberlain (1999) acknowledged that 75% of care given to pregnant women came from midwives, and that the midwifery model of care could become the dominant model for the future.

The support that midwives need when preparing to undertake new roles and responsibilities presents a significant challenge for all involved in the maternity services. 'Changing Childbirth' (DOH, 1993) has had a major influence on midwifery practice, shifting the emphasis from the medical model of care to a woman-centred approach.

The more recent publication 'Making a Difference' (DOH, 1999) also refers to the inter-professional benefits of teamworking and of role expansion, stating: 'The government wants to extend the roles of nurses, midwives and health visitors to make better use of their knowledge and skills.' The model of midwifery practice in birth centres can only emerge if midwives are empowered to use their clinical judgement and to make clinical decisions using their own responsibility and accountability.

The midwife

The existing evidence base surrounding the promotion of normality shows that the avoidance of interventions in low-risk women has positive outcomes, and the role of the midwife is central to this.

Hodnett (2002) argues that the key component in promoting spontaneous vaginal birth is the continuous presence of the midwife. Persad et al. (1996) suggest that not all midwives have the competencies to provide all elements of maternity care for low-risk women, while Rosser (2001) argues that the medicalisation of childbirth has resulted in midwives losing core midwifery skills.

Regardless of whether or not midwives have these skills, many have lost confidence in their ability to take responsibility for the care of low-risk women. Hunter (2000) describes the range of core skills required mainly by midwives to keep birth normal as follows:

- Confident in providing intrapartum care in a low-technology setting
- Comfortable using embodied knowledge and skills to assess a woman and her baby as opposed to using technology
- Able to let labour 'be' and not interfere unnecessarily

- Confident to avert and manage problems that might arise
- Willing to employ other options to manage pain without access to epidurals
- Responsible for outcomes without access to on-site specialist assistance
- Confident to trust the process of labour and to be flexible with respect to time
- Able to use available evidence to support care (one-to-one care in labour).

Evidence to support birth centres

A growing body of evidence supports the use of birth centres. According to a number of studies, birth centres reduce the levels of intervention in labour. Furthermore, women feel more empowered and midwives have more job satisfaction (Walsh, 2001). Table 6.4.2 gives a summary of supporting evidence (for a fuller literature review, see Walsh, 2001, cited in Scottish Executive, 2002).

Table 6.4.1 Birth centres in Wiltshire

Community birth centres	Miles to consultant unit	Birth numbers 2002	Home births 2002	Number of delivery beds	Water birth facilities
Malmesbury	24	94	4	2	Yes
Chippenham (Greenways)	15.5	284	14	2	Yes
Devizes	21.5	133	3	1	Yes
Trowbridge	14	355	22	3	Yes
Frome	17	235	28	2	Yes
Shepton Mallet (St Peter's)	22	105	3	1	Yes
Paulton	12	170	5	2	Yes

Table 6.4.2 Benefits of birth centres

Increased consumer satisfaction	Fewer episiotomies
High midwifery job satisfaction	Less electronic fetal monitoring
More appropriate use of midwifery skills and more autonomy	Fewer amniotomies
Women/families able to make own birth decisions	Fewer intravenous infusions
Women feel empowered	Fewer vaginal examinations
Higher normal birth rates	Lower incidence of shoulder dystocia
Lower forceps and ventouse rates	Shorter labours
Lower caesarean section rates	More likely to eat during labour
Fewer inductions	More use of hydrotherapy
Lower augmentation rates	Less fetal distress
Fewer epidurals	Less difficulty establishing respiration
Less pethidine	Increased chance of successful breastfeeding
	Cost-effective

Source: amended version of Walsh (2001), in Scottish Executive (2002).

The Wiltshire model

Protocols

All protocols have been written by multidisciplinary groups and are based on research findings where available and consensus on effectiveness. In this, as in many other areas of multidisciplinary interaction, one of the strengths is that the protocols are the same throughout the sites and are readily available in all clinical areas. They are all fully evidence-based and are referenced with a review date for revalidation. Any member of staff or professional group can put forward a draft protocol, which will be open for discussion throughout all professional groups prior to discussion at the Maternity Services Liaison Committee. A key issue is the importance of ongoing local consultation in order to offer and encourage ownership of the finished product and to increase the likelihood of its use.

Midwifery supervision, with its primary function of protecting the public from unsafe practice, cannot be separated from risk management, and the supervisor has an important role in developing and implementing protocols/guidelines for practice locally.

The Confidential Enquiry into Maternal Deaths (CEMD, 2001) highlighted the importance of good maternal history taken at booking. It stressed the importance of a risk assessment, which should be reviewed regularly. Protocols are the indispensable security net to ensure all professional groups are confident that the roles undertaken by each group are appropriate.

Midwives undertake the antenatal care for those women booked to deliver in the birth centres but also for those who are booked to give birth in the consultant unit. All midwives are based in the birth centres and are divided into teams, which provide an integrated midwifery service in the local communities. In addition, the birth centres are the first point of contact for pregnant, labouring and postnatal women across the maternity services as they are open 24 hours a day. All telephone calls are logged by the member of staff taking the call for medico-legal reasons and because of the amount of time that they can spend on the telephone. All the centres have an attached consultant who visits each for a consultant clinic on a monthly basis to prevent women having to travel to the consultant unit. Should a woman wish to have a home confinement, this will be provided by her local team of midwives working out of the birth centres. Portable water birth pools can be borrowed from the birth centres for those wishing to have a water birth at home.

Maintaining normality

The midwives actively encourage non-pharmacological labour care such as massage (and in some areas reflexology and aromatherapy) and the use of water (hydrotherapy units are available in some centres), enabling women to find their own ways of working through their labour in an active and positive way. Transcutaneous electrical nerve stimulation (TENS), pethidine and entonox are available. Epidural anaesthesia is not available in the birth centres; should a woman decide on this option she must be transferred to the consultant unit.

Experience to date in the birth centres is that very few women choose to give birth on a bed. Given the choice, the majority opt to use water or adopt vertical birth positions. As permanent water birth facilities have become available in the birth centres, so there has been a steady rise in the water birth rate. For example, Greenways' water birth rate has risen from 11% in 1999 to 41% in 2001 as women and midwives become more confident. This does not include those women who labour in water but get out for the birth. When practical, the bed will be pushed away from the centre so that it is not the focal point of the room. Birth platforms and birth mattresses are provided in most birth rooms. It is not considered good practice to have televisions in the rooms.

Transfers in labour

The overall transfer-in-labour rate remains static at 17% intrapartum, 3% maternal postpartum and 1% neonatal. A range of audits over the last five years have included intrapartum escorts, acute antenatal transfers, ambulance transfer times and failure to progress in the first and second stage, as well as looking at the actual outcomes (see Table 6.4.3 for a list of reasons for transfer in the first stage).

Table 6.4.3 Reasons for transfer in first stage: 2001

	%	n
Failure to progress	48	115
Fetal distress	18	43
Request for epidural	15	35
Meconium-stained liquor	10	23
Malpresentation (other than breech)	6	14
Raised blood pressure	5	11
Intrapartum bleeding	4	9
Breech presentation	3	7
No fetal heart heard on admission	<1 (1 client)	

Total number of women (n) = 239

Table 6.4.4 provides a detailed comparison of transfer rates. It is interesting to note that both Malmesbury and St Peter's intrapartum transfers average at about 20% which, given that they are approximately 22–24 miles from the consultant unit, suggests that their transfers-in-labour tolerance may be lower than the other birth centres. However, when trying to address rising transfer rates/trends, this needs to be carefully managed because any pressure placed on midwives not to transfer may have a detrimental effect on the safety of birth centres. Some midwives appear to have a lower transfer tolerance level than others, and this may relate directly to confidence levels. The midwives have a direct referral service to the consultant unit for advice and to arrange a transfer in labour.

One of the most difficult decisions can be when and how to transfer a woman in labour into the consultant unit, especially if she is in an advanced labour. The WWPCT does not have a policy specifying when women should be transferred in labour, as it is the responsibility of the midwife to review the individual clinical case. There is also the belief locally that it is not practical to devise a protocol for every situation without it being 'bigger than the Bible' and totally unworkable. Midwives have to rely on their clinical judgement.

Midwives in birth centres have to weigh up the risks of transfer – for example, a primigravida breech presentation with ruptured membranes arriving at the birth centre at 6 cm or a gravida four breech presentation arriving at 8 cm with membranes intact. The midwife has to undertake a risk assessment on the transfer, looking at, for example, the likelihood of the woman giving birth in the ambulance. There is also the mode of transfer to consider. For example, should a primigravida at 2 cm (not in established labour), with meconium-stained liquor, be driven by her partner on a 20-minute journey if the ambulance is at least an hour away?

Once the decision is made by the midwife to transfer a woman in labour to the consultant unit, she immediately changes from the low- to high-risk category. The midwives in the birth centres would then give the woman cimetidine (hydrochloric acid suppressant) prior to transfer. The midwives would also take any relevant blood samples prior to transfer (such as group and save and haemoglobin).

The bloods would accompany the woman into the consultant unit and be handed over at transfer. It is also beneficial to take a 'transfer-in-labour' bag for all eventualities, such as delivery equipment.

It is perhaps the biggest weakness in the maternity service as a whole that the birth centre midwife is usually unable to stay with the mother once she has been transferred. This is due to staffing arrangements, on-call cover and often the practicalities of arranging return transport for the midwife.

It is essential that there is a good working relationship with the consultant unit and the birth centre in order to provide a seamless service for the woman. If there are

Table 6.4.4 Comparison of birth centre transfer rates, 1997–2001 (total number of transfers in 2001 = 338)

		Number of births	Number of intrapartum transfers	%* intrapartum transfers	Number of neonatal transfers	%† neonatal transfers	Number of postpartum transfers	%‡ postpartum transfers	Number of other transfers	Number of total transfers
Trowbridge	2001	360	82	19	8	2	7	2	–	97
	2000	407	70	15	10	2	9	2	7	96
Frome	2001	239	35	14	4	2	7	3	–	46
	2000	306	40	12	1	0	16	5	2	59
Chippenham (Greenways)	2001	277	59	18	5	2	11	4	–	70
	2000	295	51	15	9	3	11	4	5	76
Paulton	2001	164	42	20	2	1	6	4	–	50
	2000	159	44	22	8	5	11	6	8	71
Devizes	2001	138	28	17	0	0	4	3	–	32
	2000	154	31	17	4	3	2	1	1	38
Malmesbury	2001	116	25	18	0	0	3	3	–	28
	2000	133	30	18	6	4	3	2	2	41
Shepton Mallet (St Peter's)	2001	97	11	11	1	1	3	3	–	15
	2000	107	31	22	4	4	2	2	1	38

*Number of intrapartum transfers as percentage of intrapartum transfers + total births.

†Number of neonatal transfers as percentage of total births.

‡Number of postpartum transfers as percentage of total births.

mutterings of discontent between areas then this is detrimental both to groups of staff and to the whole service. If midwives do not work at relationships, then a division could be created between those working with high- and low-risk women. The overall message should be consistent: everyone is essential to the midwifery service and no group of midwives can function without the other.

REFERENCES

Anderson RE, Murphy PA. 1995. Outcome of 11,788 planned home births attended by certified nursing midwives. A retrospective descriptive study. J Nurse Midwifery, 40: 483–492

Campbell R, Macfarlane A. 1994. Where to be Born? The Debate and the Evidence, 2nd edn. National Perinatal Epidemiology Unit, Oxford

Chamberlain G, Wraight A, Crowley P. 1997. Home births. Report of the 1994 Confidential Enquiry by the National Birthday Trust Fund. Parthenon, Carnforth

CEMD (Confidential Enquiry into Maternal Deaths). 2001. Why mothers die. Report on Confidential Enquiries into Maternity Deaths in the United Kingdom. HMSO, London

CESDI (Confidential Enquiry into Stillbirths and Deaths in Infancy). 1998. Sixth Annual Report (1 January–31 December 1997). Maternal and Child Health Research Consortium, London

Department of Health. 1993. Changing Childbirth: The Report of the Expert Maternity Group. HMSO, London

Department of Health. 1999. Making a Difference. Strengthening the Nursing, Midwifery and Health Visiting Contribution to Health and Health Care. Department of Health, London

Hodnett ED. 2002. Home-like versus conventional institutional settings for birth (Cochrane Review). In: The Cochrane Library, Issue 3. Update Software, Oxford

Hunter M. 2000. Automomy, clinical freedom and responsibilities: the paradoxes of providing intrapartum midwifery care in a small maternity unit as compared with a large obstetric hospital. Unpublished MA, Massey University, Palmerston North, New Zealand

Persad P, Hiscock C, Mitchell T. 1996. Midwives and perinatology (extended role of midwife in perinatal mortality enquiries). British Journal of Midwifery, 4(1): 20–21

Rosenblatt RA, Reinken J, Shoemack P. 1985. Is obstetrics safe in small hospitals? Lancet, i: 429–433

Rosser J. 2001. Birth centres – the key to modernising the maternity services. MIDIRS Midwifery Digest, 11(3): Supplement 2

Scottish Executive. 2002. Expert Group on Acute Maternity Services. Reference report. Scottish Executive

Walsh D. 2001. Evidence-based care series 2: free-standing birth centres. British Journal of Midwifery, 8: 6

Zander L, Chamberlain G. 1999. ABC of labour care: place of birth. BMJ, 318: 721–723

The Practising Midwife 2003; 6(5): 14–18

Birth centres in Wiltshire (2)

Vicky Tinsley

In this concluding part, I will look at the importance of educating midwives and maintaining competencies in birth centres, and how emergencies are dealt with.

Background

The West Wiltshire Primary Care Trust (WWPCT) delivers approximately 5200 babies a year, with 1800 births (37% of the total) being conducted either in birth centres or at home. The overall normal birth rate trust-wide is 68%.

The maternity service managed by WWPCT operates at seven birth centres at Malmesbury, Chippenham, Devizes, Trowbridge, Frome, Shepton Mallet and Paulton, and also at a consultant unit, the Princess Anne Wing (PAW) in Bath, where women with more complicated pregnancies give birth.

Education and maintaining competencies

Birth centres differ from other aspects of health care provision because, in the majority of cases, clients are healthy. However, this makes the identification of ill or at-risk women all the more critical. Attention needs to be paid to non-obstetric medical risk factors such as socio-economic status and domestic violence.

CEMD (2001) recommended that continuing professional development should be accepted as the responsibility of the practitioner as well as the employer, and that knowledge and skills should be regularly updated.

Midwives regularly undertake self-analysis as part of their annual supervisory review to identify their individual learning needs, and these have been addressed in a number of ways. Updating in the consultant unit has been arranged when required. Specialist practitioners and medical staff have contributed to programmes of clinical learning: for example, adult/infant resuscitation, intravenous cannulation and perineal repair. Modules appropriate to those identified needs have been accessed through the local universities: for example, midwife ventouse practitioner, examination of the newborn, normality modules, waterbirth and active birth workshops. The midwifery lecturers from Bournemouth University have been particularly proactive and visionary in developing evidence-based training delivered locally to meet these identified service developments.

A proactive interface between supervisors of midwives and providers of education is essential in commissioning training to meet local needs. Once competencies are achieved, it is vital that the level of skills and expertise are maintained. There are a variety of ways of ensuring that midwives have and maintain these essential skills, but implicit in this must be the use of evidence-based care.

Care in emergency situations

The nature and environment of a birth centre will mean that the type of risk management and decisions about care will differ from those of a midwife working in an obstetric maternity unit. All staff working in birth centres must be skilled in basic life-support techniques in maternal and infant resuscitation and the management of obstetric emergencies. It is mandatory locally for all birth centre midwives to attend the Advanced Life Support in Obstetrics (ALSO) course. This is a two-day, intensive multi-professional course using practical workshops and lectures. The WWPCT midwives have been actively involved with the initiative since its introduction in 1995–6, and there is a growing number of ALSO instructors and advisory board members working within the birth centres.

In addition to this, 'skill drills' have been introduced to ensure that midwives are able to respond in line with CESDI (1998) requirements. In all the birth centres there are manikins available to practise skill drills, particularly shoulder dystocia, malpresentations and breech deliveries. CEMD (2001) stressed the importance of managing emergencies such as severe haemorrhage. All birth centre midwives are taken through bi-manual compression in the case of a massive postpartum haemorrhage and the practical management of cord prolapse. Included in these skill drills should be the management of uncertainty.

CEMD (2001) highlights the importance of identification and support of women with higher risk pregnancies who appear unsuitable for midwife-led care and made the explicit statement that midwives should be prepared to decline to take responsibility of high-risk cases where involvement of an obstetrician is essential. However, great efforts are always made to work with the woman and her requests and, in the case of a planned inappropriate delivery in a birth centre, an individual action plan is devised for the protection of the midwives.

Integral to the provision of quality maternity services is the ability to identify and care for ill women and babies. All maternity care practitioners must have the necessary skills to recognise and initiate appropriate care for ill women and their babies.

In the event of a baby requiring resuscitation the midwife would do this, until appropriate assistance arrives. The appropriate skills would include ventilatory support by bag and mask as opposed to tracheal neonatal intubation. Particular emphasis should be paid to the recognition of the ill neonate. All staff must have the skill and competencies to assess, resuscitate and stabilise the neonatal prior to ongoing management. The midwives are not expected to intubate the baby. This has been clearly documented in the Trust's care in labour policy and agreement has been reached between midwives, obstetricians, GPs and paediatricians. The reasoning behind the decision was that effective basic resuscitation skills were thought to be more effective in emergency

situations than training several midwives to have more advanced intubation skills. It would also be more problematic to ensure that all midwives remained competent in a skill that may be needed on an occasional basis. However, an increasing number of midwives are now undertaking the Neonatal Advance Life Support (NALS) course.

The midwives' back-up in these situations would be paramedic support via the ambulance service. There are no obstetric and neonatal flying squads currently operating within this maternity service, having been disbanded around five years ago. Where emergencies arise, it is preferable to stabilise the baby prior to transfer to the consultant unit. Midwives may telephone to seek advice from senior obstetricians and paediatricians at any time, with a direct referral system.

Conclusion

Midwifery-led models of care are an increasingly important development in the future configuration of maternity services both in the UK and internationally. As traditional GP units are replaced by birth centres, any expansion of the midwives' roles and responsibilities cannot be undertaken lightly, as there must be extensive preparation and training.

The promotion of normality of childbirth is integral to a quality maternity service, but it is essential that the recognition of the ill mother and infant is paramount. The main issues appear to centre on the competencies required in caring for low-risk women and the management of recognition of obstetric emergencies within stand-alone birth centres. Supportive midwifery practice, clear protocols and ongoing clinical audit are essential for the provision of a safe, midwifery-led service. Managerial support as well as agreement and support from local obstetricians and GPs are all necessary to ensure that the midwives feel supported in birth centres. The importance of team and multiprofessional approaches to education, training and service development cannot be underestimated.

REFERENCES

CEMD (Confidential Enquiry into Maternal Deaths). 2001. Why mothers die. Report on Confidential Enquiries into Maternity Deaths 1997–99. HMSO, London

CESDI (Confidential Enquiry into Stillbirths and Deaths in Infancy). 1998. Fifth Annual Report. Maternal and Child Health Research Consortium, London

The Practising Midwife 2003; 6(6): 30–31

Questions for debate

Do you think Birth Centres are the way forward for women and midwives? If so (or if not), then why?

How do you feel about the different environments that are available for women to birth in, and in what ways do your feelings impact your practice?

Life After Birth

Exploring life after birth

If you could plan the ideal postnatal experience for a woman, what would you include? By this, I don't just mean postnatal care, or the first few days after birth: if you were given an unlimited budget to plan a Government-funded postnatal project, and there were no limits on how you could use the money, what would you make available for women and their families, and when, and how?

Postnatal care: is it an afterthought?

Julie Wray

Midwives and mothers know that after pregnancy and birth the postnatal period can be the most challenging, exciting and yet demanding, even difficult, final phase of the procreation journey. The adjustment and transition to parenthood can be a hybrid of emotions from pleasure to despair, often overwhelming mothers and fathers immediately after birth and beyond. Postnatal care should be unique, special and delivered to mothers in a sensitive and caring way so that they feel able to recover, adjust and even enjoy themselves.

Yet postnatal care is often referred to as the 'Cinderella' of maternity care. This accepted metaphor is bandied around in ordinary and everyday speech within midwifery, and I wonder why this has been sustained in our everyday discourse. What does such a negative term really mean within contemporary midwifery?

For example, is it connected to reluctance from staff (including midwives) to do this type of work? Do midwives perceive that postnatal care is dull and lacking in excitement or drama compared to antenatal care or birth? Has 'Cinderella' just become one of those words that we are all comfortable with, or does it symbolise that this aspect of the service really is an afterthought? Is it a true representation of the order of things that postnatal care is low down on the agenda?

Of course, there could be many more reasons, contentious and real, as to why this is the case. Nonetheless, it is always with regret that I feel very compromised when friends, family and neighbours approach me with their real stories about postnatal care (in its broadest sense) and their views about it. Only recently a friend shared a range of issues that demonstrated that she felt like 'Cinderella'. She described thoughtlessness and lack of attention to detail by the staff assigned to care for her during the immediate postnatal period (the first five days). For her, it was the most fundamental aspects of care and caring that were glossed over, such as access to food and drink, assistance with the baby, support and sincere help to breastfeed in the first few days. For some staff (but not all) it was a genuine effort for them to actually care for her and, as a result, she would consider painstakingly the need to ask for help before approaching anyone. This was in direct contrast to her experiences during birth. Another interesting tack she would implement on the postnatal ward was to select only staff who were known to be more caring and approachable, thereby reducing her contact and exposure to 'others'.

What my friend was describing was that her relationship with staff, some only brief encounters, affected the quality and depth of care she received – that she had to carefully 'suss out' the staff on duty. In such situations I find myself defending the midwifery community, while at the same time trying to deal with flashbacks to my own grounded experiences as a clinical midwife of 16 years and mother, where I can vividly picture the scenarios and contexts being described.

Nonetheless, it should be the case that in the UK midwifery input and postnatal care should be excellent and second to none. The scope and potential for outstanding postnatal care exists and should be the norm for both mothers and their families. In many ways it is the least territorial aspect of practice, where midwives can truly 'be with women'. So it saddens me that, too often, women feel that they are left to fend for themselves, alone and uncared for. The rhetoric is that the whole birth continuum is 'women-centred'; yet, after birth, women often report that they feel unsupported and that staff are too busy to attend to them.

A woman's stay on a hospital ward is highly dependent on the culture represented on that ward rather than anything else; in other words, the shared (or not) values and beliefs held by those midwives and other staff working on the ward. The relationships between staff and between staff and mothers, and the leadership style and support mechanisms, are an integral part of the ward culture. Consequently, these dimensions will influence mother's experiences and the birth recovery process. Furthermore, how midwifery leaders and managers prioritise postnatal care provision and how they allocate resources will further affect staffing ratios, the stability of the workforce, their attitudes and behaviours. More importantly, such issues will affect a most crucial and significant part of the birth continuum: the end bit; in other words, the postnatal experience and outcomes as perceived by the mother and her family.

Undoubtedly, both place and type of birth can impact on a mother's postnatal care, experiences and subsequent birth recovery. However, when we seek mothers' views and experiences about care after birth, it is often their hospital stays that reveal the extent to which the notions of 'care and caring' are frequently packed with tensions. This dimension has been exposed recently in a postnatal study that captured mothers' views and experiences of postnatal care (Wray, 2002).* Uniquely, local mothers and a user group were involved in the study design and construction of the questions explored so that issues that mattered to them could be examined. Very briefly, the findings highlighted profound issues about the hospital stay, including the ward environment; hygiene, cleanliness and security; rest and recuperation; privacy; and flexible visiting. Clearly, birth recovery and the transition to parenting can be hampered by what takes place in the immediate period after birth. The ward environment ought to facilitate and embrace the process and provide adequate resources to allow mothers to experience quality postnatal hospital care wherever possible. In particular, the needs of mothers who have had a difficult birth need to be taken account of, and care after birth should be designed to fully support these mothers. In contrast, mothers revealed a high regard for

care at home and their community midwives, and as such uncovered minimal areas for improvement (Wray, 2002). In 1997 the Audit Commission also found that women made more negative comments about hospital postnatal care than any other aspect of their maternity care. So what is going on within the postnatal ward environment?

Clearly, there is a body of knowledge to support the assertion that the postnatal period is an important and challenging time for a woman and her family and for the midwife providing care at this time (RCM, 2000). There are up-to-date guidelines (RCM, 2000; Bick et al., 2001) to support service delivery, facilitate evidence-based practice and promote evaluations. Such guidance on postnatal care aims on the one hand to encourage midwives to actively consider their role in connection to postnatal practice, research and education, and on the other hand to encourage them to consider the policy context. A wide set of recommendations are put forward that actively encourage midwives to participate in evaluation, critical thinking, reflection and research processes. However, it continues to be reported that research in the area of postnatal care has been neglected.

This lack of a comprehensive body of knowledge and evidence to further support midwifery practice in the postnatal period reflects perhaps the 'Cinderella' metaphor yet again. I believe, given the steeped nature of postnatal care and midwifery, that we should have an entrée of sources and approaches, including audit and a variety of research methodologies, by which to underpin postnatal practice.

Significantly, we need to explore the notion of 'caring', so that we can be sure that postnatal care is not an 'afterthought', and that mothers and their babies can expect to be cared for in a way that is conducive to satisfying them and meeting their needs.

REFERENCES

Audit Commission. 1997. First Class Delivery. Improving Maternity Services in England and Wales. Audit Commission Publications, Abingdon

Bick D, MacArthur C, Knowles H, Winter H. 2001. Postnatal Care Guidelines for Management. Churchill Livingstone, Edinburgh

RCM. 2000. Midwifery Practice in the Postnatal Period – Recommendations for Practice. Royal College of Midwives, London

Wray J. 2002. Care after birth: views of Salford and Trafford mothers – a baseline evaluation. Main Report. The University of Salford

The Practising Midwife 2003; 6(4): 4–5

*This study was commissioned by a local Maternity Services Liaison Committee and Health Authority. More detailed publications are currently being prepared.

A light in the fog: caring for women with postpartum depression

Holly Powell Kennedy, Cheryl Tatano Beck, Jeanne Watson Driscoll

It is estimated that at least one in 10 women will experience postpartum depression, yet systematic screening for it in clinical practice is too often neglected. The foggy unreality of this affective disorder leads women to believe they are losing their minds, and their efforts to find help can be elusive. Women with postpartum depression who go undetected and untreated are at risk for immediate harm and potential lifelong sequelae for themselves and their families, and especially for their children. This article provides (1) an understanding of the woman's experience of postpartum depression, (2) a review of two instruments, developed through a focused program of research to screen for the disorder, (3) triage in clinical practice, and (4) an overview of the three dimensions of treatment: psychopharmacology, psychotherapy, and psychosocial care. Practical guidance and client information are provided to assist midwives and primary care providers to incorporate systematic screening into clinical practice, to identify effective interdisciplinary treatment teams, and to muster family and community resources to help with this commonly hidden childbearing crisis.

Introduction

I started thinking death thoughts at one point. I didn't plan suicide, but I started thinking I'd be better off dead. I had never been that low in my whole life when I thought death would be the way to go. I just wanted to get out of this world. It was like everything was black.
(Beck, 1993)

The plunge into the foggy unreality of postpartum depression is an experience that 7–30% of mothers will experience (O'Hara & Swain, 1996; Parry, 1999; Kennedy & Sutterfield, 2001; Ray & Hodnett, 2001). It is an illness that regularly goes undetected and often is not shared within or beyond family boundaries, yet postpartum depression can have devastating and long-lasting effects for the mother, her infant, and her family. It is a disease that robs a woman of joy in her infant, her relationship with family, and sometimes her very life. Evidence supports vastly improved outcomes when the illness is detected and treated early (England et al., 1994). However, the knowledge base of many women's health care providers about effective care for women with postpartum depression is too often dated, inaccurate or, at worst, dangerous. An astute ability to first screen for postpartum depression and then to initiate early treatment are essential elements of caring for women during the childbearing cycle. One of the most important roles of the midwife is as a primary 'case finder' of women with this serious, and commonly hidden, childbearing crisis. This article presents an overview of postpartum depression, evidence to support the efficacy of screening for early detection, and an interdisciplinary approach to treatment.

Mood disorders in the postpartum period

Postpartum mood disorders are classically divided into three groups: maternity blues, postpartum depression, and postpartum psychosis (Arnold et al., 1999; Sichel & Driscoll, 1999). Increasing comorbid phenomena with depression are obsessive-compulsive (OCD) and panic disorders during the childbearing year (Beck, 1998a; Arnold et al., 1999). Although the focus of this article is on postpartum depression, it is helpful to understand its placement within the constellation of mood disorders during the postpartum period.

The most common experience is that of postpartum or maternity blues, which is noted in all cultures and affects as many as 25–75% of women giving birth (Miller & Rukstalis, 1999). Miller and Rukstalis prefer the term *postpartum reactivity*, because this is more descriptive of a state that is characterized by mood swings, tearfulness, irritability, and a heightened responsiveness to stimuli that peaks around three to five days postpartum (Miller & Rukstalis, 1999). Lee et al. (2000a) have found that rapid eye movement (REM) sleep is significantly altered in new mothers, which can affect mood simply from fatigue. This can heighten a woman's vulnerability to the subsequent development of depression (Sichel & Driscoll, 1999). Several reviews of the literature propose many other theories, such as psychological, social, and physiologic influences, the latter including hormone withdrawal and biologic attachment theory (Arnold et al., 1999; Miller & Rukstalis, 1999; Sichel & Driscoll, 1999). Although the cause may be unclear or multifaceted, it does appear to represent a common, but usually transient, experience for many women during the early postpartum period. O'Hara and Swain (1996) note that 25% of women with maternity blues will subsequently develop postpartum depression.

Postpartum depression is a serious condition with symptoms of a major affective disorder (Arnold et al., 1999; Parry, 1999; Sichel & Driscoll, 1999). Arnold et al. (1999) report that as many as 5.2–22% of childbearing women will experience postpartum depression, and up to 26% of adolescent mothers will be affected. Symptoms can appear soon after birth but may also be delayed for months, with the potential course lasting up to a year in length, creating confusion about accurate assignment of a diagnosis of postpartum depression (Arnold et al., 1999). This diagnostic confusion is partially related to the constraints of the *Diagnostic and Statistical Manual of Mental Disorders-IV* (DSM-IV) coding (1994) and the inconsistency of defining the postpartum time period. DSM-IV defines postpartum depression as a major depressive episode occurring within four weeks after delivery. Other sources state that postpartum depression can occur any time in the first year after birth, hence the confusion (Arnold et al., 1999; Sichel & Driscoll, 1999). The wide variation of reported ranges may also reflect common experiences of recent motherhood, such as weight loss, sleep disorders, and lack of energy, or other medical illnesses (diabetes, anemia, or thyroid disease), all potentially mimicking depressive symptoms (Arnold et al., 1999).

Women experience a variety of disabling symptoms, which may include suicidal ideation, loss of all hope, obsessive thoughts, loss of interest in life, fear and guilt, inability to concentrate, anxiety attacks, decreased libido, insomnia, self-hatred, insecurity, and fatigue (Beck, 1992, 2002a; Ray & Hodnett, 2001). The powerful and encompassing nature of this depression is frighteningly clear in the following quote of one mother:

I always knew it was crazy but I needed to do it. I would write to my baby almost as if I knew I was going to die, which is morbid. I would write what I felt about him and how much I loved him. I think that in the back of my mind I was always afraid. This is hard to say but I think I was so out of control that I was afraid that I might kill myself (quietly weeping). (Beck, 1998a)

Ray and Hodnett (2001) describe the controversies surrounding the potential etiologies for postpartum depression and categorize them into medical and psychological theories. The medical model is founded on the vast hormonal and biochemical shifts in the woman after the birth of a child, whereas the personality or psychoanalytic etiologies would point to existing factors that increase her vulnerability to depression (Sichel & Driscoll, 1999). Regardless of the cause, these women feel like they are losing their minds (Beck, 1998a) and are at risk for many future problems, including but not limited to, damaged maternal–infant interaction, psychiatric problems, marital discord, and impaired cognitive development in their children (Beck, 1995a, 1998b; Jacobson, 1999; Milgrom et al., 1999).

Recent literature suggests an increase of comorbidity of obsessive-compulsive and panic disorders during the childbearing year (Beck, 1998a; Arnold et al., 1999). Arnold et al. (1999) present a review of literature that suggests a high prevalence of obsessive thoughts during pregnancy and worsening of pre-existing symptoms. Panic disorders may improve or worsen during the pregnancy but are more likely to exacerbate during the postpartum period. Beck's (1998a) research with mothers who had experienced panic disorders describes their feelings of being paralyzed and out of control, inability to think during the attack, and subsequent exhaustion secondary to their feverish attempt to maintain composure.

Postpartum psychosis is the most severe and potentially tragic end of the psychiatric spectrum for women after childbirth, occurring in one or two women per 1000 births (O'Hara, 1995; Arnold et al., 1999). Women with postpartum psychosis lose touch with reality, cannot function, and often experience hallucinations and/or delusions. It usually occurs closer to the time of birth, although it can arise later in the postpartum period. The dramatic symptomatology makes this disorder easier to recognize; however, it can remain undetected until serious harm has befallen the mother and/or infant. Postpartum psychosis is a true psychiatric emergency. Many women with postpartum psychosis have a strong family history of depression, bipolar mood disorder, and/or alcoholism (Sichel &

Driscoll, 1999). It may be a chemically-induced illness triggered by the vast drop in estrogen, which in turn precipitates a cascade of biochemical events (Chakravorty & Halbreich, 1997; Dorn & Chrousos, 1997; Hendrick et al., 1998). Attia et al. (1999) summarize a variety of other theories that may contribute to the psychosis, including marked thyroid hormone/antibody alteration, stress-related changes in cortisol and lipid metabolism, and melatonin cycles. Although postpartum psychosis is a concerning illness, the rest of this article will focus on postpartum depression. It is this illness that is so often silent and untreated until too late, despite its serious prevalence in the population.

Historical perspectives on screening for postpartum depression

The good news is that with careful screening postpartum depression can usually be predicted and identified early (Beck, 1996a; Sichel & Driscoll, 1999). The bad news is that few women's health care providers systematically screen for vulnerability to the disorder during the prenatal period, and even more rarely is depression screening a part of preconception health care. Retrospective examination of women's lives during the prenatal period is strewn with red flags that postpartum depression is likely to occur – yet the questions are often never asked!

There are several instruments that have been used historically to screen for depression. The Beck Depression Inventory-II (BDI-II) is a well-known instrument based on the American Psychological Association criteria for diagnosing depressive disorders in adults and adolescents (APA, 1994; Beck et al., 1996). One of the concerning issues with this 21-item, self-report instrument is that its assessment of fatigue and sleep problems does not reflect the experience of a mother with a young infant (Beck & Gable, 2000). The Edinburgh Postnatal Depression Scale (EPDS) (Cox et al., 1987) is a 10-item, self-report instrument specific for postpartum depression, in which a woman responds to items that describe how she has felt in the past week. Although the EPDS has been well tested in postpartum populations, it lacks specificity because its focus reflects a general depression scale, rather than placing symptoms in the context of new motherhood. This scale also contains both positive and negative stems on the items, which may cause confusion among the responses (Schmitt & Stults, 1985; Benson, 1987; Pilotte & Gable, 1990).

Beck and Gable (2000) compared both the BDI-II and EPDS to the results of Beck's (1992, 1993, 1995b, 1996a, b, 1998a) qualitative research findings with women who were diagnosed with postpartum depression and found a lack of items specific to women's personal descriptions of the experience in both instruments. The items missing include the frequent reports of loss of control, loneliness, unrealness, irritability, fear of going crazy, obsessive thinking, difficulty concentrating, and loss of self. Their conclusion was that the BDI-II and the EPDS lacked essential factors specific to a mother's experience of postpartum depression. Based on their findings, this article will present only the Beck screening instruments in detail.

The woman's experience of postpartum depression

The most vivid descriptions of the horrifying effects of postpartum are heard best through women's voices. A number of researchers have conducted qualitative research to this end. Beck (2002a) conducted a metasynthesis of 18 qualitative studies that focused on postpartum depression to collectively examine and interpret their findings. Metasynthesis provides an organized interpretive approach to a specific group of qualitative studies (Noblit & Hare, 1988). She identified four overarching themes reflecting women's perspectives and experiences of postpartum depression: (1) incongruity between expectations and the reality of motherhood, (2) spiraling downward, (3) pervasive loss, and (4) making gains toward recovery.

Women found the reality of motherhood shattered their expectations, sometimes plunging them into despair with a downward spiral into postpartum depression (Beck, 2002a). Beck (2002a) consistently found issues of role conflict across all the studies as women struggled for perfection. As the spiral continues, anxiety mounts, creating feelings of overwhelming panic, preventing sleep, and making women believe they are losing their minds:

It's terrible. It's like the worst thing you can imagine. Think of how you would feel if your husband or child had been hit by a car and killed. Well, it would be as bad as what I felt during an anxiety attack.
(Beck, 1992)

The feelings are so powerfully physical and obsessive that women report feeling enveloped and unable to escape:

It was like every nerve in my body was exploding. Like little fireworks were going off all over my body. I felt like I was going crazy. My skin felt like it was literally crawling. I wish I could rip it off and put it on another body. I would try and wipe my skin off.
(Beck, 1993)

A part of the spiraling downward phenomenon is consuming guilt. Women report being terrified they would hurt their child, all too aware that things are terribly wrong, yet not able to get help:

I would go to my baby's room and think, put the blanket over his head. He's nothing. Then I'd start crying hysterically. I felt like the worst person in the world, the worst mother in the world. I felt tremendous guilt and just wanted to hurt myself. (Beck, 1993)

The sense of loss and anguish is tremendous and can last a lifetime. Struggling to survive, women who sought help encountered a variety of responses from providers, some positive and some not. Several examples below demonstrate some women's experiences with providers and their need for someone to recognize what is happening, to muster resources, and to be there:

I was crying as hard as I could in the shower thinking that someone was going to admit me. Who was going to take care of my baby? At that point, the nurse from my obstetrician's office called me to see how I was. I didn't feel so alone then. (Beck, 1995c)

When I stopped by my nurse-midwife's office, all she had to do is ask one or two questions and the floodgates opened, and then it became obvious to her what was going on. (Beck, 1995c)

The pleas from women are clear – they need help when postpartum depression explodes, but more importantly, they are best served if their care provider takes steps to assess, initiate appropriate interventions and referrals, and hopefully prevent their downward spiral into despair. The following sections focus on the provider's role in this process.

Assessing women for postpartum depression

It is essential to detect postpartum depression early in its course so that women can benefit from earlier treatment. Early treatment has been shown to decrease the duration of the illness (England et al., 1994). Beck has developed two instruments to help providers (Beck, 1998c, 2001, 2002b; Beck & Gable, 2000). The first is used to help predict which women are vulnerable to the development of postpartum depression and can be administered during preconception care, the prenatal course, and in the postpartum period. The second is to screen for the actual presence of postpartum depression after childbirth (Beck & Gable, 2000).

Identifying vulnerability to postpartum depression before childbirth

To develop an instrument that would assist in the prediction of postpartum depression, Beck (1996a) first conducted a meta-analysis of 44 studies that examined predictors for postpartum depression. She first identified eight predictors significantly related to postpartum depression. These include prenatal depression, childcare

stress, life stress, lack of social support, prenatal anxiety, maternity blues, marital dissatisfaction, and history of previous depression. She developed the Postpartum Depression Predictors Inventory (PDPI) based on this meta-analysis, a critical review of the literature on predictors, and her prior qualitative work (Beck, 1995b, 1996a, 1998c). An updated version identified four more predictors, including low self-esteem, low socio-economic status, marital status (single), and unplanned/unwanted pregnancy (Beck, 2001, 2002b). Other potential risk factors are noted in a recent study by Joseffsson et al. (2002), who report an increase in sick leave during pregnancy and number of antenatal visits, mostly for psychiatric or medical complications, especially hyperemesis and premature contractions.

The PDPI is for use in the preconception, prenatal, and/or postpartum periods. It is designed to identify women who are vulnerable to the development of postpartum depression; as such, it is not diagnostic but rather helps the provider identify women potentially at risk. The PDPI is meant to be used as a guide for the interview between the woman and provider, rather than as a self-report instrument (Appendix A). Although there is not a cutoff score, the checklist does provide a list of factors that can be targeted for discussion and intervention when a positive response is elicited.

Screening for postpartum depression after childbirth

Working with an expert in psychometrics, Beck's next step was to merge the results of her qualitative studies to develop the *Postpartum Depression Screening Scale* (PDSS) (Beck & Gable, 2000, 2002). This instrument is designed to screen for postpartum depression after the woman has given birth. It has been well validated, is highly sensitive and specific, and measures seven dimensions of the woman's current experience that reflect a potential diagnosis of postpartum depression. These dimensions are listed in Table 7.2.1, and the instrument is available for purchase through Western Psychological Services.

The PDSS has been compared with the BDI-II and the EPDS (Beck & Gable, 2001a). It has been found to have both higher sensitivity and specificity than the BDI-II and EPDS. The difference lay in the ability to detect sleep disturbances, cognitive impairment, and anxiety (Beck & Gable, 2001b). The PDSS places the questions of sleep disturbances within the context of new motherhood. For example, one item asks specifically about whether the woman can sleep when her baby is sleeping (Beck & Gable, 2000). The way the item is worded is discriminatory for sleep, which is disturbed beyond that of attending to a young infant (Beck & Gable, 2001a). The EPDS does not measure cognitive impairment as a symptom, and the BDI-II does not address anxiety, both of which are important aspects of the symptomatology of postpartum depression and are different from general depression, which is not temporally associated with childbirth.

Guidance for screening in clinical practice

One of the reasons that postpartum depression so often goes undetected is that women are not prepared for the possibility that this might happen to them. Postpartum care is scant at best in the United States; therefore, the crack the woman falls into can become an abyss. The reasons that care providers do not screen have not been subject to research, but one factor may be a sense of inadequacy in dealing with depression. Because midwives and all women's health care providers are in an optimal position to become case finders for potential and actual postpartum depression, knowledge of depressive disorders is an essential clinical skill. This section begins a general approach to screening and caring for women with postpartum depression, with major points for the provider highlighted in Appendix B.

The first place to begin is during prenatal care and, if possible, during preconception care. The initial assessment should include a thorough history for vulnerability to postpartum depression. In addition to using the PDPI as a guide to the interview, Sichel and Driscoll (1999) note several other areas that should be addressed. These include a family history of mood disorders/mental illness. Asking a woman about a history of depression or psychiatric illness must be more probing that just a straightforward question. Many people are reluctant to admit to any experience of mental illness or disturbance. Therefore, they may interpret a question such as 'Have you ever experienced a psychiatric illness or depression?' as one that would require a major intervention, such as drugs or hospitalization, before they would answer yes. In reality, many people have experienced depression to some extent, but obtaining that specific history takes skill and practice. Questions to probe for a prior history of depression are given in Appendix B.

Sichel and Driscoll (1999) use an earthquake analogy to describe depression to their clients. Biochemistry, genetic traits, hormonal and reproductive factors, and life events all come together to provide a framework for vulnerability. When these are misaligned, a crack or 'fault' appears. New stress, such as the birth of a baby, can create 'tremors' from that crack, or potentially a full-blown 'earthquake' – postpartum depression. Knowledge of a woman's history of prior 'life tremors' is essential to assessing her risk for a future catastrophic postpartum depression. Sichel and Driscoll (1999) also focus on the biologic and neurologic components of the illness. Any woman who has shown

Table 7.2.1 Seven dimensions of Beck and Gable's Postpartum Depression Screening Scale (PDSS)*

Dimension†	Types of questions
Sleeping/eating dimensions	Difficulty with sleeping, loss of appetite
Anxiety/insecurity	Bodily sensations, loneliness, feeling overwhelmed
Emotional lability	Experience of different emotional states
Cognitive impairment	Ability to focus and concentrate
Loss of self	Feelings of being abnormal or sense of unrealness
Guilt/shame	Sense of failure, guilt or feeling ashamed
Contemplating harming oneself	Threat to self

*The PDSS is available in short and long versions with manual for purchase for use in clinical settings from the Western Psychological Services, 12031 Wilshire Boulevard, Los Angeles, CA 90025-1251 (800-648-8857 or www.wpspublish.com).
†The reliability estimated for this scale was between 0.8 and 0.9, reflecting that it is internally consistent and actually measures essential components of postpartum depression

prior disturbance in the hypothalamic–pituitary axis should be considered at risk for postpartum depression (Amino et al., 1982; Coplan et al., 1997; Drevets et al., 1997; Duman et al., 1997; Magiakou et al., 1997).

The PDPI is most helpful during the prenatal course and the PDSS after the birth. However, these are only screening instruments; once a screen is positive, a specific and accurate diagnosis must be made. If an assessment is made during the prenatal period that the woman is at risk for developing postpartum depression, she should be referred for further evaluation and potentially for treatment. The midwife or woman's care provider should develop a working relationship with the mental health clinician to collaboratively develop a care plan through pregnancy and into the postpartum period.

Diagnosis of postpartum depression

Successful treatment of postpartum depression depends first on making an accurate diagnosis. Health care professionals skilled in working with affective disorders should be involved in making a diagnosis of postpartum depression, ideally by those experienced with postpartum depression. This does not negate the primary care provider's role but does imply that there are specific boundaries that will help to ensure a safe outcome. An ideal model of care is one that is interdisciplinary, including mental health, women's health, medicine, pediatrics, nursing, nutrition, and social work. Postpartum depression is complex and affects many people in the woman's life; therefore, a team approach is most likely going to best serve her, as well as her family.

An accurate diagnosis of depression is essential. Tragic results are correlated with cavalier treatment of women thought to have postpartum depression, when in fact they had an occult bipolar disease (Sichel & Driscoll, 1999). When such women are placed on commonly used antidepressants, they are at risk for precipitation of a manic phase, or worse, a psychotic break. Providers must (1) know their knowledge limits and boundaries in the assessment and treatment of postpartum depression, (2) provide expert referral sources for care, and (3) link the woman with support systems within her community.

Initial triage of women in the postpartum period

When a woman is assessed to be vulnerable to postpartum depression, several decisions must be made: (1) how serious is the woman's condition and (2) what is the most appropriate plan of action? A common scenario is the exhausted woman who is struggling with maternity blues and has not slept for the first three nights after the birth. Lee et al. (2000b) note that excessive fatigue and sleep deprivation, which can mimic depressive symptoms, increases susceptibility for postpartum depression. Without sleep, she will only get worse; with restorative sleep, she has the potential to recover and perhaps prevent a downward spiral. The decision breakpoint in this situation is to assess her vulnerability. Her prior history of depression should be documented in her record; if not, it should be reassessed. Questions about her sleep patterns should minimally address: (1) problems with falling asleep, even with extreme fatigue and when others are caring for the baby; (2) excessive daytime sleepiness, and (3) regularity and duration of sleep (Lee et al., 2000b). Many women will describe themselves as so 'wired' that they cannot sleep at all (Wood et al., 1997).

Appendix B provides some checkpoints to assess her safety and whether strategies and resources can be used to help her get some sleep and rest within a safe environment, with close follow-up and referral as needed. However, the guiding principle always must be *when in doubt, consult and refer.*

If an assessment is made to treat her by altering the cycle of sleep deprivation, then there are several options available. Supportive measures are helpful if the sleep deprivation has lasted only three days; if it is beyond that, medication is more appropriate. A warm bath an hour before bedtime raises the core body temperature, which will stimulate a sleep response. Other things to try are massage, relaxation and meditation techniques, and help with infant care and feeding. The use of alcohol should be discouraged because it is a depressant and can actually cause a deregulation of sleep patterns (Landolt &

Gillen, 2001). It is also addictive and can become an ineffective and dangerous crutch for a woman who is fighting depression. Diphenhydramine (Benadryl; 25–50 mg) has been used by some providers as an over-the-counter medication for sleep during these first few days. This medication is secreted into the breast milk and, although levels in breast milk have not been reported, the manufacturer does not recommend its use while breastfeeding (Briggs et al., 2002). Ito et al. (1993) found that a small percentage of infants showed symptoms of irritability with antihistamines, but none required medical treatment. As with all medications, the risks and benefits must be carefully weighed and discussed with the mother, and the pediatric provider should be involved if she is breastfeeding.

Once the sleep deprivation has gone beyond three days, the woman will be in need of thoughtful, but purposeful, pharmacologic intervention. Clonazepam (Klonopin), as an antianxiety benzodiazepine, is a good choice of medication in this situation (Hendrick & Altshuler, 1997; Llewellyn & Stowe, 1998). Dosage is usually 0.25–0.5 mg at bedtime. The goal is to keep the dose under 1 mg if she is breastfeeding. Lorazepam (Ativan; 0.25–0.5 mg), which is shorter acting, can also be considered at bedtime. Common side-effects for both include drowsiness, ataxia, and confusion (Youngkin et al., 1999). When medication is used for such a very brief time period as this, it is prudent to use short-acting agents. Some consideration can be given to formula supplementation for the feeding when medication is active in the maternal system (Byrt et al., 2001); however, recommendations are widely varied, reflecting the incomplete state of the science of medicating women while breastfeeding. A more thorough discussion of the issues of psychotropic drug use with breastfeeding is provided under 'Psychopharmacology' below.

Once the woman has achieved four or five nights of good sleep, there should be significant improvement; if not, she must be referred to specialized care. Daily phone contact is essential to assess her progress, and she and her family need ready access to their provider in case the situation suddenly worsens.

Ongoing management of postpartum depression

A holistic and family-centered framework is best in caring for women with postpartum depression. How well this episode is handled will affect many future aspects of her life, including her self-esteem, her mothering ability, her children's lives and development, her career, and her relationships with her partner and family. Each woman is an individual and must have a plan that is personalized to her needs; however, the situation can deteriorate rapidly, so astute and timely intervention is essential. A key element of care is a medical evaluation that includes screening for thyroid disease, anemia, and diabetes, which can influence, or mimic, psychiatric symptoms (Arnold et al., 1999). This evaluation should occur concurrently with specialized mental health evaluation and treatment. There are three major themes in the treatment of postpartum depression that are reviewed: psychopharmacology, psychotherapy, and psychosocial care.

Psychopharmacology

Because most major depressive disorders have a biochemical component, the first line of treatment is usually psychopharmacology (Altshuler et al., 2001). One factor to consider is whether the woman is breastfeeding. Helping her to continue breastfeeding if she desires is preferable to weaning, even with some risk of the infant being exposed to medication via lactation (Sichel & Driscoll, 1999; Buist, 2001). Unfortunately, all psychotropic medications will be secreted in breast milk. Infants' neurologic systems and body fat ratios actually enhance their uptake of these drugs, so caution is always wise. However, the benefits of breastfeeding are also very important, so the risks and benefits must be carefully weighed. Burt et al. (2001) conducted a thorough review of the use of psychotropic medication in breastfeeding women since 1955 and found no controlled studies evaluating safety. This review is an excellent resource for providing information to parents about the current knowledge of these drugs. Providers who are knowledgeable and skilled in the use of psychotropic medications should be the prescribing clinicians for women with postpartum depression because close monitoring for side-effects and effectiveness is a critical component of care. Part of the interdisciplinary team caring for this woman should include a pediatric provider who can develop a plan of care for monitoring the infant.

The first drug of choice should be one that she may have used effectively in the past without adverse effects (Cohen, 2001). Women with a prior history of depression may have positive experiences with medications that can guide treatment postpartum (Sichel & Driscoll, 1999). The next choice is to consider tricyclic antidepressants. There are substantial data available for these medications and their relationship to long-term outcomes in children who were breastfed (Wisner et al., 1996; Nulman et al., 1997; Burt et al., 2001); therefore, this class of medication is often a good choice despite some of their side-effects. Side-effects of tricyclic antidepressants can include dry mouth, urinary retention, constipation, diarrhea, postural hypotension, nervousness, blurred vision, tachycardia, anxiety, nervousness, and sexual dysfunction (Youngkin et al., 1999). Because these drugs can take up to three to four weeks to become fully effective, it is helpful to combine them with an antianxiety medication such as clonazepam (Klonopin) or lorazepam (Ativan), especially because anxiety is a common symptom of postpartum depression. Antianxiety drugs act quickly and can provide the woman with initial relief and a sense of positive movement toward recovery.

The selective serotonin reuptake inhibitor (SSRI) agents have recently been found to be helpful in the treatment of postpartum depression, especially for those women with heightened anxiety. Data have been reported that the antidepressants sertraline (Zoloft) and paroxetine (Paxil) and their metabolites are either undetected or detected at very low serum concentrations in the baby's blood (Stowe et al., 1997; Hendrick et al., 2000; Misri et al., 2000). Misri et al. (2000) studied serum concentrations of paroxetine in 25 breastfed infants, finding levels below quantification with no short-term side-effects. Fluoxetine (Prozac) has been found to be in low serum concentrations in infant's blood. The dilemma with the use of Prozac is the long metabolic life of the medication, requiring more time for the drug to clear the system.

Data on the use of psychotropic medications and lactation are changing rapidly; therefore, clinicians must stay up to date with the latest recommendations. Although Buist (2001) urges caution, she states 'given the data on the adverse effects of depression and psychosis on mother–infant interaction and infant development, there is increased recognition of the importance of aggressively treating maternal depression postpartum'. She recommends an informed and shared decision between the mother and clinician, with input from the partner, and takes into consideration the age and health of the infant and the mother's desire to breastfeed. The infant should be carefully followed for sedation, weight gain, and developmental milestones. As with all medications, the risks, benefits, length of time until the drug becomes effective, and side-effects of the treatment (for mother and infant) regimen need to be carefully reviewed so the woman and her family can make an informed choice. The conversation should also be well documented in the medical record.

Psychotherapy

A concurrent dimension of treatment is psychotherapy, preferably with mental health clinicians skilled in caring for women with postpartum depression (Sichel & Driscoll, 1999). There are multiple approaches, but it should be aimed at supporting the woman through the crisis of the postpartum depression and then moving forward to help her deal with any underlying issues that might affect her full recovery. A significant factor for women with postpartum depression is a feeling of loss and grief. Women feel robbed of what was supposed to be a joyful time in their life; sometimes they can barely remember their child's infancy. They talk about the loss of their relationships, their ability to mother, and their own identity (Beck, 2002b). One woman summed it up succinctly by stating:

I feel robbed of the first six months of my daughter's life. I never really got to hold her as a baby and I feel cheated. (Beck, 1993)

Therapy must address this grief for women to heal. Therapeutic sessions should be frequent early in the illness, sometimes with daily phone calls. Because most psychiatric inpatient options in the United States do not offer overnight mother–baby care, outpatient care is preferable, unless the woman's safety is a major risk.

Psychosocial care

The third dimension of care is attending to the psychosocial factors in the woman's life. A woman with postpartum depression needs multidimensional supports to help her get well. It is this dimension in which the midwife or primary care provider can often be of most assistance. The establishment of a relationship and rapport during the prenatal period can provide continuity and connection in the postpartum period. This knowledge can help to identify resources that will meet the woman's and family's needs.

The family also becomes a client in postpartum depression; they too are at risk of destruction. Meighan (1999) conducted a phenomenologic study of fathers' experience with postpartum depression. Fathers described how their wives seemed to become alien. They also described their despair and anger as their world and dreams collapsed:

It amazed me to see my wife change overnight. It wasn't her … I knew it wasn't her. (Meighan, 1999)

I felt pushed to the edge – didn't know how to express it. I didn't like it … I was angry at the situation, angry at depression, angry at her for being depressed. (Meighan, 1999)

Like the woman with postpartum depression, fathers also felt lost, fearful, alone, and too often unsupported. Half of the sample described their fear of their wife's potential suicide:

… I might find her dead. I had to condition myself every day when I got home … if you go in and she's on the floor call 911 … (Meighan, 1999)

I felt like I was out there on my own, without anybody to guide me, or anybody to talk to. (Meighan, 1999)

The overriding goal is to get the woman with postpartum depression into a mentally healthy place to live and provide support to her and her family. Sometimes these are simple measures, such as mobilizing friends, family, and community for meal preparation and child care. Other times, more sophisticated measures are needed, such as a Temporary Disability Insurance (TDI) extension to provide more recovery time without depleting the family's finances.

Supportive measures for women experiencing depressive symptoms have been developed to guide the psychosocial care by Sichel and Driscoll (1999) and are referred to by the acronym 'NURSE'. The elements include nourishment and needs, understanding, rest and relaxation, spirituality, and exercise. The key is to draw on all that is known to help with depression; this includes attending to basic needs, as well as what is understood about mind–body physiology. Emphasis is given to fully supporting the family to help her recover. They should also be reminded to apply these same principles to themselves, as the helpers who are also in need of care.

Attending to a woman's nutrition is crucial, particularly because the combination of depression and coping with a new baby are likely to preclude her from eating well. A nutritional assessment should be conducted with recommendations as needed. If poor nutrition is a concern, a multivitamin per day should be encouraged, and the woman (or a member of her family) should be referred for nutritional counseling. Some promising research indicates that alpha-omega-3 fatty acids are implicated in nerve cell membrane health and can play a role in protecting against depression (Severus et al., 1999; Sichel & Driscoll, 1999; Barclay, 2002). These can be prescribed as supplements individualized to the woman's specific need and can also be obtained in foods rich in this food source. Barclay (2002) suggests tuna, salmon, algae, and limiting fish to 12 cooked ounces per week, as well as avoiding shark, swordfish, king mackerel, and tilefish to prevent mercury contamination.

Helping a woman to understand the multifaceted components of the illness can alleviate the guilt and shame she may experience with postpartum depression. A woman does not cause her postpartum depression; she is not to blame. Psychotherapy helps her to gain insight into the illness and to learn to cope and to grow beyond it. Sichel and Driscoll (1999) use spirituality as a way of understanding what helps the woman to feel uplifted and joyful. Working with the woman to reconnect with her spirituality can help her to draw on her inner strengths. Regular exercise will increase the body's mood-enhancing endorphins and will elevate T cells, which are part of the brain's immune function (Sichel & Driscoll, 1999). All of these combined can aid her recovery.

Summary and future directions

It is clear that postpartum depression is a serious and prevalent illness affecting a wide range of women for whom we provide care. Previous research indicates that it is predictable and treatable and that treatment is enhanced when it is identified early. The following quote summarizes the disappointment when a provider is not attentive to the woman's experience of PPD:

My doctor never told me about other women with postpartum depression. I was in the total dark the whole time. It wasn't until I started coming to the support group that I realized, for God's sake, that other women went through this! (Beck, 1993)

Women's health care providers must make judicious decisions about their role in the care of women with postpartum depression. The ideal approach is interdisciplinary, drawing on mental health, medicine, pediatrics, social work, nursing, family, and community support systems. All have potential to work collaboratively to enable the woman to heal.

There is a shocking lack of national progress toward humanistic and holistic care for women with postpartum depression. The frequent and appalling headlines that expound the devastating and violent ends when women drop over the edge and murder their children are usually condemning. However, a review of most of the cases reveal striking clues that the woman was in trouble and was, in fact, close to the edge – but no one noticed. Not only are health care providers in the United States slow to recognize and treat postpartum depression, specialists in the field and facilities geared specifically to its

treatment are almost nonexistent. Compare this to Great Britain, where recognition of severity of the condition resulted in the passage of a law in 1865 preventing women from being charged with infanticide in the first year postpartum (Semprevivo, 1990; Hamilton & Harberger, 1992; Brockington, 1996). Support for postpartum women in Great Britain is extended to mother–baby specialized care in further recognition that recovery for a mother is essential to maintain an intact family unit (Milgrom et al., 1999).

Midwives and women's health care providers must be the case finders and at the forefront of advocating for this group of women. It is too prevalent and significant a problem to ignore any more and must be on the national agenda. That comes from grass roots efforts, as well as political and professional mandates. However, it starts with us saying, 'Women deserve more'. One way to increase the strength of that voice is to design intervention research that provides evidence for improving outcomes by implementing consistent screening for postpartum depression, in addition to initiating an interdisciplinary and specialized treatment plan. The charge is ours to make a difference in the lives of these vulnerable women, to be the light in the fog.

Acknowledgements

The authors thank Judith Buongiorno Ellison for her thoughtful review of this manuscript, and for her pioneering work in establishing postpartum support groups in Rhode Island.

REFERENCES

Altshuler LL, Cohen LS, Moline ML, Kahn DA, Carpenter D, Docherty JP. 2001. Treatment of depression in women. The Expert Consensus Guideline Series. A Postgraduate Medicine Special Report: 2001. Postgrad Med, March, Spec. No.: 1–107

American Psychiatric Association. 1994. Diagnostic and Statistical Manual of Mental Disorders, 4th edn. American Psychiatric Association, Washington, DC

Amino N, Mori H, Iwatani I, Tanizawa O, Kawashima M, Tsuge I, Ibaragi K, Kamahara YP, Miyal K. 1982. High prevalence of transient postpartum thyrotoxicosis and hypothyroidism. N Engl J Med, 306: 849–852

Arnold AF, Baugh C, Fisher A, Brown J, Stowe ZN. 1999. Psychiatric aspects of the postpartum period. In: Miller LJ (ed.), Postpartum Mood Disorders, pp. 99–113. American Psychiatric Press, Washington, DC

Attia E, Downey J, Oberman M. 1999. Postpartum psychoses. In: Miller LJ (ed.), Postpartum Mood Disorders, pp. 99–117. American Psychiatric Press, Washington, DC

Barclay L. 2002. DHA fatty acids may reduce postpartum depression. MedscapeWire (Internet), cited 23 May. Available from: http://www.medscape.com?viewarticle/431587_print

Beck CT. 1992. The lived experience of postpartum depression: a phenomenological study. Nurs Res, 42: 166–170

Beck CT. 1993. Teetering on the edge: a substantive theory of postpartum depression. Nurs Res, 42: 42–48

Beck CT. 1995a. The effects of postpartum depression on maternal–infant interaction: a meta-analysis. Nurs Res, 44: 298–304

Beck CT. 1995b. Screening methods for postpartum depression. JOGNN, 24: 308–312

Beck CT. 1995c. Perceptions of nurses' caring by mothers experiencing postpartum depression. JOGNN, 24: 819–825

Beck CT. 1996a. A meta-analysis of predictors of postpartum depression. Nurs Res, 45: 297–303

Beck CT. 1996b. A concept analysis of panic. Arch Psych Nurs, 10: 265–275

Beck CT. 1998a. Postpartum onset of panic disorder. Image J Nurs Scholars, 30: 131–135

Beck CT. 1998b. The effects of postpartum depression on child development: a meta-analysis. Arch Psych Nurs, 12: 12–20

Beck CT. 1998c. A checklist to identify women at risk for developing postpartum depression. JOGNN, 27: 39–46

Beck CT. 2001. Predictors of postpartum depression. An update. Nurs Res, 50: 275–285

Beck CT. 2002a. Postpartum depression: a metasynthesis. Qual Health Res, 12: 469–488

Beck CT. 2002b. Revision of the postpartum depression predictors inventory. JOGNN, 31: 394–402

Beck CT, Gable RK. 2000. Postpartum depression screening scale: development and testing. Nurs Res, 49: 272–282

Beck CT, Gable RK. 2001a. Comparative analysis of the performance of the postpartum depression screening scale with two other depression instruments. Nurs Res, 50: 242–250

Beck CT, Gable RK. 2001b. Further validation of the postpartum depression screening scale. Nurs Res, 50: 155–164

Beck CT, Gable RK. 2002. Postpartum Depression Screening Scale Manual. Western Psychological Services, Los Angeles, CA

Beck CT, Steer R, Brown G. 1996. BDI-II Manual. Psychological Corporation, San Antonio, TX

Benson J. 1987. Detecting item bias in affective scales. Educ Psychol Meas, 47: 55–67

Briggs GG, Freeman RK, Yaffe SJ (eds). 2002. Drugs in Pregnancy and Lactation: A Reference Guide to Fetal and Neonatal Risk, 6th edn. Lippincott Williams & Williams, Philadelphia

Brockington IF. 1996. Motherhood and Mental Health. Oxford University Press, New York

Buist A. 2001. Treating mental illness in lactating women. Medscape Women's Health eJournal (Internet), 6: 1–7, cited 22 May. Available from: http://www.medscape.com/viewarticle/408939_print

Burt VK, Suri R, Altshuler L, Stowe Z, Hendrick VC, Muntean E. 2001. The use of psychotropic medications during breastfeeding. Am J Psych, 158: 1001–1009

Chakravorty SG, Halbreich U. 1997. The influence of estrogen on monoamine oxidase activity. Psychopharmacol Bull, 32: 229–233

Cohen L. 2001. Drugs, pregnancy, and lactation: treating postpartum depression. OBGYN News, 1 February

Coplan JD, Pine DS, Papp LA, Gorman JA. 1997. A view of noradrenergic hypothalamic–pituitary–adrenal axis and extrahypothalmic corticotrophin-releasing factor function in anxiety and affective disorders: the reduced growth hormone response to clonidine. Psychopharmacol Bull, 33: 193–204

Cox JL, Holden JM, Sagovsky R. 1987. Detection of postnatal depression: development of the 10-item Edinburgh Postnatal Depression Scale. Br J Psych, 150: 472–476

Dorn LD, Chrousos GP. 1997. The neurobiology of stress: understanding regulation of affect during female biological transition. Semin Reprod Endocrinol, 15: 19–35

Drevets RS, Price JL, Simpson JR, Todd RD, Reich T, Raichel ME. 1997. Subgenual prefrontal cortex abnormalities in mood disorders. Nature, 386: 824–827

Duman RS, Heninger GR, Nestler EJ. 1997. A molecular and cellular theory of depression. Arch Gen Psychiatry, 54: 597–606

England SJ, Ballard C, George S. 1994. Chronicity in postnatal depression. Eur J Psych, 8: 93–96

Hamilton JA, Harberger PN. 1992. Postpartum Psychiatric Illness: A Picture Puzzle. University of Pennsylvania Press, Philadelphia

Hendrick VC, Altshuler LL. 1997. Management of breakthrough panic symptoms during pregnancy. J Clin Psychopharmacol, 17: L228–L229

Hendrick V, Altshuler LL, Suri R. 1998. Hormonal changes in the postpartum and implications for postpartum depression. Psychosomatics, 39: 93–101

Hendrick V, Stowe ZN, Altshuler LL, Hostetter A, Fukuchi A. 2000. Paroxetine use during breastfeeding. J Clin Psychopharmacol, 20: 587–589

Ito S, Blajchman A, Stephenson M, Eliopou C, Koren G. 1993. Prospective follow-up of adverse reactions in breast-fed infants exposed to maternal medication. Am J Obstet Gynecol, 168: 1393–1399

Jacobson T. 1999. Effects of postpartum disorders on parenting and on offspring. In: Miller LJ (ed.), Postpartum Mood Disorders, pp. 119–139. American Psychiatric Press, Washington, DC

Josefsson A, Angelsiöö L, Berg G, Ekström CM, Gunnervik C, Nordin C, Sydsjö G. 2002. Obstetric, somatic, and demographic risk factors for postpartum depressive symptoms. Obstet Gyenecol, 99: 223–228

Kennedy B, Sutterfield K. 2001. Postpartum depression. Medscape Psychiatry and Mental Health eJournal (Internet), 6: 1–7, cited 22 May. Available from: http://www.medscape.com/viewarticle/408688_print

Landolt HP, Gillen JC. 2001. Sleep abnormalities during abstinence in alcohol-dependent patients: aetiology and management. CNS Drugs, 15: 413–425

Lee KA, Zaffke ME, McEnany G. 2000a. Parity and sleep patterns during and after pregnancy. Obstet Gynecol, 95: 14–18

Lee KA, McEnany G, Zaffke ME. 2000b. REM sleep and mood state in childbearing women: sleepy or weepy? Sleep, 23: 877–885

Llewellyn A, Stowe ZN. 1998. Psychotropic medications in lactation. J Clin Psych, 59(Suppl. 2): 41–53

Magiakou MA, Mastorakos G, Webster E, Chorousos GP. 1997. The hypothalamic–pituitary–adrenal axis and the female reproductive system. Ann NY Acad Med, 816: 42–56

Meighan M. 1999. Living with postpartum depression: the father's experience. MCN, 24: 202–208

Milgrom J, Martin PR, Negri LM. 1999. Treating Postnatal Depression: A Psychological Approach for Health Care Practitioners. John Wiley, New York

Miller LJ, Rukstalis M. 1999. Beyond the "blues". Hypotheses about postpartum reactivity. In: Miller LJ (ed.), Postpartum Mood Disorders, pp. 3–19. American Psychiatric Press, Washington, DC

Misri S, Kim J, Riggs KW, Kostaras X. 2000. Paroxetine levels in postpartum depressed women, breast milk, and infant serum. J Clin Psychopharmacol, 61: 828–832

Noblit GW, Hare RD. 1988. Meta-ethnography: Synthesizing Qualitative Studies. Sage, Newbury Park, CA

Nulman I, Rovet J, Steward DE, Wolpin J, Gardner HA, Theis JGW, Kulin N, Koren G. 1997. Neurodevelopment of children exposed in utero to antidepressant drugs. N Engl J Med, 336: 258–262

O'Hara MW. 1995. Postpartum Depression: Causes and Consequences. Springer-Verlag, New York

O'Hara MW, Swain AM. 1996. Rates and risk of postpartum depression – a meta-analysis. Int Rev Psych, 8: 37–54

Parry BL. 1999. Postpartum depression in relation to other reproductive cycle mood changes. In: Miller LJ (ed.), Postpartum Mood Disorders, pp. 21–45. American Psychiatric Press, Washington, DC

Pilotte WJ, Gable RK. 1990. The impact of positive and negative item stems on the validity of a computer anxiety scale. Educ Psychol Meas, 50: 603–610

Ray KL, Hodnett ED. 2001. Caregiver support for postpartum depression (Cochrane Review). In: The Cochrane Library, Issue 3. Update Software, Oxford

Schmitt N, Stults DM. 1985. Factors defined by negatively keyed items: the result of careless respondents? Appl Psychol Meas, 9: 367–373

Semprevivo DM (ed.). 1990. Postpartum Depression. NAACOG Clinical Issues in Perinatal and Women's Health Nursing. Lippincott, Philadelphia

Severus WE, Ahrens B, Stoll AL. 1999. Omega-3 fatty acids – the missing link? Arch Gen Psychiatry, 56: 380–381

Sichel D, Driscoll JW. 1999. Women's Moods: What Every Woman Must Know About Hormones, The Brain, and Emotional Health. William Morrow, New York

Stowe ZN, Owens MJ, Landry JC, Kilts CD, Ely T, Llewellyn A, Nemeroff CB. 1997. Sertraline and desmethylsertraline in human breast milk and nursing infants. Am J Psych, 154: 1255–1260

Wisner KL, Perel JM, Findling RL, Hinne RL. 1996. Nortriptyline and its hydroxymetabolites in breast-feeding mothers and newborns. Psychopharmacol Bull, 33: 249–251

Wood AF, Thomas SP, Dropplemann PG, Meighan M. 1997. The downward spiral of postpartum depression. MCN, 22: 308–317

Youngkin EQ, Sawin KJ, Kissinger JF, Israel DS. 1999. Pharmacotherapeutics: A Primary Care Clinical Guide. Appleton & Lange, Stamford, CT

Appendices

Appendix A: Postpartum Depression Predictors Inventory (PDPI) – revised and guide questions for its use

During Pregnancy

Marital status	Check one	
1. Single	☐	
2. Married/co-habitating	☐	
3. Separated	☐	
4. Divorced	☐	
5. Widowed	☐	
6. Partnered	☐	

Socio-economic status		
Low	☐	
Middle	☐	
High	☐	

Self-esteem	Yes	No
Do you feel good about yourself as a person?	☐	☐
Do you feel worthwhile?	☐	☐
Do you feel you have a number of good qualities as a person?	☐	☐

Prenatal depression		
1. Have you felt depressed during your pregnancy?	☐	☐
If yes, when and how long have you been feeling this way?		
If yes, how mild or severe would you consider your depression?		

Prenatal anxiety		
Have you been feeling anxious during your pregnancy?	☐	☐
If yes, how long have you been feeling this way?		

Unplanned/unwanted pregnancy		
Was the pregnancy planned?	☐	☐
Is the pregnancy unwanted?	☐	☐

History of previous depression		
1. Before this pregnancy, have you ever been depressed?	☐	☐
If yes, when did you experience this depression?		
If yes, have you been under a physician's care for this past depression?		
If yes, did the physician prescribe any medication for your depression?		

	Yes	No
Social support		
Do you feel you receive adequate emotional support from your partner?	☐	☐
Do you feel you receive adequate instrumental support from your partner (e.g. help with household chores or babysitting)?	☐	☐
Do you feel you can rely on your partner when you need help?	☐	☐
Do you feel you can confide in your partner?	☐	☐
(repeat same questions for family and again for friends)		
Marital satisfaction		
Are you satisfied with your marriage (or living arrangement)?	☐	☐
Are you currently experiencing any marital problems?	☐	☐
Are things going well between you and your partner?	☐	☐
Life stress		
Are you currently experiencing any stressful events in your life such as:		
financial problems	☐	☐
marital problems	☐	☐
death in the family	☐	☐
serious illness in the family	☐	☐
moving	☐	☐
unemployment	☐	☐
job change	☐	☐
After Delivery, Add the Following Items		
Child care stress		
Is your infant experiencing any health problems?	☐	☐
Are you having problems with your baby feeding?	☐	☐
Are you having problems with your baby sleeping?	☐	☐
Infant temperament		
Would you consider your baby irritable or fussy?	☐	☐
Does your baby cry a lot?	☐	☐
Is your baby difficult to console or soothe?	☐	☐
Maternity blues		
Did you experience a brief period of tearfulness and mood swings during the first week after delivery?	☐	☐

COMMENTS:

Appendix B: Essential strategies for identification and management of postpartum depression

Preconception, prenatal, and postpartum assessment for vulnerability for postpartum depression

Key points	Resources
• Women with prior history of depression, depression during pregnancy, child care stress, life stress, lack of social support, prenatal anxiety, maternity blues, marital dissatisfaction, low self-esteem, low socio-economic status, single, and an unplanned or undesired pregnancy have the greatest vulnerability. • Assist the woman to garner resources to help her manage sources of stress. • Referral for mental health care if she has a history of depression or is currently depressed.	Postpartum Depression Predictors Inventory (PDPI) (see Appendix A) Probing questions to elicit a history of depression: Have you had … • Any history of depression, requiring medication or not? • Episodes of emotional changes such as tearfulness? • Extreme feelings of high and low? • Problems sleeping, such as not being able to fall asleep, or awakening in the night and not being able to go back to sleep? • Feelings of anxiety or panic? • Problems with headaches or stomach disorders? • Constant fatigue that was not related to a medical problem? • Counseling or therapy? • Stressful times in your life? • Thoughts of harming yourself?

Specific screening for postpartum depression

Key points	Resources
• Screening is an ongoing process and should be conducted by all clinicians who come into contact with a woman with a young infant. • If a woman is assessed to be vulnerable to the development of postpartum depression she should be formally screened. • Referral for diagnostic evaluation if she screens positive, including mental health evaluation by clinician, experienced in postpartum depression, and a medical evaluation.	Postpartum Depression Screening Scale (Beck & Gable, 2002) Available from: Western Psychological Services, 12031 Wilshire Boulevard, Los Angeles, CA 90025-1251 (800-648 8857 or www.wpspublish.com). This comes with manual and short and long versions. Client handout

Triage and care for women with sleep deprivation in the early postpartum period

Key points	Resources
• Assessing the difference between maternity blues (which can be complicated by sleep deprivation) and actual postpartum depression is critical. • Lack of sleep can mimic symptoms of depression, as well as increase a woman's vulnerability for moving into a depressive episode. • Breaking the cycle of sleep deprivation is essential in helping her restore normal functioning. • Enlisting the support of family is very important.	Postpartum Depression Predictors Inventory (PDPI) (see Appendix A) Checkpoints to assess her safety: • Is she safe? • Can someone remain with her at all times? • Is she at risk for suicide or homicide? • Who and what are her resources? • Can her family, partner, friends provide the care she needs, and will they call for help if they feel they cannot handle the situation?

Management of postpartum depression

Key points	Resources
• Should be under the guidance of an experienced mental health clinician. • Midwives and women's health clinicians are essential for helping woman maintain breastfeeding and family support. • Can include pharmacology, psychotherapy, and psychosocial care, or combination.	Client handout ACNM website for resources and bibliography on postpartum depression (www.midwife.org) American Psychiatric Association (www.psych.org) Books: • Sichel D, Driscoll JW. 1999. Women's Moods: What Every Woman Should Know About Hormones, The Brain, and Emotional Health. William Morrow, New York. Videotapes: • *Fragile Beginnings, Diapers and Delirium* – Driscoll JW • *Postpartum: A Bittersweet Experience* – Driscoll JW Support groups: Depression After Delivery (DAD) Telephone: 800-944-4773 Website: www.depressionafterdelivery.com Postpartum Support International Telephone: 805-967-7636 Website: www.postpartum.net

Journal of Midwifery and Women's Health 2002;
47(5): 318–330

Hands off! The Breastfeeding Best Start project (1)

Sally Inch, Susan Law, Louise Wallace

Human milk has evolved over many thousands of years to meet the specific needs of human infants ... not surprisingly, therefore, the more that is known about the nutritional, immunological and other properties of breast milk, the more superior it appears in comparison with all other available milks for human babies.
(RCM, 2002)

Fundamental to successful breastfeeding is the mother's ability to attach her baby to her breast in a way that results in pain-free feeding for her and effective milk removal by her baby.

The extent to which this is not achieved by many of the women who want to breastfeed is catalogued every five years in the Infant Feeding reports. The major reasons mothers give for ceasing to breastfeed earlier than they had intended are sore nipples and an apparent insufficiency of milk.

In 2000, 69% of all those who gave birth in the UK started to breastfeed. One in five of these women had given up within two weeks of the birth, citing sore nipples (28%) and insufficient milk (40%) as reasons (Hamlyn et al., 2002). In the vast majority of cases, the underlying cause of both conditions is poor attachment.

The challenge for health professionals is to reduce this huge attrition rate by assisting mothers to acquire, as speedily as possible, the skills necessary to carry out this learnt, manual task.

This article reports on the Breastfeeding Best Start (BSB) project, which sought to identify whether midwives could be successfully trained in a 'hands-off' technique, and whether that would translate into a higher number of women continuing to breastfeed.

The current situation

In order to support new mothers, the midwife needs to have a clear understanding of how a baby breastfeeds. She needs to appreciate the contribution that the position of the baby's body relative to the mother's makes to the mother's ability to attach her baby to her breast correctly. She also needs to know in detail how the mother should bring the baby to the breast in order to attach in a manner that will result in pain-free, efficient feeding.

However, there is currently no mandatory requirement for the knowledge and skills necessary to enable women to breastfeed successfully to be included in midwifery training, either as part of the EU Midwives Directive EEC 891594 or the (now defunct) ENB/UKCC. The quality and amount of teaching on breastfeeding depends entirely on the teaching institution. This deficiency is now being addressed in part by the Unicef UK Baby Friendly Initiative's Best Practice Standards for breastfeeding education provided to midwifery and health visiting students, which was launched in the summer of 2002 (Radford, 2003).

The Unicef UK Baby Friendly Initiative proposed that sufficient breastfeeding training and learning outcomes should be included within the core curriculum to equip students with the knowledge and skills to implement the 'Ten Steps to Successful Breastfeeding' and/or the 'Seven Point Plan for Protecting, Promoting and Supporting Breastfeeding in Community Health Care Settings' and to support informed decision-making.

A minimum of 18 hours training would be required for all student midwives and health visitors. At least 80% of sampled students should be able to answer basic questions on breastfeeding correctly.

The case for 'hands-off' help

Ultimately, a mother needs to be able to attach her baby to her breast herself. However, what frequently happens in hospital when a mother asks for help is that the midwife attaches the baby for her. Sometimes, this is because the mother is demonstrably unable to attach her baby herself yet, but often it is easier and quicker than teaching her.

Box 7.3.1 Training programme

This training programme enabled the experimental group of midwives to deliver the required practical education.

(a) Verbal interaction with mothers

All mothers involved were asked to call a midwife when their baby was ready for his/her first feed on the postnatal ward. If the mother was allocated to a midwife from the experimental group, that midwife would then go to her bedside and:

- Greet the mother and introduce herself.
- Give her an explanation of the sequence of events and purpose of the intervention, which would last about 45 minutes.

The midwife would explain that:

- The session would be a practical instruction to enable the mother to correctly position and attach her baby to her own breast.
- A verbal check would be made to ensure that the mother knew that the baby was correctly attached (see below).
- A written information sheet would be given as a reminder (see below).

At the end of the session, the mother was given a feed diary and asked to fill it in every day for the next six weeks. The midwife also reminded the mother that a researcher would contact her at home when her baby was six weeks old.

(b) Midwives' training

In order to be able to deliver this verbal intervention, midwives who had been randomly allocated to the experimental group took part in a four-hour training programme. This consisted of:

1 A 10-minute session to hone their verbal skills. For example, a pair of midwives would sit back to back. One was given a picture of rectangles and circles and asked to describe it to the other midwife in a way that would permit her to draw it without seeing it.

2 An anatomy and physiology update to increase understanding of how a baby breastfeeds, using acetates and video:

- The internal anatomy of the breast.
- The action of a baby's tongue when milking the breast.
- The way in which a baby gapes to receive the breast.
- The external appearance of a well-attached and poorly attached baby.
- The average amounts of milk taken per feed, in each 24-hour period from birth.
- The average feed frequency from birth to seven days.
- The variation in the rates of milk transfer and therefore feed length.

3 Explanation of positioning for the mother and the baby, using acetates, video and other aids to emphasise:

- The position of the mother (sitting up only for the purposes of the study).
- The relationship of the baby to the breast.
- The relationship of the baby to the mother's body:
  across lap – same arm as breast
  across lap – opposite arm as breast
  underarm – on side of bed
  underarm – using two chairs at right angles.

4 Teaching the mother how to attach her baby to her breast by herself. The following aspects were included:

- Supporting the breast (if necessary).
- Extending the baby's head slightly.
- Keeping the breast still and moving the baby's mouth against the mother's nipple to elicit the gape reflex.
- Moving the baby to the breast as the baby responds.
- Bringing the baby to the breast with the chin leading.
- Aiming the baby's bottom lip as far from the base of the nipple as possible.

5 An 11-point checklist (viewed as an acetate), in answer to the question, 'How do you know if it's right?' This would help the mother and the midwife to know when attachment was correct. This was also reproduced in the written information sheet that would be left with the mother at the end of the session:

- 'It should not hurt. If your nipple hurts when you are feeding it is probably not quite right. Take your baby off the breast and start again. If you leave your baby on the breast when your nipple is hurting, your nipple will become sore.
- Your baby starts to suckle almost immediately.
- Your baby's sucking pattern changes from quick, short sucks to slow, deep sucks.
- Your baby is relaxed and will remain so until the very end of the feed.
- Your baby will pause from time to time during feeding and then start sucking again without having to be prodded or coaxed.
- Your baby can breathe easily without the need for you to press your breast away from your baby's nose.
- Your baby's chin is in close contact with your breast.
- Your baby's mouth looks wide open.
- If you can see any of the dark part on your breast, there is more visible above your baby's top lip than below the bottom lip.
- Your baby will let go of the breast spontaneously when he has finished, or can be encouraged to fall away if the breast is gently raised.
- When your baby has come off the breast, your nipple should be the same shape as it was before the feed started. If your nipple has been compressed it was not far enough back in the baby's mouth.'

6 The trainers also went through the wording on the information sheet to be left with the mother (this was further clarified in the training session by means of video clips):

- 'Sit yourself comfortably, preferably in a chair so that you have some back support, and so that your back is straight and your lap almost flat. You may need to put your feet on a footstool.
- If it is helpful to wrap your baby, wrap him so that his arms are lying at his side, not across his chest, so that he can get closer to your breast.
- Support your baby, on a pillow if necessary, in such a way that his nose, not his mouth, is in line with your nipple before the feed begins.
- Hold your baby's body in such a way that he is able to come up to the breast from below, so that his top eye could make contact with yours.
- If you need to support your breast, do so by placing your fingers flat on your ribcage, at the junction of your breast and ribs, with your thumb uppermost. Remember to keep your breast still.
- Support your baby's head and shoulders in such a way that his head is free to extend slightly as he is brought to the breast – so that his chin and lower jaw reach the breast first.
- Move your baby against the breast so that his mouth touches the nipple, in order to elicit the gape. Do not move your breast against your baby's mouth.
- Aim your baby's bottom lip as far away as possible from the base of the nipple when he gapes, so that he scoops in as much breast as possible with his tongue.'

It has been suggested that mothers who have 'hands-off' help in the early days are more likely to be breastfeeding at six weeks postpartum than those who have 'hands-on' support (Benjamin, 1999; Carson, 1999; Napier, 2000; Fletcher & Harris, 2000; Ingram et al., 2002).

When the project began, the only previous randomised controlled trial that had been conducted to test this hypothesis was Christine Carson's unpublished study (Carson, 1999). In 1997, Carson began a pilot study of 60 mothers, randomly allocating them to receive 30 minutes of verbal guidance on positioning and attachment at their bedside within 36 hours of birth. She subsequently found that, compared with the control group who received 'normal care', the mothers for whom she provided hands-off care, at a time when the baby was ready to feed, were more than twice as likely to be still breastfeeding at two weeks postpartum – the study's end point.

(Immediately prior to this, Carson had been a breastfeeding specialist. She was also able to provide the intervention free of the usual constraints attendant on midwives working on a busy postnatal ward.)

The launch of the BSB project

The purpose of the project was to see if midwives who were not employed in a specialist role could replicate these results in a standard clinical setting. Commissioned by the Department of Health's Infant Feeding Initiative, the project was launched at a major conference for National Breastfeeding Awareness Week in 2001 entitled 'Inequalities in Breastfeeding – Bridging the Gap'. The research questions (see below) were formulated by the Initiative (Carson, 2001). Following a competitive tendering exercise, advertised Europe-wide, a team from Coventry University, led by Louise Wallace, were awarded the funding to conduct this trial.

Research questions

Because the quality and amount of pre-registration training is currently so variable, it was not possible to assume a minimum level of prior knowledge of breastfeeding of participants. The study was thus designed to answer two questions:

1. Can midwives be skilled to educate mothers who have chosen to breastfeed in the first 24 hours of the postnatal period?

In order to answer this question, the experimental group completed the training programme described in Box 7.3.1.

2. If a knowledgeable midwife gives practical education within the first 24 hours postnatally, will this increase the duration of breastfeeding?

(Results for this question have been published elsewhere and are not reported here.)

Acknowledgement

This work was supported by the Department of Health Infant Feeding Initiative.

REFERENCES

Benjamin M. 1999. Survey of Infant Feeding Practices in Warwickshire 1997/98. Audit Report, p. 23. Conducted by the Clinical Effectiveness Department, Warwick Hospital. Available from: South Warwickshire Dietetic Service Health Promotion Dept, 19 Waterloo Place, Warwick Street, Leamington Spa

Carson C. 1999. Investigation into the use of a planned educational intervention on the duration of breastfeeding in primiparous mothers. Unpublished Masters thesis, Faculty of Health and Community Care, University of Central England, Birmingham

Carson C. 2001. How is the government going to raise breastfeeding rates? British Journal of Midwifery, 9(5): 292–293

Fletcher D, Harris H. 2000. The implementation of the HOT program at the Royal Women's Hospital. Breastfeeding Review, 8(1): 19–23

Hall Moran V, Dinwoodie K, Bramwell R, Dykes F, Foley P. 1999. The development and validation of the Breastfeeding Support Skills Tool (BeSST). Clinical Effectiveness in Nursing, 3: 151–155

Hamlyn B, Brooker S, Oleinikova K, Wands S. 2002. Infant Feeding 2000: A Survey Conducted on Behalf of the Department of Health, the Scottish Executive, the National Assembly for Wales and the Department of Health, Social Services and Public Safety in Northern Ireland. TSO, London. Reported in: Brooker S. 2002. Infant Feeding Survey 2000. The Practising Midwife, 5, 24–26

Ingram J, Johnson D, Greenwood R. 2002. Breastfeeding in Bristol: teaching good positioning, and support from fathers and families. Midwifery, 1(2): 87–101

Moran VH, Bramwell R, Dykes F, Dinwoodie K. 2000. An evaluation of skills acquisition on the WHO/Unicef Breastfeeding Management Course using the pre-validated Breastfeeding Support Skills Tool (BeSST). Midwifery, 16(3): 197–203

Napier D. 2000. Breastfeeding initiation: benefits of the hands off technique. BMJ, 321: 467e (electronic letter)

Radford A. 2003. Baby friendly education standards. The Practising Midwife, 6(1): 32–33

The Practising Midwife 2003; 6(10): 17–19

Hands off! The Breastfeeding Best Start project (2)

Sally Inch, Susan Law, Louise Wallace

Design

Four hospitals in three trusts took part. Approval was obtained from all three of the relevant ethics committees. Eligible midwives at each site were invited to take part. They were then randomly allocated to receive (or not to receive) breastfeeding training. Those who received the training were the 'experimental arm' and those who did not were the 'control arm'. Midwives allocated to the control arm, and midwives who declined to take part in the study, were offered the training course at the end of the trial.

Eligible midwives were all those likely to work on the postnatal ward in any of the hospitals between May and October 2001. These formed the first wave. When the recruitment period was extended, a second wave was included with the same criteria, so that the inclusion period matched the length of the period of mother recruitment. There were about 320 midwives eligible at the first wave of the trial and approximately a further 45 at the second wave. Ultimately, 108 midwives took part.

The midwives were treated as research participants. They were stratified for grade as a proxy for experience (E grade and below versus F and above), full- or part-time contract, permanent or temporary, and working nights or not. Once a midwife had consented to enter the trial, the University of Birmingham Clinical Trials Unit randomly allocated her to either the control or the experimental arm, with no input from midwives, managers or researchers. Once allocated, midwives could not change groups. Randomisation was blind. Allocation was not blind to midwives once allocated, since staff needed to know the group assignment to ensure at least one from each arm was available to a mother at randomisation. Mothers, however, were blind to allocation.

When the midwives in the experimental group had received their training, new mothers (who had consented antenatally to participate) could be randomly allocated to receive help with their first feed on the postnatal ward from either an experimental or a control group midwife.

Procedure

The midwives were given an outline of the trial procedure. They were told that:

1. Mothers and babies would be assessed as eligible for the trial as they were admitted to the postnatal ward. The study included all first-time mothers who wished to breastfeed, and who were likely to be well enough to sit up to breastfeed. (This excluded those whose babies were in special care baby units or women who had had a general anaesthetic and/or caesarean.) Eligible mothers would be asked by the midwife to confirm their consent. The midwife would then enter their names into the computer.

2. All trial mothers would be asked by the admitting midwife to call her when they were ready to breastfeed.

3. When the mother called, the admitting midwife would find the midwife allocated (experimental or control group) by pressing a button on the computer to trigger randomisation. She would then inform the relevant midwife.

4. If an experimental group midwife was selected, she would collect a sealed envelope containing the data and information sheets, pick up a feeding diary for the mother and follow the protocol.

5. If a control group midwife was selected, she would follow her normal practice. Once the first feed was complete, she would give the mother a copy of the feeding diary.

6. Once the first feed was over, the mother would receive all other care from the midwife to whom she had been allocated for the shift.

7. Midwives in the experimental group would be asked to complete a simple checklist (data sheet) to indicate how far the new approach had been applied, and any special circumstances that needed to be taken into account.
8. All midwives with trial mothers would ask them to keep a daily breastfeeding diary for six weeks.

At the end of the training session, the experimental group midwives were each given a hard copy of the information sheet, the feeding diary and the data collection sheet.

It was stressed that to avoid 'contamination' they should not discuss training, protocol, the data collection sheet or the information sheet with colleagues in the control group. Only the feeding diary would be common to both groups.

Devising, administering and scoring

The programme

The training programme was devised by Sally Inch (John Radcliffe Hospital site, Oxford Radcliffe Trust), in collaboration with Naomi Morton (Horton site, Oxford Radcliffe Trust), and the package was taken for discussion with all the trainers before being distributed.

The programme was repeated until all the recruited midwives had been trained. At the completion of the trial, the training programme was offered to all the midwives in the control group.

The trainers

There were seven trainers on the project, who instructed the experimental group midwives (sites are in brackets):

- Beth Graham and Alison White (John Radcliffe Hospital site, Oxford Radcliffe Trust)
- Naomi Morton and Collette Fisher (Horton site, Oxford Radcliffe Trust)
- Sue Aucutt and Majella Johnston (University Hospitals, Coventry and Warwickshire NHS Trust)
- Sally Davies (Warwick Hospital, South Warwickshire General Hospitals NHS Trust).

At all sites, the trainers had completed the 18-hour Unicef UK Baby Friendly Initiative's training programme within the last three years, all had considerable experience in dealing with breastfeeding mothers and were currently leading in-service training in breastfeeding management.

The number of midwives present in each training group session varied from two to eight, depending on the site. This slightly affected the way in which the package was taught, with more or less time spent on different aspects in response to the perceived needs of the trainees.

Scoring system

In order to answer the first of the questions ('Can midwives be skilled to educate mothers who have chosen to breastfeed in the first 24 hours of the postnatal period?'), the researchers needed a previously validated method of determining whether the training had increased the knowledge base of the midwives.

This was kindly provided by Victoria Hall Moran who, along with co-workers at the University of Central Lancashire (UCL), had developed and validated a questionnaire, to be used in conjunction with video clips, to assess the effectiveness of the BFI training programme (details of the assessment tool and the validation process can be found in Hall Moran et al., 1999 and Moran et al., 2000).

Nine of the 11 (open-ended) UCL questions were directly applicable to the Breastfeeding Best Start (BSB) training. The remaining two related to practice issues beyond the scope of the four-hour programme, so two alternative questions were asked. The participants were asked to fill in the questionnaire both immediately before and immediately after they received training.

The completed (anonymous) 'pre' and 'post' questionnaires from each training session were sent to an independent assessor for marking – Susan Law at Coventry University – using the UCL scoring system devised by Hall Moran et al. (1999). Following the initial scoring, a random sample of 20% (22/108) was second-marked by a colleague. This showed only one discrepancy out of 704 mark pairs considered (less than 0.15% disagreement), which was immediately resolved between the markers and the score adjusted. This demonstrated a high level of inter-rater reliability.

Eliminating the 'practice' effect

To ensure that the differences between the pre- and post-training scores were not simply due to the effect of being presented with the same questionnaire for a second time, a group of 27 volunteer student midwives filled in the questionnaire twice, with an interval of four hours between each attempt, but with no other additional breastfeeding instruction or information.

The difference in score rating between the two exposures without any intervening training was compared with that obtained before and after the training programme. This demonstrated that the 'practice effect' of completing the questionnaire twice was minimal, but the effect of the training was to produce a highly significant increase in the post-training score.

In summary, the scores obtained after exposure to the training package showed a large mean increase for participants at all sites, irrespective of experience, clinical grade, qualifications or post-registration study.

Full details of the statistical analysis of the data from the questionnaire will be published elsewhere.

Implications for practice

The overall results of this part of the BSB project show that the study participants did achieve significantly higher breastfeeding knowledge scores following exposure to the training package. It can be concluded that all groups of midwives can be trained with a short and focused training workshop to improve their skills for support of breastfeeding women. It also suggests that the training package is sufficiently robust not to be affected by differences in the teaching environment or by the trainers' individual teaching styles.

What remains to be established (pending the results) is whether providing hands-off care at the time of the first feed on the postnatal ward has any impact on the subsequent duration of breastfeeding (Henderson et al., 2001), or whether the apparent correlation between early hands-off care (Benjamin, 1999) and increased breastfeeding duration is an artefact of maternal recall or a marker for innate manual dexterity. It is also necessary to determine whether withholding hands-on care at this early stage adversely affects breastfeeding outcome.

Acknowledgement

This work was supported by the Department of Health Infant Feeding Initiative.

REFERENCES

Benjamin M. 1999. Survey of Infant Feeding Practices in Warwickshire 1997/98. Audit Report, p. 23. Conducted by the Clinical Effectiveness Department, Warwick Hospital. Available from: South Warwickshire Dietetic Service Health Promotion Dept, 19 Waterloo Place, Warwick Street, Leamington Spa

Hall Moran V, Dinwoodie K, Bramwell R, Dykes F, Foley P. 1999. The development and validation of the Breastfeeding Support Skills Tool (BeSST). Clinical Effectiveness in Nursing, 3: 151–155

Henderson A, Stamp G, Pincombe J. 2001. Postpartum positioning and attachment education for increasing breastfeeding: a randomized trial. Birth, 28, 236–242

Moran VH, Bramwell R, Dykes F, Dinwoodie K. 2000. An evaluation of skills acquisition on the WHO/Unicef Breastfeeding Management Course using the pre-validated Breastfeeding Support Skills Tool (BeSST). Midwifery, 16(3): 197–203

The Practising Midwife 2003; 6(11): 24–25

'White blood': dose benefits of human milk

Suzanne Colson

Human milk, like blood, is a living, vital substance. Because it is considered similar to the placental blood of intrauterine life, Riordan and Auerbach (1997) coined the term 'white blood' to describe human milk. It could be said that white blood takes over from cord blood and that the mammary gland takes over from the placenta to nourish the offspring. This switch represents a potential nutritional continuum from fetus to neonate.

Metaphorically, human milk nourishes the infant's blood – the supposed seat of passion, temperament and mettle. Traditionally, human milk has offered succour, comfort, nutrition, warmth and peace.

Biologically, breastfeeding is a blueprint for enhanced health. Although the constituents of mammalian milks are roughly similar, the type and amount of proteins, fats, sugars, minerals and vitamins vary from mammal to mammal to meet the changing nutritional and developmental needs of the offspring for each species (Lawrence, 1997). This is called biospecificity. Many of the components are multifunctional. For example, the proteins in human milk prevent infection and inflammation, promote growth, transport trace minerals, catalyse reactions and synthesise nutrients (Institute of Medicine, 1991). Lawrence (1997) highlights that the constituents of human milk represent a 'delicate balance of macro nutrients and micro nutrients, each in proper proportion to enhance absorption'. This is termed bioavailability.

Mammalian milk is easily obtained, produced in species-appropriate quantities, at body temperature. No preparation is needed. It is delivered fresh, warm and alive when ingested by the offspring. What is unique to mammalian milk is a biological design that promotes nutritional efficacy.

What is nutrition?

In simple terms, nutrition is a three-way relationship between food, the body and health. It consists of five parts:

- Ingestion
- Digestion
- Absorption
- Metabolism
- Excretion.

Efficient nutrition concerns the ease with which food is obtained (ingestion), and how complete and accessible the nutrients are for digestion and absorption (bioavailability) so that they can be converted to use as building blocks or for energy to meet the body's needs (metabolism). Efficient nutrition is also reflected in the percentage of food ingested that cannot be utilised and is therefore excreted.

For nutrition to be effective, the right nutrient needs to be available in a usable form, in the right amount, at the right time. For example, human milk and sea fish are unique as they are the only foods for human consumption that contain pre-formed, very-long-chain polyunsaturated fatty acids such as docosahexaenoic acid (DHA 22:6) in the omega-3 family (Lawrence, 1997). Because they are building blocks for the central nervous system and the human brain, these have been called the 'neural fatty acids' (Crawford & Marsh, 1989).

This is an eloquent example of biospecificity and bioavailability. In the first year of life, the infant's brain triples in size. According to nature's blueprint, pre-formed DHA (the right nutrient) is easily and rapidly absorbed into the brain in just the right quantities, at just the right time, throughout the baby's first year. In contrast, DHA is not normally found in bovine milk. The process of adding medium-chain fatty acids one by one – such as alpha-linolenic acid, the parent omega-3 molecule – which the body can then convert into DHA, results in an artificial milk feed that only mimics human milk. This guarantees neither digestion nor absorption (Lawrence, 1997). It is an educated guess that informs how much DHA should be added to enrich bovine milk

197

to feed the brains of human infants. Too much or too little at any one time could have negative consequences.

After weaning, milk from any species is no longer a large part of the mammalian diet. It is only in recent human history that children and adults have drunk large quantities of another mammal's milk. Encouraging massive ingestion of bovine milk was probably an expedient public health measure initiated when dietary habits were poor and a range of foodstuffs was either scarce or expensive. Bovine milk provides many essential nutrients and there was always at least one cow available in each village. At best, bovine milk can be thought of as a human convenience food.

Getting the best from the breast

Successful nutritional postnatal adaptation relies on two conditions. First, to ensure unlimited access to the mammary gland, the baby needs to remain close to the mother's body contour. I call this biological nurturing, and preliminary results of research examining the mechanisms involved suggest that biological nurturing positions trigger ingestion.

The second condition concerns exclusivity of breastfeeding. Exclusive breastfeeding from birth is defined as giving the baby no other food or liquid but human milk (World Health Organisation, 2001). That means no sugar water or plain water, no juice, no teas, no honey, no cereals.

Problems in consistency of breastfeeding definitions and poor research design have misled many health professionals to believe that supplementation with artificial milks is a reasonable response to common breastfeeding problems if the mother chooses, or is in agreement, to do so. Recent feeding statistics show that 28% of breastfeeding babies are given at least one bottle of artificial milk feed while in hospital (Hamlyn et al., 2002). This early supplementation is highly associated with unintended breastfeeding cessation during the first two weeks (Hamlyn et al., 2002). On the postnatal ward, the slogan 'breast is best' often appears to be an unattainable ideal.

Raisler et al. (1999) point out that, throughout this health debate, little attention has been paid to breast milk dose. In its usual context, dose quantifies the amount, the frequency and the duration of any treatment.

In relation to feeding, dose response can be interpreted in two ways. The first concerns the amount of human milk or the amount of infant formula ingested; the latter weakens the 'combination event' effect or nutrient-to-nutrient interaction that characterises species specificity and bioavailability (Lawrence, 1997). Furthermore, foreign protein (bovine, goat, soy, etc.), non-lactose disaccharides and vegetal

fats are basic constituents of human milk substitutes. Any dose or amount ingested, even one bottle, sensitises the baby's system to non-human components and may decrease potential health benefits. The effects may be irreversible.

The second interpretation of breast milk dose concerns the amount of milk ingested over a period of time. Exclusive breastfeeding as opposed to mix-feeding over any number of months increases the dose, the amount of human-specific milk that a baby ingests and, as a result, enhances breastfeeding health benefits.

The early days

Human milk and infant formula are not metabolised in the same way. When healthy babies are breastfed, they generate ketone bodies. These result from the beta oxidation of fats (from human milk and from adipose tissue stores) and are now recognised to be an alternative fuel for the neonatal brain during the first three postnatal days (Hawdon et al., 1992). This is called suckling ketosis and is recognised as a protective and counter-regulatory mechanism that offers an alternative brain fuel when neonatal blood glucose (BG) concentrations are in the lower ranges (Hawdon, 1999). Recent research has shown that suckling ketosis does not occur when infants are formula fed (DeRooy & Hawdon, 2002). There is a clear dose response: any supplementation of breastfed infants reduces ketone body concentrations in an inverse relationship to the amount of artificial formula feed given (Hawdon et al., 2000).

Some would argue that underpinning practice with the physiology associated with non-human milks should remain the gold standard because it has been 'good enough'. Yet, in the short term, we know that giving bottles of infant formula does not always raise BG concentrations (Hawdon & DeRooy, 2002). When healthy infants who are at risk of neonatal hypoglycaemia are given artificial milk feeds, no alternative fuel supply is synthesised when their BG concentrations are borderline. These babies often require intravenous glucose and are admitted to special care.

Breast milk dose and diabetes

The incidence of early-onset insulin-dependent diabetes (IDD) among children up to the age of four doubled over a 10-year study period in Oxford (Gardner et al., 1997). Although causes are unknown, the researchers postulated that factors associated with early postnatal life may be responsible. Five to six children per thousand may be born with this genetic predisposition (Tarn & Thomas, 1988); unless there is a family history of diabetes, it is impossible to know which babies could be affected. The British Paediatric Association (1994) highlights a reduction in juvenile IDD associated with breastfeeding. This appeared to be a dose response. Other studies have identified associations between the early introduction of bovine milk protein and IDD in genetically predisposed children (Akerblom et al., 1993; Gerstein, 1994). And, as early as 1996, Henshel and Inch wrote that giving just one bottle of artificial milk feed may increase the risk for those babies who are genetically susceptible.

Bigger is not always better...

Childhood obesity in Britain has reached epidemic proportions (Chinn & Rona, 2001). Fat babies appear to have an increased risk of becoming obese teens and adults (Kramer, 1981). One study revealed an association between exclusive breastfeeding for three to five months and a 35% reduction of obesity or being overweight in school-aged children (Von Kries et al., 1999). A clear dose–response effect for the duration of breastfeeding was demonstrated; this protective effect was not attributable to differences in social class or lifestyle. A protective programming effect was theorised: babies fed artificial milk from birth have significantly higher plasma concentrations of insulin (Lucas et al., 1980). These higher concentrations would be expected to stimulate fat deposition (Von Kries et al., 1999).

There is evidence that, even though they grow more rapidly during the first two months, breastfed (BF) babies gain less weight, on average, during the first year than formula-fed (FF) babies, even after solids are introduced (Dewey, 1998). There is also evidence that BF infants self-regulate their energy intake at a lower level than FF infants (Dewey, 1998). Although the mechanisms are unclear, Dewey (1998) poses a key question: why do FF infants consume more energy than BF infants? Body temperature and minimal observable metabolic rate have been reported as lower in BF than FF babies (Butte, 1996). Although this may be part of the explanation, it cannot explain these differences in fatness (Dewey, 1998). These adverse consequences may be caused by the excessive protein intake found in infant formula (Dewey, 1998) – yet another dose response.

Other dose benefits

In the long term, some important health differences have been found that may be associated with breast milk dose. A retrospective study examining health risks for cardiovascular disease compared method of feeding during the first postnatal week. Subjects who were formula fed had significantly higher glucose tolerance test results at 120 minutes and higher prevalence of impaired glucose tolerance than those who were exclusively breastfed. Formula-fed subjects also had higher fasting insulin concentrations (Ravelli et al., 2000).

There is an increasing body of scientific evidence that demonstrates other dose risks associated with formula feeding, even in industrialised countries (MIDIRS, 2003). For babies, exclusive breastfeeding confers dose protection against gastroenteritis, respiratory infection and urinary tract infections (Lawrence, 1997). For mothers, exclusive breastfeeding is strongly associated with a reduction in pre-menopausal breast, ovarian and endometrial cancers. Exclusive breastfeeding is now advised for the first six months of life (WHO, 2001).

Conclusion

Taken together, the above evidence suggests the following practice recommendations to support exclusive breastfeeding:

- Inform mothers concerning dose risks associated with formula feeding
- Carry out risk/benefit assessments before offering any artificial milk supplements to breastfeeding mothers experiencing difficulties
- Sharpen clinical skills associated with breastfeeding assessments and, in particular, criteria concerning breast milk transfer (i.e. clinical indications that the baby is getting enough milk)
- Underpin feeding practices with an entirely human nutritional continuum from fetus to neonate.

Diseases of civilisation such as obesity, diabetes and cardiovascular disease are increasing at endemic proportions. Although they seem remote from giving birth and breastfeeding, there is an increasing need to understand and to promote the biological blueprint to enhance health.

REFERENCES

Akerblom HK, Savilahti E, Saukkonen TT et al. 1993. The case for elimination of cow's milk in early infancy in the prevention of type 1 diabetes: the Finnish experience. Diab/Meta Rev, 9(4): 269–278

British Paediatric Association. 1994. Is breast feeding beneficial in the UK? Arch Dis Child, 71: 376–380

Butte NF. 1996. Energy requirements of infants. Eur J Clin Nutr, 50(Suppl.): 24–36

Chinn S, Rona RR. 2001. Prevalence and trends in overweight and obesity in three cross-sectional studies of British children 1974–94. BMJ, 322: 24–26

Crawford M, Marsh D. 1989. The Driving Force. Mandarin Paperbacks, London

DeRooy L, Hawdon JM. 2002. Nutritional factors that affect the postnatal metabolic adaptation of full-term small and large for gestational age infants. Pediatrics, 109(3): E42 www.pediatrics.org/cgi/content/full/109/3/e42

Dewey KG. 1998. Growth characteristics of breast-fed compared to formula-fed infants. Biol Neonate, 74: 94–105

Gardner SG, Bingley PB, Sawtell PA, Weeks S, Gale EAM. 1997. Rising incidence of insulin dependent diabetes in children aged under 5 years in the Oxford region: time trend analysis. BMJ, 315: 713–717

Gerstein HC. 1994. Cow's milk exposure and type I diabetes mellitus, a critical overview of the clinical literature. Diabetes Care, 17(1, January): 13–19

Hamlyn B, Brooker S, Oleinikova K, Wands S. 2002. Infant Feeding 2000 – Office for National Statistics. Stationery Office, London

Hawdon JM. 1999. Hypoglycaemia and the neonatal brain. Eur J Paediatr, 158(11, Suppl. 1): S9–S12

Hawdon JM, Ward Platt MP, Aynsley-Green A. 1992. Patterns of metabolic adaptation in term and preterm infants in the first postnatal week. Arch Dis Child, 67: 357–365

Hawdon JM, Williams AF, Lawrence SM, Colson S, Thurston JG. 2000. Formula supplements given to healthy breastfed preterm babies inhibit postnatal metabolic adaptation: results of a randomised controlled trial. Arch Dis Child, 82(Suppl. 1): Conference Abstract G102, April

Henschel D, Inch S. 1996. Breastfeeding: A Guide for Midwives. Books for Midwives, Cheshire

Institute of Medicine. 1991. Nutrition During Lactation. National Academy Press, Washington

Kramer MS. 1981. Do breast-feeding and delayed introduction of solid foods protect against subsequent obesity? J Pediatr, 98(6): 883–887

Lawrence RA. 1997. A Review of the Medical Benefits in Contraindications to Breastfeeding in the United States – Maternal and Child Health Technical Information Bulletin. National Centre for Education in Maternal and Child Health, Arlington, VA

Lucas A, Adrian TE, Blackburn AN, Sarson DL, Aynsley-Green A, Bloom SR. 1980. Breast vs bottle: endocrine responses are different with formula feeding. Lancet, 1: 1267–1269

MIDIRS Midwifery Digest. 2003. National Electronic Library for Health Informed Choice Leaflets; Informed Choice for Professionals Breastfeeding or Bottle Feeding, No. 7; online at http://www.midirs.org/nelh/nelh.nsf/TOPICVIEW?OpenForm&id=3BC0 176B5FE32F3380256B8F00512A84

Raisler J, Alexander C, O'Campo P. 1999. Breast-feeding and infant illness; a dose–response relationship. Am J Pub Health, 89(1, January): 25–30

Ravelli ACJ, Van der Meulen JHP, Osmond C, Barker DJP, Bleker OP. 2000. Infant feeding and adult glucose tolerance, lipid profile, blood pressure and obesity. Arch Dis Child, 82: 248–252

Riordan J, Auerbach K. 1997. Breastfeeding and Human Lactation. Jones & Bartlett, London

Tarn AC, Thomas JM. 1988. Predicting insulin-dependent diabetes. Lancet, 1: 845–850

Von Kries R, Koletzko B, Sauerwalk T et al. 1999. Breast-feeding and obesity: cross sectional study. BMJ, 319: 147–150

World Health Organisation. 2001. Child and Adolescent Health and Development, Exclusive Breastfeeding; online at http://www.who.int/child-adolescent-health/NUTRITION/infant_exclusive.htm

The Practising Midwife 2003; 6(10): 11–13

Mother and baby – a good start

Sarah J Buckley

Introduction

Labour and birth are profound and major events, providing a transition to motherhood and to life outside the womb that is designed to be safe and fulfilling for mother and baby. This paper describes the transition for mother and baby in terms of the first hour after birth, the first days after birth and the first weeks after birth.

The hour after birth – don't disturb mother and baby

The hour after birth is a precious and unique time, hormonally and physiologically, for mother and baby. The hormones that have catalysed the processes of labour and birth are at peak levels for the mother, with parallel hormonal peaks for the baby. Together they produce an ecstatic state for both partners, enhancing early attachment and assisting with the physical transitions of this time (Buckley, 2004).

These ecstatic hormones include: oxytocin, the hormone of love; beta-endorphin, the hormone of pleasure and transcendence; adrenaline/noradrenaline (epinephrine/norepinephrine), hormones of excitement and fight or flight; and prolactin, the hormone of tender mothering and milk production.

The ecstatic hormones of the first hour

Oxytocin, the hormone of love, reaches peak levels for the new mother – the highest in her life – during the hour after birth, and is highest as she births her baby's placenta (Nissen et al., 1995). Maternal oxytocin release is enhanced when mother and baby are skin-to-skin and eye-to-eye with each other (Uvnas-Moberg, 2003), and through the newborn's early pre-breastfeeding and breastfeeding behaviours (Nissen et al., 1995; Matthiesen et al., 2001).

The baby also experiences a peak of oxytocin at birth, with neonatal levels elevated for the first four days (Leake et al., 1981). Oxytocin is also present in breast milk (Takeda et al., 1986). Oxytocin catalyses feelings of love and connectedness, and reduces the response to stress (Uvnas-Moberg, 2003).

Beta-endorphin, a naturally occurring opiate (and therefore related to drugs such as morphine and pethidine), is secreted from the pituitary under conditions of stress. In labour, beta-endorphin assists the mother-to-be to transcend pain and to enter the altered state of consciousness that characterises a normal birth. Beta-endorphin reaches peak levels in the minutes after birth for mother and baby, and maternal beta-endorphin levels decline slowly to normal one to three days after birth (Bacigalupo et al., 1990). Beta-endorphin contributes to the euphoria of the early postnatal period and is recognised as an important hormone of bonding and mutual dependency.

Like oxytocin, beta-endorphin is present in breast milk (Zanardo et al., 2001) and is released by the mother with each breastfeeding episode (Franceschini et al., 1989).

Adrenaline and noradrenaline (epinephrine and norepinephrine), collectively known as the catecholamine hormones, also peak at birth for mother and baby, although levels decline more rapidly than the other hormones. For the mother, peak levels of catecholamines in the second stage help to catalyse a quick and easy birth through activation of the fetal ejection reflex (Odent, 1990, 1992). Maternal adrenaline levels are back to normal within 15–30 minutes after birth (Lederman et al., 1977), which is a necessary decline – ongoing elevation would inhibit oxytocin release and increase the new mother's risk of postpartum haemorrhage (Saito et al., 1991; Odent, 2004).

Newborn catecholamine levels remain elevated for the first 12 hours (Eliot et al., 1980). These fight-or-flight hormones assist with the major circulatory adjustments that are necessary for the transition from fetal to neonatal life (Lagercrantz & Slotkin, 1986). Noradrenaline (norepinephrine) is recognised as an important element in maternal bonding: mice bred to be deficient in noradrenaline (norepinephrine) do not care for their young or tend their nests (Thomas & Palmiter, 1997).

Prolactin, the hormone of tender mothering, also peaks with the birth of the baby (Fernandes et al., 1995), and helps the new mother to enact her instinctive mothering behaviours (Grattan, 2001). Prolactin is present in breast milk (Kacsoh et al., 1993; Ellis & Picciano, 1995) and is thought to play an important role in newborn brain development (Grattan, 2001).

Mother–baby connection

This unique and brief hormonal situation is, according to Odent (2002), '… one of the most critical phases in the life of human beings'. Mother and baby are adjusting – biologically, psychologically and emotionally – to their new states, and establishing a relationship of 'biological nurturance' (Colson, 2002), which includes the establishment of breastfeeding. Separation of mother and baby is a major intervention at this time, with significant short-, medium- and long-term sequelae.

For example, separation will reduce the new mother's opportunities to release oxytocin, as above, and may therefore increase her risk of bleeding. Separation is also harmful to the baby. Separated babies display more stressed behaviours – increased crying, shorter sleep and less organised neurobehaviour (Ferber & Makhoul, 2004) – compared to babies allowed uninterrupted skin-to-skin contact with the mother for the first hour. A 'separation distress call' has been recognised in newborns, equivalent to that in other mammalian species, signalling the evolutionary need for continuous mother–infant contact for our species (Christensson et al., 1995).

Skin-to-skin contact, and the oxytocin that is released through this and through breastfeeding, also causes a vasodilation of the blood vessels on the mother's chest wall, creating a natural warming mechanism for her newborn, or older baby (Uvnas-Moberg, 2003).

The establishment of breastfeeding and early mothering behaviours are, in many studies, more difficult when the first contact between baby and breast is delayed. For example, in one study, mothers whose babies' lips had touched their nipple in the first hour kept their infants with them for an extra 100 minutes daily, compared to mothers who had not had this experience (Widstrom et al., 1990). Other research has suggested that a delay in maternal–infant contact (in this study due to operative delivery) has a negative impact on maternal mood and wellbeing, even up to eight months after birth (Rowe-Murray & Fisher, 2001).

The mother's ecstatic hormones, augmented by contact with her baby, also help her to birth her baby's placenta, and protect her from postpartum haemorrhage (PPH) by ensuring ongoing release of oxytocin. This keeps her uterus well contracted. Efficient oxytocin release requires low maternal catecholamine levels; therefore, it is important to keep the new mother feeling warm, safe and undisturbed in her interactions with her newborn (Buckley, 2005).

Odent (2001) believes that disruption of the time after birth has become almost universal because it interferes with the bond between mother and baby, and with the development of the offspring's capacity for love and altruism, which are related to the oxytocin system. Such deficits in love and altruism allow an individual, a tribe or a society to more easily wage war, and the more aggressive the individuals, the more likely the group is to survive and to vanquish its opponents. He attributes, for example, the globally widespread belief that colostrum is harmful to the newborn to the more aggressive attitudes that a society may foster through separating mother and baby because of this belief (Odent, 2001).

Implications for carers

Midwifery best practice aims to keep mother and baby together, ideally skin-to-skin, for this time. Observations and monitoring of mother and baby can be done unobtrusively, and interventions, including separation, can be reserved for emergencies.

When this time is undisturbed, the mother is likely to deliver her baby's placenta without complications during the first hour (Odent, 2002; Buckley, 2005) and breastfeeding is likely to be established with more ease.

The days after birth – lotus birth and the golden orb

The enormous adjustments that mother and baby make at birth – physiologically, hormonally, neurologically and emotionally – continue for the days and weeks to follow. In particular, the physiological shift from transplacental nutrition to breastfeeding requires many new skills for both partners, and is aided by the hormones of this period, especially oxytocin, the hormone of love and milk ejection (which is also enhanced through skin-to-skin contact with the baby), and prolactin, the hormone of tender mothering and milk production, which is increased by carrying and caring for infants (Roberts et al., 2001; Soltis et al., 2005).

Rest and support

In modern times, these early days are often not recognised as unique and important, and many postpartum women find themselves back to cooking, cleaning and caring for their families within a few days of giving birth. This may reflect our cultural ignorance of the importance of this time for mother and baby, as well as our expectation of the 'supermum' who is supposed to give birth and be back on her feet within hours.

Davis (1988) notes also our cultural difficulties with surrender and vulnerability, and with taking a 'respite from our social obligations'. Also, the loss of the extended family, early hospital discharge and inadequate paternal leave result in many new mothers having little practical support at a time when it is most needed.

However, this is a very important time, and the new mother requires rest and support so that she can honour this process, emotionally integrate her birth experiences and begin her new role as a breastfeeding mother. The special and delicate nature of this time has been described as 'the golden orb of the babymoon' (Lennox, 2002).

According to this model, keeping mother and baby safe and secluded will keep the orb intact. Conversely, if not honoured (for example, through venturing out at an early time, having too many visitors, insufficient rest), the orb can develop cracks, which dissipates the magical energy of this time and can leave the new mother and baby without a protective buffer. Lotus birth can be helpful in maintaining this 'golden orb', practically and energetically.

Lotus birth

Lotus birth is essentially non-severance of the baby's cord, so that baby and placenta remain attached until natural cord separation occurs at the umbilicus. Typically the 'breaking forth' time, before separation, lasts four to seven days, although it can be as short as 36 hours or as long as 12 days. During this time, mother and baby are together at home.

Lotus birth honours the sacredness of the early days, and gives the newborn a gentle transition from attachment to the placenta in the womb, to attachment to mother and breast. Lotus birth gives the mother (and family) an enhanced awareness of the uniqueness and brevity of this time, and allows the baby to set the pace of the early days. Lotus birth imprints trust in the natural processes, and helps to maintain the 'golden orb' by keeping visitors away during the breaking forth time.

Lotus birth is a simple concept and requires no technical equipment. The baby's placenta is usually washed, to remove clots, in the early hours and can then be left to drain in a sieve or colander for 12 hours or so, which keeps the placenta as dry as possible.

After draining, parents can place the baby's placenta in a container, with or without a lid – for example, a ceramic bowl or an ice-cream carton with a corner cut off for the cord. The placenta is usually covered in salt or powdered herbs for preservation. Some parents choose to wrap their baby's placenta in a cloth, towel or nappy, or in a specially made placenta bag.

The baby's placenta is then attended to every 12–24 hours by drying and removal of clots, and, if desired, salting and rewrapping. The cord dries from the umbilical end, becoming hard and brittle. The placenta also dries and, if treated with salt, shrinks. Treatment does not stop some degree of decay of the placenta, especially in a hot climate or if breaking forth takes many days, and some families use lavender or other essential oils on the placenta or coverings. Note that cooling the placenta is not recommended as a means of preservation: babies may become unsettled when their placenta is cold.

The baby and placenta can be cared for on the bed, with mother in close attendance, or alternatively the placenta may be bundled up, with the baby, in a blanket or shawl. As the mother of three lotus babies, I have noticed that the more quiet and still I am, along with my baby, the shorter the breaking forth time.

Some parents have reported that their baby cried loudly and/or for the first time around the time of separation, which some have experienced as akin to a second birth. For example, a friend danced around the house, when her daughter's cord separated, exclaiming, 'We've got her, we can keep her!' Others have felt that their baby became more present after separation. Another lotus mother of twins expressed understandable relief at not having to carry two placentas around!

It is interesting to note that, in many traditional cultures, the timing of postnatal rituals, and of the re-entry of mother and baby into society, is counted from the dropping off of the baby's cord stump (Priya, 1992).

In summary, the early days after birth require an ongoing awareness and attention to rest for mother and baby. This can usefully be imagined as preserving the 'golden orb of the babymoon'. Lotus birth creates a sacred space for rest and integration. Lim (2001) observes: '… mother lays-in, close to the baby and placenta, breastfeeding is established in this sacred circle of quiet, restful seclusion … It is during this space out of time that family may be invented, that the new mother reinvents herself'.

The weeks after birth – babymoon

Lying-in traditions

Davis (1988) suggests that the new mother may be more able to 'take charge' at around postnatal day 11, but it is important to remember that she is still in a vulnerable and unique state during the weeks that follow.

Most traditional cultures recognise this, and have traditions to ensure that the new mother has close care, comfort and company during these early weeks. The new mother is absolved from social and family obligations for this period, which lasts typically 40 days or around six weeks (Priya, 1992; Rice, 1993; Kitzinger, 2000).

Also, there are usually strong prohibitions, proscriptions and rituals at this time, with the aim of protecting mother and baby from harm, including harm from unseen spirits. Special nourishing foods are provided, in order to give the new mother strength and a good milk supply.

The new mother's 'lying-in period' often incorporates ritual seclusion, because the new mother, with her postpartum blood and lochia, is said to be unclean and dangerous to men. As a result of this belief, the new mother and baby are attended by female relatives and helpers, and enjoy a period of feminine nurturing and celebration (Kitzinger, 2000).

A common cross-cultural practice at this time is massage. A traditional midwife will visit the mother daily, even twice daily, to massage the mother and often the new baby also. This helps the mother's body to recover, helps the baby to grow straight and strong, and helps with any digestive or other upset (Kitzinger, 2000).

Many cultures also have beliefs and practices designed to keep the new mother warm. Some south-east Asian countries practise 'mother-roasting': building a fire in the birth hut to keep the new mother and baby warm, and prohibiting cold environments and cold foods. This is recognised as important preventative medicine amongst these traditions – for example, one mother reported: 'If we touch cold water [after birth], when we get old then we will be sick with cold bones, our bones will feel painful' (Rice, 1993).

Priya (1992) notes:

Once the exclusion period is finished, mothers usually have few problems. They do not suffer the isolation of the modern woman or, usually, the full responsibility of bringing up their baby ... In the close network of relationships and support, there are rarely problems for the new mother in adjusting to her role.

Western cultures

Western cultures have also, in the recent past, acknowledged this need for a period of postnatal withdrawal and support through the ritual of 'churching'. Churching is a ceremony of thanksgiving and purification that occurs when mother and baby go to church for the first time after birth. In Eastern orthodox churches, this ceremony occurs on the 40th day (Knodel, 1995).

The babymoon

The rest and support that many cultures provide can be difficult for modern women to access. Extended families are often geographically distant, and may be emotionally or philosophically distant as well. And the early weeks, even more so than the early days, may be hard to 'island' – to create a space of quiet and rest.

However, when the new mother does not gain the opportunity to rest and recuperate, she risks her physical health, her breastfeeding ease and the smooth integration of her new role, and new baby, into the household. As a mother of four, I have found that resting at this time builds a store of energy and nourishment that sustains me for the first six to 12 months postpartum. This accords with the traditional Chinese medicine (TCM) belief that postnatal rest is essential to rebuild the Qi (life energy) lost during pregnancy and birth (Betts, 2005).

A well-planned babymoon is crucial to the postpartum and ongoing well-being of mother and baby, and best practice midwifery care involves discussion, encouragement and planning for this practice. The following is a list of ideas for new mothers to consider, with support from their midwife and families, which will help to create rest and nourishment for mother and baby in the early weeks.

Suggestions for a blissful babymoon

General
- Arrange leave for partner for at least two weeks, if possible.
- Negotiate support from other friends and relatives for six weeks.
- Consider hiring household help, either live-in or visiting, for two to six weeks. Ask prospective gift-givers to sponsor this help.
- Ask friends to help with other children, especially driving to school and other activities, for two to six weeks.
- Consider keeping your own and family activities in the bedroom, alongside the baby, for the first week or so.
- Stay in your pyjamas for as long as you need to, ideally one to two weeks.
- Consider staying at home, not driving or being driven, for two to six weeks.

Food
- Ensure plenty of grocery supplies – buy two or more of everything in the last few weeks of pregnancy.
- Ensure at least one week of easy main meals in the freezer or pantry.

- Consider asking friends to donate a frozen meal or baking before the birth.
- Consider asking a friend to organise a meal roster – a list of friends to bring fresh home-cooked meals for the family – for a week or so, beginning soon after the birth.
- Stock up on snacks, cakes, etc. for morning and afternoon tea.

Household
- Do any major cleaning and reorganising before the birth.
- Ideally have household help for the first six weeks.
- Arrange a nappy-wash service, if necessary.
- Give yourself at least 10 days free from any household tasks – laundry, cleaning, cooking, etc.
- Have a friend or partner do your essential shopping for the first six weeks.
- Ask friends to help with errands and unexpected needs for two to six weeks.

Rest
- Prioritise your own needs for this time. Rest is essential and is a vital ingredient for later energy and ongoing health.
- Ask friends and relatives to arrange visits with you in advance. Scheduling a general visiting time (e.g. Sunday afternoon) at least 10 days after the birth may be helpful. Ask visitors to bring food.
- Limit visitors for the first week or so and always say no (even at the last minute) if you are tired.
- Hang a sign on the front door – 'Mother and baby resting'.
- Keep phone calls to a minimum – use a message on your answering machine to let people know about your baby and your visiting arrangements.

In summary, the postnatal period is often neglected in modern cultures, but is very important in ensuring a smooth transition for mother, baby and family. Midwifery care, with sensitive attention to, and planning for, the first hour after birth, the early days and the first six weeks can assist with this process.

REFERENCES

Bacigalupo G, Riese S, Rosendahl H et al. 1990. Quantitative relationships between pain intensities during labor and beta-endorphin and cortisol concentrations in plasma. Decline of the hormone concentrations in the early postpartum period. Journal of Perinatal Medicine, 18(4): 289–296

Betts D. 2005. Postnatal acupuncture. Journal of Chinese Medicine, 77: 5–15

Buckley SJ. 2004. Undisturbed birth: nature's hormonal blueprint for safety, ease and ecstasy. MIDIRS Midwifery Digest, 14(2): 203–209

Buckley SJ. 2005. Leaving well alone – a natural approach to third stage. Medical Veritas, 2(2): 492–499

Christensson K, Cabrera T, Christensson E et al. 1995. Separation distress call in the human neonate in the absence of maternal body contact. Acta Paediatr, 84(5): 468–473

Colson S. 2002. Womb to world: a metabolic perspective. Midwifery Today Int Midwife, 61: 12–17

Davis E. 1988. Energetic Pregnancy. Celestial Arts, Berkeley, CA

Eliot RJ, Lam R, Leake RD et al. 1980. Plasma catecholamine concentrations in infants at birth and during the first 48 hours of life. J Pediatr, 96(2): 311–315

Ellis LA, Picciano MF. 1995. Bioactive and immunoreactive prolactin variants in human milk. Endocrinology, 136(6): 2711–2720

Ferber SG, Makhoul IR. 2004. The effect of skin-to-skin contact (kangaroo care) shortly after birth on the neurobehavioral responses of the term newborn: a randomized, controlled trial. Pediatrics, 113(4): 858–865

Fernandes PA, Szelazek JT, Reid GJ et al. 1995. Phasic maternal prolactin secretion during spontaneous labor is associated with cervical dilatation and second-stage uterine activity. J Soc Gynecol Investig, 2(4): 597–601

Franceschini R, Venturini PL, Cataldi A et al. 1989. Plasma beta-endorphin concentrations during suckling in lactating women. Br J Obstet Gynaecol, 96(6): 711–713

Grattan DR. 2001. The actions of prolactin in the brain during pregnancy and lactation. Prog Brain Res, 133: 153–171

Kacsoh B, Veress Z, Toth BE et al. 1993. Bioactive and immunoreactive variants of prolactin in milk and serum of lactating rats and their pups. J Endocrinol, 138(2): 243–257

Kitzinger S. 2000. Rediscovering Birth. Little, Brown, London

Knodel N. 1995. The Thanksgiving of Women after Childbirth, commonly called The Churching of Women. University of Oxford, Online. Available at: http://users.ox.ac.uk/~mikef/church.html, 20 July 2005

Lagercrantz H, Slotkin TA. 1986. The "stress" of being born. Scient Am, 254(4): 100–107

Leake RD, Weitzman RE, Fisher DA. 1981. Oxytocin concentrations during the neonatal period. Biol Neonate, 39(3–4): 127–131

Lederman RP, McCann DS, Work B Jr et al. 1977. Endogenous plasma epinephrine and norepinephrine in last-trimester pregnancy and labor. Am J Obstet Gynecol, 129(1): 5–8

Lennox S. (2002). Master of Arts thesis, Victoria University, Wellington

Lim R. 2001. Lotus birth... asking the next question. Midwifery Today, 58: 14–16

Matthiesen AS, Ransjo-Arvidson AB, Nissen E et al. 2001. Postpartum maternal oxytocin release by newborns: effects of infant hand massage and sucking. Birth, 28(1): 13–19

Nissen E, Lilja G, Widstrom A et al. 1995. Elevation of oxytocin levels early post partum in women. Acta Obstet Gynecol Scand, 74(7): 530–533

Odent M. 1990. Position in delivery (letter). Lancet, 335(8698): 1166

Odent M. 1992. In: The Nature of Birth and Breastfeeding, pp. 29–43. Ace Graphics, Sydney

Odent M. 2001. The Scientification of Love, Revised. Free Association Books, London

Odent M. 2002. The first hour following birth: don't wake the mother! Midwifery Today Int Midwife, 61: 9–12

Odent M. 2004. Putting an end to women's global slaughter. Primal Health Research, 12(2): 1–7

Priya JV. 1992. Birth Traditions and Modern Pregnancy Care. Element, Longmead, Shaftesbury, UK

Rice PL. 1993. My Forty Days: A Cross-cultural Resource Book for Health Care Professionals in Birthing Services. Centre for the Study of Mother's and Children's Health, Melbourne

Roberts RL, Jenkins KT, Lawler T et al. 2001. Prolactin levels are elevated after infant carrying in parentally inexperienced common marmosets. Physiol Behav, 72(5): 713–720

Rowe-Murray HJ, Fisher JR. 2001. Operative intervention in delivery is associated with compromised early mother–infant interaction. Br J Obstet Gynaecol, 108(10): 1068–1075

Saito M, Sano T, Satohisa E. 1991. Plasma catecholamines and microvibration as labour progresses. Shinshin-Thaku, 31: 381–389

Soltis J, Wegner FH, Newman JD. 2005. Urinary prolactin is correlated with mothering and allo-mothering in squirrel monkeys. Physiol Behav, 84(2): 295–301

Takeda S, Kuwabara Y, Mizuno M. 1986. Concentrations and origin of oxytocin in breast milk. Endocrinol Jpn, 33(6): 821–826

Thomas SA, Palmiter RD. 1997. Impaired maternal behavior in mice lacking norepinephrine and epinephrine. Cell, 91(5): 583–592

Uvnas-Moberg K. 2003. The Oxytocin Factor. Da Capo Press, Cambridge, MA

Widstrom AM, Wahlberg V, Matthiesen AS et al. 1990. Short-term effects of early suckling and touch of the nipple on maternal behaviour. Early Hum Dev, 21(3): 153–163

Zanardo V, Nicolussi S, Carlo G et al. 2001. Beta endorphin concentrations in human milk. J Pediatr Gastroenterol Nutr, 33(2): 160–164

Where might we go from here?

At the beginning of this section, I invited you to dream up a postnatal project, given unlimited funding and no restrictions. Having read the articles in this section, did your project include any of the suggestions made in here, or would you go for different priorities? If your budget was more limited, and you could offer a few things, but not everything, what would you prioritise?

Focus on...
Diversity (2)

SECTION CONTENTS

Adolescent motherhood in an inner city area in the UK: experiences and needs of a group of adolescent mothers

An examination of the issues faced by young pregnant women

Maria Barrell

It appears that there is a sense of crisis related to adolescent motherhood in the United Kingdom (Social Exclusion Unit, 1999). This crisis focuses not only on the increase in adolescent births but the socio-economic context in which those births occur and the cultural ideology they challenge. Lawson and Rhode (1993) argue that adolescent motherhood challenges traditional assumptions about the boundaries of youth and sexual independence at a time when adolescents cannot readily achieve financial independence. In the UK there is a convergence of related trends.

Trends include:

- Increased levels of sexual activity, especially outside of marital relationships
- More unplanned pregnancies, resulting in more abortions
- Higher rates of non-marital childbirths and single parenting
- Greater numbers of young female headed families living in poverty, dependent on the State and subject to all the disadvantages accompanying that status.

British attitudes to adolescent motherhood have been viewed as constituting a 'subdued moral panic' (Henshaw et al., 1989). One major criticism of some of the research undertaken in adolescent motherhood is it has a tendency to be labelled as unplanned, unwanted and outside of marriage. Macintyre and Cunningham-Burley (1993) suggest that this form of analysis is narrow and limited, as it does not take into account wider societal issues. The increase in sexual activity, abortions, non-marital childbirth, single parenting and female poverty is also apparent among the older population as well as younger, and in many cultures some of these trends are viewed as relatively unproblematic. High levels of sexual activity, frequency of abortion and non-marital childbirth provoke little concern in some countries, e.g. Sweden. In the UK, where overall rates of

adolescent fertility are lower than the USA, the proportion of non-marital childbirth is higher (Vinovskis, 1988; ONS, 2002). It is suggested that there is in fact no consensus as to whether adolescent motherhood is a serious social problem.

Research suggests that the vast majority of adolescent mothers are eventually able to complete their education (Waite & Moore, 1978), secure full-time employment, and avoid state dependency. Not all are, in any case, dependent upon the state. The achievements of many adolescent mothers and their children should not deflect attention from the hardships they confront or from the substantial number who experience enduring difficulties. Not only has popular research in the area of adolescent motherhood misrepresented the problem, it has also misjudged the prescription (Lawson & Rhode, 1993). Pearce (1993) argues that the common characterisation of 'children bearing children' disempowers adolescents and suggests that adolescents lack maturity in decision-making. Lawson and Rhode (1993) suggest childbirth is one of the few avenues available to satisfy needs to love and be loved for many adolescents from disadvantaged backgrounds.

In the literature there seems confusion in relation to adolescent decision-making and who should be making decisions. With regard to motherhood the popular view focuses on the maturity of the adolescent and the inability to make a rational choice. However, Ruddich (1993) suggests that this is not always the case: adolescent choices can be viewed as rational but in many of the studies undertaken in this area this choice has failed to be acknowledged. Adolescents are confronted with three choices: whether to engage in sexual activity, whether to use contraception and whether to bear a child. It is apparent that sex education in schools is inadequate and does not equip adolescents with the necessary knowledge to make an informed decision. Interestingly, anecdotal evidence suggests that truancy rates amongst adolescents within inner city areas are significant; therefore, their knowledge base related to sex education is questionable. Government policy has advocated adolescents to 'just say no', but what policy fails to recognise is that adolescents need to be empowered to 'just say no' and the source of this empowerment is through education (Lawson & Rhode, 1993).

Decisions to bear a child are probably best viewed as a complex mix of individual needs and social forces. Lawson and Rhode (1993) suggest that adolescents are influenced less by the desire to have a child than by family and peer pressures; motherhood becomes a way to punish parents, to please grandparents or male partners, or to gain status. Early research into pregnancies among low-income adolescents suggested that many mothers were not motivated to have a child but were insufficiently motivated to avoid it: the economic opportunities sacrificed through early motherhood did not appear sufficiently great to justify deferring childbirth (Bowerman, 1966). This interpretation of adolescent motherhood could still have currency in today's society.

Summary

It may well be that a considerable gap exists between adolescent mothers' needs and experiences and Government policy about them and social perceptions of them. This study provides an opportunity to explore the ideologies that inform Government policy (Social Exclusion Unit, 1999) and uphold social stereotypes of adolescent mothers. An important aspect of the study will be its focus upon the social, educational and economic expectations of a group of adolescent mothers and the coping strategies that they adopt.

Aims of the study

- To generate a grounded theory of adolescent motherhood drawn from the experiences of a group of adolescent mothers.
- To contribute to midwives' understanding of the lives and experiences of adolescent mothers.

Study sample

This study has provided an opportunity to explore issues identified in the literature from the experiences of a group of adolescent mothers ($n = 35$) as they participate in a specially designed educational programme to allow them to complete their compulsory education. This is a qualitative study, which adopts a grounded theory approach set within an interactionist framework (Strauss & Corbin, 1990).

The limitations of the study are recognised in that the findings are not generalisable, but a range of issues are highlighted that may inform midwifery practice and point to the need for a multidisciplinary approach to provide seamless care and support for adolescent mothers.

Study setting

The group of adolescent mothers were attending a Pupil Referral Unit exclusively designed for adolescent mothers to facilitate the completion of compulsory education.

Ethical consideration

The proposal was presented to the Pupil Referral Unit and considered by the Local Education Authority, where approval was granted. Consent was gained from all the mothers in the study and confidentiality has been maintained throughout.

Data collection

Over a four-month period, one day per week was spent in the Pupil Referral Unit. During this time a reflective diary was kept, observing the mothers in the Unit and recording the observations. Combined with the literature, the observation period provided the themes for the development of the research methodology.

Four central themes were developed:

- The educational experiences of the mothers at the Pupil Referral Unit
- Social and economic experiences of the mothers and the coping strategies they employ
- Perceptions of the support systems offered in the Pupil Referral Unit
- Feelings related to motherhood.

Focus group interviews

The next stage of this study involved focus group interviews (Krueger, 1997a, b, c; Krueger & King, 1997). Five dates for the interviews were agreed. An adapted data analysis technique was developed, guided by the methodology advocated by Strauss and Corbin (1990).

The analysis of the data prompted further development of the initial themes with the emergence of lines of enquiry. The emerging six themes and lines of enquiry are as follows:

THEME 1
What does motherhood mean to an adolescent mother?
Lines of enquiry
- Shock and fear

- Reduction in freedom and choices
- Age, maturity, responsibility, loss of independence and freedom
- Having a social life and feelings of guilt
- The caretaker role
- Labelling and stereotypes.

THEME 2
Fathers of the children and relationships with men
Lines of enquiry
- Mixed reactions
- Negative status
- Having a child was the mother's problem
- The paternal role
- The provider
- Supporter
- Relationships with other men
- Maternal grandparents' reactions to the father
- Marriage.

THEME 3
Relationships
Lines of enquiry
- Relationship with parents
- Relationships with friends.

THEME 4
Stigmatisation
Lines of enquiry
- Being part of a stigmatised group
- Perceptions that motherhood ruins adolescent females lives.

THEME 5
Support
Lines of enquiry
- Support from the family
- Support from the State
- Support from the Pupil Referral Unit
- Support from peers.

THEME 6
Education
Lines of enquiry
- Truancy and dislike of school
- Pressure to attend school
- Attendance at the Pupil Referral Unit
- Availability of childcare facilities
- Educational achievement and career aspirations.

Findings

Using a grounded theory data analysis (Strauss & Corbin, 1990) of the themes and lines of enquiry has revealed that adolescent motherhood comprises a complex range of issues with opposing and overlapping dimensions:

Dimensions of adolescent motherhood
- Maturity versus immaturity
- Caring for a child versus being cared for
- Responsibility versus freedom
- Fatherhood versus motherhood
- Dependence versus independence
- Aspirations versus acceptance.

Figure 8.1.1 illustrates the interconnecting dimensions of adolescent motherhood.

The next stage of the study involved undertaking semi-structured interviews ($n = 15$). The semi-structured interviews allowed for the further exploration of the opposing dimensions, incorporating and further developing the themes and lines of enquiry.

Maturity versus immaturity

Within this paper one dimension of the study, maturity versus immaturity in adolescent motherhood, will be explored. The issues surrounding this dimension are multifaceted and not easily untangled.

Whilst the mothers perceive themselves as being mature because of their maternal status, there are aspects of their lives where they are dependent for assistance and support, dependent upon their families, in particular, the father of the child, the Pupil Referral Unit, their peers and the State.

Motherhood was an experience all the mothers shared. Without exception, none of the mothers had planned pregnancy. The reasons for becoming pregnant were alluded to and included:

Figure 8.1.1 Interconnecting dimensions of adolescent motherhood

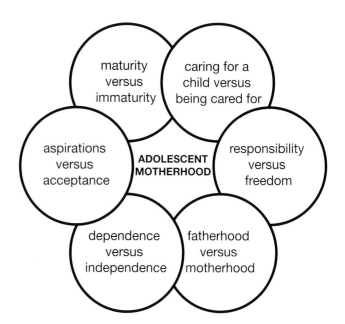

- To be sexually active was the norm
- Not sufficient known about sex and contraception
- Knowledge of sex and contraception was often based on folklore and ineffective practices
- Lack of motivation to use contraception
- 'I thought it would never happen to me'
- 'It was only a one-night stand'.

Chronic truancy was an issue for the majority of the mothers. Pregnancy was not the reason for truancy, but pregnancy was a consequence. Recent Government initiatives (Social Exclusion Unit, 1999) have advocated sex education programmes within schools, but for those adolescents who do not attend school, this initiative is ineffective.

The adolescents, when pregnancy was confirmed, did return to education, but the reasons for the excellent attendance at the Pupil Referral Unit were much more than the education the unit offered. The unit offered the mothers a structure to their lives and broadened their traditional perception of education. The mothers felt the unit was not like mainstream school, they were allowed to take their child with them and were responsible for the care of their child during the education process. The mothers received individual tuition and were allowed to work at their own pace. The environment was baby friendly, the mothers were brought to the unit by minibus at 9.30 a.m. and then returned home at 2.30 p.m. for the babies to have an afternoon sleep. It is interesting to note that the mothers felt they were perceived differently and given a different, more mature status because they were 'mothers at school'. Pupil Referral Units, whilst adapting to the specific needs of adolescent mothers, may also contribute to the mothers' feelings of maturity by offering them an alternative environment reflecting their status as mothers.

The mothers at the unit represent only the tip of the iceberg. Many mothers do not return to school; they have tuition at home or drop out of the educational system altogether. From an educational perspective the mothers referred to the unit have been advantaged in many ways, as attendance at the unit is 100%.

For the majority of the mothers, termination of pregnancy was not an option. Many had concealed their pregnancy and therefore it was too late to consider a termination. The mothers accepted pregnancy as their responsibility. Maternal grandparents were supportive; most of the mothers lived with their parents, often in overcrowded conditions. Some of the mothers lived in their own home and some lived with a boyfriend or the father of the child, but they were still supported and relied on their parents. Parents were initially shocked when they found their daughter was pregnant, but they stood by them regardless. Maternal grandmothers in particular appeared to act as gatekeepers and, for some of the mothers, ties to the father of the child were broken. The decision to break ties with the father was a 'trade-off' by mothers to secure the support of parents.

The role of the father of the child was not clear from the data. Some of the mothers still had contact with the father and allowed access to the child, although they were not dependent on the father for support. Some mothers were living with the father and appeared to have a stable relationship. For many of the mothers the father was no longer a part of their lives. The mothers perceived the father of the child as a means of financial support and if the father was not financially stable then he was excluded. Consequently, many of the fathers of the children were afforded no status as a parent. Some of the mothers had boyfriends and it appeared from the data that some boyfriends were happy to assume the role of father even if the child biologically was not their own.

Age of mother

The actions and reactions of the mothers imply that motherhood was not a state that was planned or desired. The mothers were all pregnant during the ages of 14 and 15 years. Some mothers had attempted to conceal the pregnancy, not wanting to inform their parents or face the reality of pregnancy and the impact it would have on their lives. Some parents had suspected pregnancy but did not broach the subject initially with their daughters. All of the mothers reported that, after the initial shock, their parents had been supportive.

Perceived maturity

The majority of the mothers felt they had matured since having the baby. Actually having the baby marked a process of maturity. The baby brought with it a reality in the mothers' lives and with it the status of motherhood, which could not be concealed. The Pupil Referral Unit reinforced their status as mothers, being specifically designed for this purpose.

Those interviewed that were pregnant reacted differently. In the early stages of pregnancy they felt they had not changed; as pregnancy progressed and body image changed then they perceived themselves maturing, getting ready for the baby.

What appears obvious from the mothers' comments is that, during the latter stages of pregnancy and motherhood itself, the mothers themselves appeared to change. They assumed responsibility for the child and made changes to their lives. Change and responsibility were linked to maturity. Age was also a contributing factor for the mothers; with motherhood, they felt older.

Responsibility of caring for a child

Many of the mothers in the study had younger brothers and sisters and were therefore exposed to and engaged in childcare.

Most of the mothers had assumed responsibility for the care of their child. Many had experience in caring for children, although there was recognition that it was different with their own child. The mothers did receive support from family members. They seemed accepting of their maternal responsibility. Caring for the child appeared to focus on the physical care; there was little discussion of emotional responsibility.

Relationships with friends

Relationships with friends played a significant role in the mothers' feelings of maturity. Many of the mothers had lost contact with their pre-pregnancy friends, the main reason for this being motherhood and the sense that they had nothing in common with their friends anymore. For some of the mothers, attendance at the Pupil Referral Unit had meant losing touch with friends.

In general, the mothers all agreed that their lives had changed with motherhood and attendance at the Pupil Referral Unit. A number of reasons were presented by the mothers to support the changes to their lives; however, all of these reasons centre on their status as mothers. The responsibilities they assume, their reliance on their families for support, finance and care of the child appear to place restrictions on their lives. The mothers did not appear to resent motherhood; there appeared to be a sense of acceptance of their position, which underpinned their notions of maturity, a maturity which appears to be enforced.

Conclusion

It is apparent from the findings that the mothers struggle with many aspects of motherhood, the struggle focusing on emotional expectations of the family, peers and the Pupil Referral Unit. In many ways society perceives adolescent mothers as being immature. Regardless of this perception, they are expected to aspire to the role of mother and are actively scrutinised in their effectiveness within this role.

The process of female reproduction is associated with the maturing of the female body. The normal female body becomes fully functional after bearing a child: all of the reproductive functions designed for childbearing are utilised. Within this narrow definition the female body matures after bearing a child. The adolescent female who becomes a mother has assumed the status of physical maturity through motherhood. It is unclear if a process of emotional maturity accompanies reproduction or if this has to be learned by the mother, perhaps through experience.

Many of the mothers perceive maturity through childbearing as complete in all aspects. Many of the mothers are used to caring for siblings and have little problem in adapting to the physical care of their child. From the data there seems to be a void between physical and emotional maturity. The mothers are able to care for their child but need support for the emotional and operational impact of motherhood on their lives.

The mothers relate having a child as a rite of passage to maturity through motherhood. For some of the mothers, perhaps their pre-pregnant lives had little meaning or value, so they have aspired to the status of motherhood unconditionally. The mothers fully accept the responsibility of motherhood and are able to provide the physical care and nurture of their child, but they are ill-prepared for the realities that motherhood brings to their lives. Many of the mothers reported they had lost contact with their pre-pregnancy friends, having nothing in common with them any more. As mothers they place the child at the centre of their lives but they need the support and assistance to mature emotionally. Attendance at the Pupil Referral Unit emphasises this perceived maturity. The unit does not operate as a traditional school. Attendance at the unit is excellent, but the mothers get more than a formal education; they are recognised as mothers and this reinforces feelings of maturity.

The mothers' need of support is perhaps a hallmark of their immaturity. They have adapted to the role of mothers and this is reinforced, but they still have aspirations for their future, aspirations that perhaps mirror the hopes and dreams of their non-pregnant contemporaries. From the mothers' comments, it appears that with motherhood comes a suppression of individuality and an acceptance of 'their lot'. The Pupil Referral Unit provides them with an avenue of protection and escape, where they can complete their education and adapt to motherhood, the price being a loss of their individual aspirations.

The initial results of this small study are significant to midwifery and health, as they portray adolescent motherhood as a complex issue that involves all aspects of an adolescent's life. Midwives are in a prime position to support adolescent mothers through recognition of their needs as mothers and adolescents.

REFERENCES

Bowerman CE. 1966. Unwed Motherhood: Personal and Social Consequences. Institute for Research in Social Science, North Carolina

Henshaw K, Kenney AM, Somberg D, Van Vort J. 1989. Teenage Motherhood in the United States: The Scope of the Problem and the State Response. Guttmacher Institute, New York

Krueger RA. 1997a. Analysing focus groups. In: Morgan DL, Krueger RA (eds), The Focus Group Kit. Sage, London

Krueger RA. 1997b. Developing questions for focus groups. In: Morgan DL, Krueger RA (eds), The Focus Group Kit. Sage, London

Krueger RA. 1997c. Moderating focus groups. In: Morgan DL, Krueger RA (eds), The Focus Group Kit. Sage, London

Krueger RA, King JA. 1997. Involving community members in focus groups. In: Morgan DL, Krueger RA (eds), The Focus Group Kit. Sage, London

Lawson L, Rhode DL (eds). 1993. The Politics of Pregnancy. Yale University Press, New Haven, CT

Macintyre S, Cunningham-Burley S. 1993. Teenage motherhood as a social problem: a perspective from the United Kingdom. In: Lawson L, Rhode DL (eds), The Politics of Pregnancy. Yale University Press, New Haven, CT

ONS. 2002. Birth Statistics: Births and Patterns of Family Building, England and Wales, 2001. Series FMI no. 30. HMSO, London

Pearce DM. 1993. Children having children: teenage motherhood and public policy from the woman's perspective. In: Lawson L, Rhode DL (eds), The Politics of Pregnancy. Yale University Press, New Haven, CT

Ruddich S. 1993. Procreative choice for adolescent women. In: Lawson L, Rhode DL (eds). The Politics of Pregnancy. Yale University Press, New Haven, CT

Strauss A, Corbin AJ. 1990. Basics of Qualitative Research. Sage, London

Social Exclusion Unit. 1999. Teenage Pregnancy. The Stationery Office, London

Vinovskis MA. 1988. An Epidemic of Adolescent Motherhood? Some Historic and Policy Perspectives. Oxford University Press, Oxford

Waite L, Moore K. 1978. The impact of an early first birth on young women's educational attainment. Social Forces, 56: 845–865

BIBLIOGRAPHY

Burgess A. 1997. Fatherhood Reclaimed. Vermilion, London

McCue Horwitz S, Klerman LV, Sung Kuo Jekel JF. 1991. School-age mothers: predictors of longterm educational and economic outcomes. Pediatrics, 87(6): 862–868

Morgan DL. 1993. Successful Focus Groups: Advancing the State of the Art. Sage, London

Morgan DL. 1997. The focus group guidebook. In: Morgan DL, Krueger RA (eds), The Focus Group Kit. Sage, London

Phoenix A. 1993. The social construction of teenage motherhood: a black and white issue. In: Lawson L, Rhode DL (eds), The Politics of Pregnancy. Yale University Press, New Haven, CT

Robinson S, Thompson AM. 1989. Midwives Research and Childbirth, Vol. I. Chapman & Hall, London

Stewart DW, Shamdasani PN. 1990. Focus Groups: Theory and Practice. Sage, London

The Practising Midwife 2003; 6(3): 21–24

Why choose motherhood?
The older teenage client's perspective

Is the term 'teenage pregnancy' an example of lazy labelling, branding older teenage mothers as irresponsible?

Claire Beckinsale

Picture the scene. There are two women waiting at a General Practitioner's surgery. They have both recently discovered they are pregnant.

The first woman has been in a stable, healthy relationship for two years and this is a planned pregnancy. She currently lives with her fiancé in well-maintained accommodation. She has an accessible and extensive support network.

The second woman has become pregnant as a result of a short relationship. Her social status and well-being is integrated in her career, which involves a lot of travel, long hours and total commitment. Her lifestyle does not adapt well to the inclusion of a child. She did not include motherhood in her long-term future. She will request a termination.

Both of these women are going to be made to feel irresponsible and victimised. Why? Because the first woman is 'only just 18 years old', and because the second is 38 years old and 'this may be her only chance of fulfilling her role of a mother'.

I want to explore the issues surrounding teenage pregnancy from the viewpoint of teenagers aged 17–19 years who welcome or choose to become pregnant. I will adopt a positive viewpoint to support the important decision that thousands of young mothers have made.

To understand the experience of these mothers we need to consider the factors influencing society's attitudes. I will consider issues of age and when a child becomes adult, the power of language and labelling. I will then explore the political incentives and research, and the schemata of society and influences on stereotype formation.

I shall consider why teenagers choose motherhood, and how improvements can be made in health services, society and education.

'What are you going to do when you grow up?'

Adolescence begins 'at the onset of puberty, when sexual maturity, or the ability to reproduce, is attained'. An adolescent is challenged to resolve the issues of sexuality, social relationships with parents and peers, and occupation selection (Zimbardo, 1992). Finding resolve to these issues is a complex task that would render a huge proportion of our adult population as adolescents!

Box 8.2.1 shows Levinson's (1986) stages of adulthood, which recognises that we leave adolescence to enter early adult transition at the age of 17–22 years.

Age has many facets that contribute to the overall perception of oneself. Factors include appearance (biological age), how old we feel (subjective age) and our life experiences and status (functional age) (Kastenbaum, 1979).

It is recognised that our perception of optimum age is directly influenced by our own age (Gross, 1992). The majority of society will be older and this could be a negative factor in the perception of teenage pregnancy. Teenagers themselves are rarely the voices that speak out against this issue. Phoenix (1991) found that teenage mothers did not regard themselves as 'too young' and 92% felt they were coping well or very well.

The power of language

The label 'teenage' encompasses both adolescents and adults, without respecting chronological age or considering biological, functional and subjective attributes. It does not promote individualism or holistic attitudes, yet the comparison between a 13-year-old mother and a 19-year-old mother and their ability to parent may well highlight tremendous differences.

Box 8.2.1 Levinson's stages of adulthood

Ages 17–22	**Early adult transition** Leave adolescence, make preliminary choice for adult life	
Ages 22–28	**Entering the adult world** Initial choices in love, occupation, friendship, values, lifestyle	
Ages 28–33	**Age 30 transition** Change in life structure. Either a moderate change or, more often, a severe and stressful crisis	
Ages 33–40	**Settling down** Establish a niche in society, progress on a timetable, in both family and career accomplishments	
Ages 40–45	**Midlife transition** Life structure comes into question. Usually a time of crisis in the meaning, direction and value of each person's life. Neglected parts of the self (talents, desires, aspirations) seek expression	
Ages 45–50	**Entering middle adulthood** Choices must be made and a new life structure formed. Person must commit to new tasks	
Ages 50–55	**Age 50 transition** Further questioning and modification of the life structure. Men who did not have a crisis at age 40 are likely to have one now	
Ages 55–60	**Culmination of middle adulthood** Build a new life structure. Can be time of great fulfilment	
Ages 60–65	**Late adult transition** Reappraisal of life. Moments of pride in achievement are interspersed with periods of despair	
Ages 65–80	**Late adulthood** Make peace with oneself and others. Fewer illusions, broader perspective on life	
Ages 80+	**Late late adulthood** Final transition. Prepare for death	

Phoenix (1991) found that when the words 'teenage' and 'pregnancy' are put together it immediately implies a lack of the necessary maturity. This leads to negative views that she believes to be unfounded.

In recent years there has been huge interest in reducing teenage pregnancy rates within government, the media and social structures. The use of the term 'teenager' is used in government initiatives such as *The Health of the Nation* (Department of Health, 1992) and the paper 'Teenage pregnancy' (presented by parliament in 1999). These initiatives propose to reduce the number of teenage pregnancies by 50%. The aims could be viewed as conflicting with Article 12 of the Human Rights Act (1998), which states:

Men and women of marriageable age have the right to marry and found a family.

Eighty-two thousand of the 90,000 pregnancies to teenagers were conceived in women aged 16–19 ('Teenage pregnancy', 1999). Therefore, the majority could have been viewed as exercising their human rights. Many of the teenage mothers addressed have also been granted the right to vote, drive, drink alcohol, take on mortgages and financial loans, and commit to marriage. Are the women that I am considering only able to make the life decisions that society permits, regardless of consequence?

It is clear that many research articles and government initiatives are focusing on pregnancies in women under

18 years old and the majority on pregnancy in under 16 years old (see Box 8.2.2). The generic term 'teenage' is used in the title of the works but the findings only apply to 9% of teenage pregnancies (where girls are under 16). Therefore the label 'teenage' is used to address the issues of the minority and misused in ideologies.

Box 8.2.2 Use of the label 'teenage' excludes older teenage mothers

Literature reference	Age of subjects
Bachman J. 1993. Self-described learning needs of pregnant teen participants in an innovative university/community partnership. Maternal–Child Nursing Journal, 21(2): 65–72	< 16
Kalmuss D, Namerow P. 1994. Subsequent childbearing among teenage mothers. Family Planning Perspectives, 26(4): 149–153	< 17
Lobb M. 1987. Teenage Pregnancies, pp. 624–628	< 16
Maternity Alliance. 2000. Pregnant Teenagers, Young Mothers and Benefits. Maternity Alliance, London	< 18
Millar W. 1997. A perspective on Canadian teenage births. Canadian Journal of Public Health, 88(5): 333–336	< 17
Peckham S. 1993. Preventing unintended teenage pregnancies. Public Health, 107(2): 125–133	< 16
Piyasil V. 1998. Anxiety and depression in teenage mothers. Journal of the Medical Association of Thailand, 91(2): 125–129	< 18

The older teenage mothers appear to be a voiceless group within society, silenced by the ingrained guilt they may feel for shaming society by becoming young parents. After all, if you saw enough media coverage and government effort put into preventing you from becoming pregnant, then surely for you to be pregnant is wrong?

I consider the unnecessary and misplaced labelling lazy and inconsiderate, but perhaps created by the need for sensationalist headings and impressive statistics. As little perceived offence is recognised from older teenage mothers there may be no incentive to correct this inaccuracy.

It would create uproar in society if the government decided to tackle 'reducing the number of conceptions in women over 40 years old', for example. Women in this age group are thought to have specific risks that could apply to their pregnancy and the health of their children, but such campaigns would be an infringement of their rights. In fact, technology is aiding women over the age of menopause to become mothers, so why is the issue of teenage pregnancy so acceptably bad in our society?

A dystopic account of teenage pregnancy and parenthood is depicted in society but is not necessarily representational. Focus is put on young mothers' lack of maturity, limited childcare and lack of parenting skills. This is influential in creating stereotypical and judgemental attitudes in society. The family of Zoe Joynson would not allow anyone to criticise her mothering abilities. Zoe, aged 19, tragically died during a house fire whilst using her body to shield her baby from the flames. Baby Bradley survived unhurt because of his mother's ultimate act of love (Joynson, 2001).

Research findings challenge many of the sweeping assumptions of teenage pregnancy outcomes. The heavily quoted 'increased incidence of low birth weight babies to teenage mothers' seems to have an outdated and questionable basis (Satin et al., 1994; Reichman & Pagnini, 1997; Jolly et al., 2000).

Studies have shown that teenage mothers actually have a higher rate of normal vaginal deliveries with no intervention and lower incidence of caesarean section deliveries (Makinson, 1985; Jolly et al., 2000). In isolation of other factors a pregnancy in teenage years does not equate to a high-risk pregnancy. Niven (1992), in *Psychological Care for Families*, felt it necessary to state that she was not including teenage mothers in the chapter titled 'Problems' as this is not a group recognised as experiencing more problems before, during or after birth. Lilley (1990) found that infant care practices of unmarried teenage mothers were similar to a random sample of mothers living in the same area.

Why is teenage motherhood so bad?

The predominant image of the teenage mother as the 'schoolgirl mother' is statistically inaccurate and non-representational of the majority of teenage mothers. The image creates powerful responses in society that could be due to the discomfort of considering the 'child' as a sexual being. Parents often perceive their offspring as vulnerable and child-like even when they are well into adulthood (just ask my mother!). We are motivated to nurture and protect our children. To acknowledge that they have made the transition into developing a sexual identity independent of our influence may create disharmony in our inner selves. Blame may be placed on the parents as they have directly failed to protect their 'child'.

Pregnancy is a visual message that enables any witnessing person to draw on one true and accurate conclusion – the pregnant person is no longer a virgin and has had sexual intercourse at least once. Attempts to conceal pregnancy may be a way of preventing shame on families and loved ones.

People need to make their mental worlds 'cognitively comfortable' (Festinger, 1957). Acknowledgement that a group previously considered as needy and dependent are taking control over their futures may produce dissonance and negative feelings of disapproval and hostility, creating a need to suppress the 'threatening group'.

Attitudes to sexuality must also be a factor in our responses. Sex is presented to us by many media throughout our lives. The media make us sexually aware in magazines, videos and films in a way that encourages the expression of sexuality; being 'sexy' is a desirable state. During our fundamental years we are formally taught by authorities (i.e. schools) of the negative consequences of sexual activity, with little attention given to the spiritual individuals that we all are. Indeed, this focus is continued in the initiatives to discourage teenagers becoming pregnant. Information is provided of:

- The 90% chance that a teenager has of becoming pregnant in the first year of being sexually active and not using contraception
- The risks of sexually transmitted infections if condoms aren't used.

These factors are very important issues that directly affect all sexually active people, not isolated to teenagers alone as presented in the literature. Attributing such universal issues in a way that suggests ownership by a minority group promotes further social marginalisation.

The struggle against patriarchal suppression by feminists may indirectly add to social disapproval of teenage parenthood. Beauvoir (1953) believed that from the beginning of history women were doomed to domestic work and 'prevented ... from taking part in the shaping of the world ... her enslavement to the generative function'. Teenage mothers could be seen as entering into the 'role' that feminists have campaigned against, consolidating the suppression of their potential.

Why are teenage women choosing motherhood?

Educating myself about the reasons why motherhood is desired has fascinated me. I am a mother of two beautiful children. I have known since I was 17 years old that I would welcome and cherish motherhood. Diana Birch (1999) describes my longing for motherhood as a 'magical belief'. It is an 'intrinsic idea with high emotional content, a feeling of instinct and intuition and which may have no perceivable basis on current reality'. Ann Phoenix (1991) found that 20% of young mothers aged 16–19 had wanted to conceive, with 25% of women not minding being mothers. So what may have influenced the decisions of these women?

The nature–nurture debate

Stanworth (1988) believes that women are biologically determined to reproduce. Hubbard (as cited by Walton, 1994) maintains that there is no biological desire to reproduce, but that it is a social construction to keep women in a domestic role. I feel that an element of both theories is applicable. We are given potentials by our genetic make-up but our destinies are extrinsically determined.

The genetic element could partially account for the fact that the mothers of teenage mothers were often teenage parents themselves (Chaplin & McDiarmid, 1992; McVeigh & Smith, 2000).

An interesting theory could also be that the reduced chance of undergoing major abdominal surgery during childbirth in our teenage years is motivational for these women. Our instinct for survival may have adapted to reduce the risks created by the interventionalist medical experience of modern childbirth!

More focus is given to the socio-economic characteristics of teenage mothers, with more teenage mothers coming from middle-class than affluent backgrounds. Two-thirds of teenage women from affluent areas have abortions in comparison to a quarter from deprived areas (Wallace, as cited by Carroll, 2001). The issue of self-esteem is raised by this social difference, with Wallace believing that 'less well-off girls have few social and educational alternatives ... Middle-class girls have other options for achieving self-esteem'. Class also influences how we perceive pregnant teenage women,

with middle-class women being viewed as 'victims' and black working-class women being 'deviants' (Chaplin & McDiarmid, 1992).

Traditionally, young people were seen to become adult when they married and/or went out to work (Walton, 1994). In our present economic climate, working-class women may choose motherhood for their own personal development. Motherhood could be a realistic and achievable goal that facilitates an entrance into adulthood.

Matsuhashi and Felice (1991) found that teenage women in the third trimester of pregnancy had clearer self-identity, more positive body image and higher self-esteem than non-pregnant teenagers. The positive status of pregnancy and motherhood in society may have been an influence in the findings. The capacity to reproduce confirms that she can fulfil her biological 'function'. Further proof could be attributed to this theory when we consider the feelings of inadequacy and failure that women experience when they are unable to become pregnant, along with the extent of the testing, procedures, and emotional and financial costs that families undergo.

Pregnancy may be the first time a teenage woman is in a valued role, independently belonging to a positively perceived group in society. The admission into the group named 'mother' is not reliant on academic ability, social grouping or financial contribution.

I strongly believe that pregnancy and motherhood can be a means of self-healing and opportunity for growth. The positive aspect of parenting for young survivors of abuse/neglect was explored in research conducted by Williams and Vines (1999). The pregnant woman can identify with her baby and identify with her own 'inner child' (Birch, 1999), a time where she is now a force and can influence a situation. She can become the mother that she needed to have as a child, putting right the failures of her own parents. Phoenix (1991) recognised that a large percentage of young mothers have divorced parents. Pregnancy and parenthood to young mothers have been considered as a catalyst to reconnecting with families (Williams & Vines, 1999), aiding integration back into the family network (Toberer et al., 2000).

How can we help?

Pregnant teenage women are often associated with late booking for antenatal care. This confirms to many health professionals the lack of responsibility, commitment and maturity of the teenage mother. This creates a negative circle of poor communication that increases the alienation felt by teenage mothers. Health professionals must accept some responsibility for creating an environment that is perceived as threatening by this group of clients. Rozette et al. (2000) reported that teenage mothers 'were afraid that health staff could force them to have an abortion' and 'afraid or ashamed of the medical staff's likely reaction'.

Health professionals are not blank slates, we are influenced by social constructions and create our own stereotypes and prejudices accordingly. It is important that we are given the opportunity to analyse, recognise and adapt/accommodate our schemata to prevent negative transmission to clients. We promote holistic and individualised care for women and families; I believe we need to adopt the same attitude to members of our profession.

Midwives are individuals with a whole lifetime of experiences that make us human. Self-recognition can uncover underlying conflicts. If health professionals with a positive attitude and interest are identified in maternity units a referral system could be implemented. An open-minded and non-threatening manner could transform the image that teenage mothers have and positively influence their experience of our service.

Traditional professional education and working environments do not promote the opportunity for self-analysis. My experience of preparing this paper is proof of this fact. When I realised that my thoughts and concepts were fundamental, encouraged and acknowledged, I had to transform my attitude to accommodate and 'allow' myself this freedom. The successful academic is usually one that can be objective and professional, with the ability to cite the theories of a range of experts without considering their own subjective, emotional and personal opinions based on life experiences and 'magical beliefs'.

In reality, however, teenage mothers are unconcerned about the academia surrounding them, but are affected by what is directly attributed to their personal experience – attitudes of staff. We can present ourselves as 'judgemental and patronising', treating teenage mothers 'differently' to older mothers and failing to treat them as 'normal'. One young mother urged health professionals to:

Respect us as young mothers and not judge us.
(Rozette et al., 2000)

Western social and political systems need to recognise the wider picture when considering teenage pregnancy rates rather than just allocate blame and attempt to eradicate. Society needs to be more accepting and acknowledge the reasons why teenagers are entering into parenthood. A percentage of teenage mothers come from disadvantaged backgrounds. Addressing the needs of these people when they are children could enable the process of healing to begin earlier, raising self-esteem and preventing them entering into motherhood prematurely.

Teenage parents have to accommodate the transition to becoming parents. This can be a traumatic period of adjustment for any parent, as Kate Figes' book *Life After Birth* (1998) demonstrates. Isolation can consolidate negative feelings; therefore, a supportive social network in an environment where mothers feel respected and valued is imperative. Friends and family can provide this as well as schemes such as peer support groups and Sure Start initiatives.

Some teenage mothers may feel comfortable in antenatal and postnatal education programmes aimed at all mothers, but if this is not the case we may need to adapt our current ideas to provide specific classes for young parents. If this is heavily led by the requirements of individual groups it could ensure that the needs of the parents/parents-to-be are met and provide a supportive social link.

If young women from working-class backgrounds are becoming mothers to gain self-esteem, the education system may be failing them. Do we put too much emphasis on academic achievements rather than practical life skills? How can we prevent teenage women becoming self-fulfilling prophecies who, given opportunities to develop self-esteem by other means, would have chosen to do so?

An education programme designed to inform pupils of the realities of parenting, and the teaching of parenting and life skills, could educate pupils enough to facilitate informed choice. If or when they become parents it should be at the right time of life for them. In teaching programmes attention is given to a diverse range of subjects – for example, drama skills – yet the percentage of pupils that become actors is fractional to the percentage that will become parents. Education needs to be more grounded and applicable to real life to be a worthwhile foundation for adulthood.

I have found the issues surrounding teenage motherhood fascinating and complex. The exploration of the broader issues, such as attitudes towards age and motivations for motherhood, has been useful for my self-awareness.

In conclusion, it has not been my aim to advocate pregnancy for young women. I feel that the transition occurring during these years from adolescence to early adulthood is often not acknowledged in society's attitudes towards teenage pregnancy. I do not believe that being a teenage mother per se equates to poor motherhood, just as not every 20-year-old and older mother has the ability to effectively parent and convey positive values to their children.

REFERENCES

Beauvoir S. 1953. The Second Sex. Jonathon Cape, London

Birch D. 1999. Psychological issues in teenage pregnancy. Journal of Adolescent Health and Welfare, 12(2): 5–12

Carroll H. 2001. Nice girls like these. Real, 14 May, 12–16

Chaplin J, McDiarmid P. 1992. Teenage parenthood – myth and reality. Community Health Action, 25: 3

Department of Health. 1992. The Health of the Nation – A Strategy for Health in England. HMSO, London

Festinger L. 1957. A Theory of Cognitive Dissonance. Harper & Row, New York

Figes K. 1998. Life After Birth. Penguin, Middlesex

Gross R. 1992. Psychology: The Science of Mind and Behaviour, 2nd edn. Hodder & Stoughton, London

Jolly M et al. 2000. Obstetric risks of pregnancy in women less than 18 years old. Obstetrics and Gynaecology, 96(6): 962–966

Joynson K. 2001. I'll be a great mum, you'll see. That's Life, 21: 26–27

Kastenbaum R. 1979. Growing Old – Years of Fulfilment. Harper & Row, London

Levinson D. 1986. A conception of adult development. American Psychologist, 41: 3–13

Lilley J. 1990. The infant care practises of young unmarried mothers. Journal of Reproductive and Infant Psychology, 8: 277–278

Makinson C. 1985. Young age per se does not make a high-risk pregnancy. Family Planning Perspectives, 17: 132

Matsuhashi Y, Felice M. 1991. Adolescent body image during pregnancy. Journal of Adolescent Health, 12: 313–315

Niven C. 1992. Psychological Care for Families Before, During and After Birth. Butterworth-Heinemann, Oxford

Phoenix A. 1991. Young Mothers? Policy Press, London

Reichman N, Pagnini D. 1997. Maternal age and birth outcomes: data from New Jersey. Family Planning Perspectives, 29(6): 268–272

Rozette C et al. 2000. A profile of teenage pregnancy. The Practising Midwife, 3(10): 23–25

Satin A et al. 1994. Maternal youth and pregnancy outcomes: middle school versus high school age groups compared with women beyond the teen years. American Journal of Obstetrics and Gynecology, 171(1): 184–187

Stanworth M. 1988. Reproductive Technologies: Gender, Motherhood and Medicine. Basil Blackwell, Cambridge

Toberer S et al. 2000. Teenage Pregnancy and Choice. Abortion or Motherhood: Influences on the Decision. York Publishing Services, York

Walton I. 1994. Sexuality and Motherhood. Books for Midwives, Cheshire

Williams C, Vines S. 1999. Broken past, fragile future: personal stories of high-risk adolescent mothers. Journal of the Society of Pediatric Nurses, 4(1): 15–23

Zimbardo P. 1992. Psychology and Life, 13th edn. HarperCollins, New York

The Practising Midwife 2003; 6(3): 10–13

Beating disability, embracing motherhood

Simone Baker

I was born in 1962, a year when many women had mixed feelings about being pregnant and having babies. Thalidomide had hit the headlines, and newspapers were reporting 'monster' babies being born around the UK and in Europe with horrific congenital deformities: babies with no arms and shortened legs; and, in severe cases, with a tiny head attached to a limbless trunk.

On 27 September, after a traumatic breech delivery, I was whisked away to the nursery, despite my mother's pleas to see her newborn baby. Doctors decided how to break the news to her. I was one of those 'monster' babies. Twenty-four hours later, she unwrapped the blanket to study me for the first time. She touched the tiny malformed arms, shortened to elbow length, the three fingers on flipper hands and the legs shortened at the femur, and said a silent prayer: 'God, if this child is going to suffer any pain, please take her now before I grow to love her any more'.

When one plans to have children, I think it is fair to say that one expects it to happen immediately! But I now know that for many women this isn't the case, and indeed it wasn't for me. After a year, I was referred to a fertility clinic. Two and a half years later it was discovered that I had a 'unicornate' uterus – only half-formed. One of my fallopian tubes wasn't connected to my uterus, and taking into account my age at the time (33) my chances of conceiving were drastically reduced.

A month later, and without any fertility treatment, I discovered I was pregnant!

My midwife said she could help and advise on every aspect of pregnancy and birth, but would probably not be able to offer much support in problems presented by my disability. I hadn't even considered potential problems. I had coped with everything else life had put my way, including finding employment, passing my driving test and living independently. I hadn't considered this new challenge to be any different.

I made some enquiries about sources of help. I discovered the Mary Marlborough Centre in Oxford, and was referred there by my GP for an assessment. This was carried out by an occupational therapist, who took me through every stage of caring for a newborn: bathing, dressing, feeding, changing, etc. There were useful items of equipment to see and try, such as a cot with a gate-opening side, a changing mat with a harness on it and a life-size, live-weight doll, which I used to try out different slings and other items.

Visits to the antenatal clinic were a bit of a challenge. As my bump grew larger, I found it nearly impossible to climb on to the examination couch. I would often have to remind the midwife or GP to pull my trousers back over my bump after examination, as I could no longer reach to do this with my shortened arms.

Halfway through my pregnancy, I was prescribed a course of steroids in case the baby should be born prematurely. I was naturally concerned about possible side-effects for either myself or the baby, but I was told that 'any side-effects are far outweighed by the benefit of the steroids for the baby'. Of course, I experienced virtually every side-effect: insomnia and restlessness, a bright red face once a week, sugar in my urine and, worst, no fetal movement the day after I'd taken the dosage – worrying weeks that seemed to last forever.

A difficulty I knew I'd have in hospital following the birth would be the height of the cribs. I am only five feet tall, and because my arms are short I have very limited reach. I pointed this out to the staff in the maternity unit, and enquired whether I might bring in a Moses basket on a stand. I was told that, because of infection control and fire regulations, this wouldn't be possible – the crib needed to be on wheels in case of an evacuation. I accepted this, but no alternative was offered.

I had a planned caesarean at 40 weeks under regional anaesthetic. Lois Nicole Baker was delivered eight minutes after the operation had started, weighing in at a healthy 6 lb 14 oz.

I had been keen to have my husband in the hospital with me to provide essential personal assistance, such as lifting the baby, bathing and reaching things. I knew that the ward staff would be very stretched, and felt I couldn't justify summoning assistance for passing drinks or cutting up food. Provision was made but, again, not in an ideal way. My husband slept on a Z-bed which was folded up every day as the room was so tiny. He was instructed to go home to shower, as he couldn't use the maternity ward facilities. He would collect my breakfast for me each morning, and was embarrassed at the strange looks he got from the postnatal women all collecting their breakfasts in their dressing gowns.

I couldn't wait to get home – I felt so 'disabled' in the hospital. Breastfeeding in hospital got off to a shaky start; I didn't feel comfortable trying to breastfeed on the bed, and the floor wasn't comfortable or clean enough for me to try feeding that way. My sister and I had designed and constructed a beanbag of enormous proportions to help me with breastfeeding, which was waiting for me at home.

Three days later, I was thrilled to be at home again, where breastfeeding proved much easier. I could place the beanbag around my waist while seated on the floor. We had included fabric handles to assist with pulling the beanbag into place. This beanbag became Lois's world

for the next few weeks, and an essential tool in enabling me to breastfeed. It provided a safe and comfortable raised surface on which I could place my newborn baby while I got into position on the floor.

I used a muslin cloth folded into a strip behind Lois's back, pulling the two ends underneath her arms to the front. Using my teeth to take the weight, I would lift her stork-like. I use my mouth and teeth a lot to assist me with daily living tasks, and I have developed considerable strength in my neck and jaw. This system worked well for breastfeeding, as I could lift and turn her from breast to breast to feed. At five months, Lois's weight prevented the use of this method, but by then she had developed a degree of head control.

Lois adapted quickly to me. As a baby, she would cling like a limpet when I carried her. At 20 months, she could climb confidently up and down the stairs, climb up and down from her high chair, strap herself into her pushchair, and climb into her car seat. Her deftness with clothing and footwear impressed everyone. I couldn't easily cuddle Lois on my lap, so she cuddled me, climbing on to the seat behind me and encircling my shoulders and neck in a huge embrace.

Is being a mum with a disability hard work? Being a mum is hard work, full stop! Being a disabled mum presents everyday challenges, but Lois and I face them together and head on.

The Practising Midwife 2003; 6(7): 16–17

Post-traumatic maternity: a time for healing or wounding?

Mindy Levy

Women who have survived traumas experience maternity in a different light than other women. They have fears, insecurities and doubts that set them apart. They are plagued by frightening memories, guilt and feelings of victimisation. They yearn to regain normality, social acceptance and optimism; often, they turn to maternity in hope of achieving these goals. As midwives, we come face to face with their plight during pregnancy, birth and puerperium.

Birth changes women

Birth transforms women into mothers. Some are exhilarated by the experience of pregnancy and birth, by the discovery of their physicality, by the awareness of their power and by their victories. They seem to be transported to another sphere of reality, as if they are floating on air. Other women are disappointed and angry with themselves and their caretakers, bewildered, weakened and dismayed by the events that surround the birth of their children. These women require time to gain perspective on the meaning of these confusing and overwhelming experiences. Rarely is a woman apathetic to the memory of her birth. Birth seems to change each and every woman in many different ways.

Women who have been emotionally wounded by traumatic experiences approach pregnancy, birth and mothering with a mixture of hope and fear. Remnants of shadowy experiences leave them wounded, terrorised and helpless; these dark memories linger deep inside their bodies. Their hope is that the baby, which is good, pure and uncontaminated, will arrive and light up the darkness that pervades their inner selves. They fear failure, inadequacy, mistreatment, injury and pain.

Zohar's story

Recently I heard the story of Zohar, a woman whose shattered life was changed significantly by her pregnancy. One morning, while riding in a public bus, she was traumatised by the blast of a terrorist bomb. She was the mother of a six-month-old baby at the time, and was critically injured and hospitalised for over a month and a half. She came home broken physically but full of hope for a good recovery. Her baby didn't recognise her and refused to even approach her. What was left of her life before the bombing fell completely apart. She became fearful, sleepless, agitated, dependent and distraught. For months she wandered around listlessly looking for a way to feel whole again, to regain her physical health, to re-establish her motherhood, to recreate a semblance of her life before the bombing as a woman, as the mother to her baby and as a partner to her husband who had become her primary caregiver.

Several months later she became pregnant, and her pregnancy became the trigger that eventually led her through a process that promoted emotional healing. She was, in a literal sense, reborn together with her developing fetus.

I had lost 20 kilo. I didn't believe that my body could sustain life. Something inside me had dissolved. After the initial shock wore off and my belly started to show, I realised that I was going to become a woman again, a mother. I have a fetus growing in my uterus; everything is normal, and I am becoming feminine and round. I suddenly understood that if my body was strong enough to nurture a developing fetus, then my soul was strong enough to nurse itself back to health. I took control again and found myself a therapist.

This woman's story added new substance to my belief that pregnancy and birth are experiences that are of such great significance in women's lives that they can trigger and promote healing processes in the emotionally wounded. Birth can empower women; it has the potential for transformation, for implementing change. A positive, empowering birth can be the experience that helps a woman discover her power and her capabilities and can change her forever.

Post-traumatic maternity

Mothering is a common denominator among women across cultures and time. Most women define themselves through their pregnancies, births and the mothering of their children. It is what the female body knows best; mothering is what women do. In the eyes of women, losses that involve the ability to mother are losses that are critical, irreplaceable and unbearable. The woman who is wounded physically and emotionally is anxious about maintaining her ability to procreate and care for her children. The woman who has been traumatised fears that she may never be the same and that she may never properly fulfil her role as mother.

Women come to their births traumatised from a wide variety of past experiences: sexual abuse, domestic violence, rape, sudden or premature loss of loved ones, natural disasters, perinatal loss, terrorism and previous births. As midwives we tend to underestimate the number of women who have suffered from traumatic experiences in their lives; it is almost impossible for us to fathom the extent of this phenomenon. We know little about the personal histories of the women we work with beyond what they choose to share with us. Often, the most pertinent details are those that are missing from their stories.

When a woman suffers a traumatic experience, that event becomes a chapter in her history and a part of her body, a vague and often elusive portion of her memory. Her body remembers what happened, even though her cognitive recollections may play tricks with the chain of events. Powerful but imperfect sensory memories linger: the smells, the sights, the sounds and the touch. The feelings and emotions associated with these sensations are tucked away deep within the self. On a conscious level, she may even forget what happened.

During pregnancy, birth and lactation, as a result of hormonal changes, women tend to open up and become super-sensitive to the environment and to themselves. Emotions are exaggerated and often clarified. Sensitivity to others is heightened, exposure to memories is increased and past traumatic experiences are brought to light. Forgotten or hidden materials surface unexpectedly and transform routine maternity experiences into retraumatising events. Triggers that are unknown to the woman may set off unpredictably powerful reactions.

Lessons learned

After hearing Zohar's story, I set out on a journey as a midwife and a woman to learn as much as possible from other women who suffered similar experiences. I eagerly listened to eight women who agreed to share their distressing stories with me. They explained what it was like to be terrorised by sudden and extreme trauma. They told me how they gathered together shattered parts of their selves, became pregnant, gave birth and became mothers, each under the shadow of her own trauma.

Each woman reacted differently. The events of her life changed her forever, as she continued to maintain a life that was hers alone. Today life goes on for all of them, each with her history, personality, identity, body and self that enable her to cope and grow from these experiences in a manner that is uniquely hers.

The lessons I learned from the shared experiences of these women were numerous. Similarities between their stories and those of sexual abuse and birth trauma survivors were revealed. Some of the collective themes that emerged reflect issues that may be specific to this particular type of trauma. Others may be generalised more broadly. Further research is needed in order to better understand additional sources of women's traumas and their effect on maternity experiences.

Post-traumatic pregnancy

Post-traumatic pregnancy is an experience filled with extreme ambivalence, fear, self-doubt and anxiety. The death-like darkness of the trauma remains within the consciousness of the post-traumatic woman, while a fresh new life is developing in her pregnant womb. The inherent contradictions are enormous.

Although she is hopeful for a new beginning, she is also deeply aware of the dangers that life can bring. She experiences the power of her body as it creates and nourishes her fetus. Fetal movements remind her that she is about to become a mother, and that her life is moving forward. On the other hand, as the pregnancy progresses, her fears mount; she dreads going to the hospital. She is afraid to feel pain again, to see blood, to feel helpless and to be dependent on others. She is afraid to go to the place that is likely to remind her of her trauma. She is afraid of losing control, being hurt and being surrounded by strangers again. Her experiences have damaged her sense of basic trust.

Post-traumatic birth

As labour begins, the pain of the contractions reminds the woman of other pain and the trauma that she has felt in the past. She is weakened by her doubts and fears. She may feel that she is incapable of coping with this highly arousing experience. She feels that she is different from other birthing women. She has special needs; she has unique fears that no one can anticipate. She may lose the ability to cope with the challenge of labour because memories of her trauma intertwine with the sensory experiences of pain and create an intensely confusing and difficult experience. From the start, she may request a caesarean section in order to avoid the intensity of the birth and achieve a sense of control.

The last few months of the pregnancy were filled with fears. I wanted the baby, but I was scared to death. I was scared of going back to the hospital, of seeing blood, of being cut. My fears were totally out of control; most of them were unwarranted. Somehow, the bombing attached itself to the birth and got stuck. In the ninth month the fears peaked. I was afraid of seeing green uniforms, of being at the mercy of others, of being dependent on their decisions and the touch of their hands. I was afraid of the blood, the operating room, the anaesthesia and the needles. I was convinced that a C-section would be easier for me, that it would hurt less and that there would be less blood than in a regular birth. Everything would be sterile; I would go in and come out with a baby.

Post-traumatic mothering

Mothering is a difficult undertaking for all women. Those who have suffered losses of confidence and security as a result of trauma approach the task from a perspective of apprehension and weakness. Post-traumatic mothering is filled with fears and anxieties concerning basic safety. Fortunately, newborn babies are sources of hope, light, optimism and innocence; they represent the goodness in human nature and the renewal of life. Women are reborn as mothers when they give birth to their babies. Young children force their mothers forward into the reality of the here and now and prevent them from dwelling on their dark pasts. They help heal their mothers from their traumas but pay the price of being overprotected by them.

Care of post-traumatic mothers

Midwifery care of post-traumatic women begins with identifying them. Some women will come forth and share the stories of their traumas. Some will shy away from the difficult task of exposing their weaknesses. These women often feel voiceless and are accustomed to keeping their traumas to themselves. They quickly learn that no one can really understand their pain or is interested in hearing about it. Although they may beg to scream out desperately for help, they silence themselves in order to survive within their social contexts.

All midwives work with post-traumatic women, and we must make a concerted effort in order to successfully pick them out of the crowd. How can we learn to identify them? See Box 8.4.1.

If communication with caregivers is effective, the unique needs of the post-traumatic woman will be identified before, during and after labour. If she receives care that answers her specific needs, she may have a positive and empowering birth experience. If a safe place

Box 8.4.1 Identifying the woman who has been traumatised

Is she the woman with fear in her eyes?
Is she the woman who incessantly asks questions?
Is she the woman with needle phobia?
Is she the woman who is silent and distant?
Is she the woman who screams?
Is she the woman who requests a C-section?
Is she the woman who refuses to be examined by a male caregiver?
Is she the woman who freezes up or dissociates during a vaginal examination?
Is she the woman who demands total control over every detail?
Is she the woman who refuses all interventions?
Is she the woman who cries?
Is she the woman who doesn't want to be touched?
Is she the woman who trusts no one?

is provided for her, she may feel strong, secure and able to cope. The significance of a good birth experience is far-reaching; it boosts her confidence, reaffirms her belief in herself and helps her to reconnect with the wisdom and power of her body. It provides her with a new memory that will empower her in subsequent times of distress and enable her to connect to her capable self. This may be the time when healing begins for her (see Box 8.4.2).

If the needs of the post-traumatic woman are ignored, missed or wrongly identified, or they are treated coldly and insensitively by midwives or doctors, she may suffer a disempowering and re-traumatising birth experience. Routine tasks in the delivery room are far from mundane for her. She may suffer losses concerning her body's abilities to perform the basic female functions of pregnancy, labour, birth and lactation. She may come away from birth with new traumatic memories that will make mothering a newborn baby a complex task. Even if she succeeds in achieving maternity, normality may still remain unattainable for her (see Box 8.4.3). Trauma is a very personal and subjective experience; only the traumatised can feel and sense it.

Conclusion

Pregnancy, birth and mothering are the exclusive experiences of women, and may be among the most significant events in their lives. Past experiences play vital roles in shaping the course of these events and in determining their impact and significance. A woman's perception of her maternity experiences will affect the future of her mothering, her relationships, her children and her children's children. Each woman carries, along with her own history, the history of her mother's pregnancies and births; likewise, her birth experiences will inevitably become a part of her children's histories.

Box 8.4.2 Promoting healing in the post-traumatic mother

Accept her just the way she is

Help her to identify and state her needs

Communicate with her empathetically

Remember how much pain she has already suffered

Respect her special requests

Encourage her to concentrate on the here and now

Provide information regarding physiological processes

Avoid unnecessary medical interventions

Provide rationale and explanations for all actions

Avoid surprises

Receive permission before touching her body

Give her a feeling of control in decision-making

Prepare her for the possibility of emergency procedures

Protect her privacy fiercely

Provide her with a permanent caregiver

Help her to identify and express her approach to pain relief

Encourage her to express her fears as they arise

Encourage upright positions during labour

Remind her of the final goal – the baby

Box 8.4.3 How can we inadvertently hurt and retraumatise women?

By providing inadequate support

By assuming that we know what is best for them

By ignoring the signs and signals that they send us

By assuming that routine procedures are harmless

By not listening

By using words that remind them of their trauma

By not respecting their privacy

By violating the boundaries of their bodies without their explicit permission

By forcing them to lie on their backs

By bullying them

As midwives, we find ourselves intimately involved in the pregnancies, births and postpartum experiences of women. We touch their bodies and souls in many ways; we are witnesses to their pain and to their weaknesses. We are with them during moments of great apprehension and fear, and we share with them the exhilaration of their births. Our words and actions can be soothing and empowering; the memory of the care we provide may nurture a woman for the rest of her life.

For women who live in the shadow of trauma, routine prenatal exams, seemingly normal births and postpartum visits may unpredictably turn into terrifying nightmares. We must constantly be sensitive to the possibility that our words and actions can cause traumatic materials to surface; our awareness of that possibility is the key to prevention. As women, we too may have suffered traumas of our own which may challenge our ability to support the women with whom we work.

Pregnancy, birth and mothering are opportunities for change, growth and transformation. We must keep in mind the knowledge that there is vast potential for both wounding and healing during this time. We are more often than not among the catalysing factors for both of these very powerful processes. We cannot shy away from the enormous significance of our words and actions during this very vulnerable time.

Pregnancy filled up a hole in me, not only from the bombing, but also from my past. Now I am a mother, and everything is going to be fine. I was raised to believe that motherhood is a wonderful thing and that it doesn't come easily. I'm happy because I am OK, I am alive and I am a mother.
(Zohar)

Questions for debate

How easy is it for women with disabilities to access the place from which you offer maternity care? Could you negotiate the area blindfolded? In a wheelchair? With limited movement? If you couldn't hear anything? Is there anything that could be done to improve the experiences for women whose needs might differ?

How might your needs differ if you were a teenager? If you invited some teenagers to visit your place of work/read the leaflets you give out to women/comment upon their experiences of health care, do you think they would feel positively or negatively about the service offered in your area?

Stories and Reflection

Creating a scene: the work of Progress Theatre

Kirsten Baker

It's a wet Wednesday and a roomful of midwives is tackling some of the thornier problems that beset contemporary midwifery culture. They are looking at how midwives behave, not only with each other but with the women in their care.

A pretty dismal picture emerges. The midwives under review do not seem to be 'with women' at all. In fact, far from it. A glance around the room reveals that these midwives perceive themselves to be separated from women – separated from providing the sort of care that enhances both the giver and receiver.

One of the factors in this separation is represented by Hannah, a member of the audience. She has just been asked by her colleagues to play the role of a bladder – a full bladder – and there is a brief debate as to where in the emerging picture Hannah should place herself. The process of building this picture – the who, why, what and how of it – is lively: sometimes there is a wide-ranging consensus, and sometimes heated debate.

While Hannah's position is being discussed, Geraldine temporarily stops strangling Lou. Geraldine is acting out the role of 'policy' and Lou is 'guidelines'. Maggie is standing on a table with arms outstretched, eyes on a distant horizon: she is 'medicine'. Paula is outside the door, ear cupped in hand, but looking away: she is 'central government'. The pregnant or labouring woman may be behind or among all of these, and the relationship between her and her midwife is clearly a messy, unsupportive affair.

These are sad, difficult realisations. However, not only do the realisations keep coming, but there is also a great deal of laughter in the room. Humour provides a safety valve: as the comedian and playwright Trevor Griffiths said, 'We work through laughter, not for it'. On this wet Wednesday, agents that are associated with pain, blame or shame are all brought out into the open and given physical form by members of the audience. The demons are there for all to see.

'Theatre of the Oppressed'

Progress Theatre uses a methodology called 'Theatre of the Oppressed', based on the work of Brazilian dramaturg Augusto Boal. Progress was conceived in 1999 by Mavis Kirkham, Professor of Midwifery at the University of Sheffield, and has been gestating since then in a group of midwife actors. We have worked across the country, providing theatre workshops for a wide range of midwives and student midwives, examining aspects of our practice and culture.

Offshoots of Progress have appeared, although of course the use of some form of drama within midwifery education has been around since midwives began to pass on their skills to the next generation. From the animated storyteller demonstrating the behaviours of a woman in labour to her young apprentice, to the use of role play in the classroom and the ritualised conduct of the lecture theatre – all are theatrical forms.

So why use Theatre of the Oppressed? Isn't it a bit heavy for a bunch of midwives just getting on with their work? And won't it just make people dissatisfied? After all, it isn't always that bad, is it?

There are two significant points here. The first is the notion of midwives as an oppressed group. The second is the importance of finding a methodology that illuminates and challenges this rather than reinforces it.

Setting the scene

Since the organisation of maternity care has placed medical institutionalisation at its centre, the default position for midwives has arguably been 'with institution' rather than 'with woman'. Institutions may appear to offer society a place of certainty and safety within the dangerous world of childbearing, where birth, sex and death coexist. Institutions are also based on complex systems of (dis)organisation and on hierarchies that can be more or less visible. This tends to breed alienation: a sense experienced by individuals within it of powerlessness and disaffection. In institutions where the hierarchies are strong (and the fear great), the 'normal' assumptions readily become those of the most dominant group. When other groups internalise these values, even when their interests are not best served by them, there can be a resultant experience of oppression.

When Progress first began, we worked with a group of student midwives in Sheffield and asked them to show us 'pictures' of their clinical practice, built with their own bodies, such as the one described above. We also asked them to tell us why they had chosen to be midwives. The words they used to describe their images were harsh: conflict, frustration, powerlessness and bewilderment, to name but some examples. The way in which they had described their desire to become midwives, meanwhile, was heartwarming: to be with women; for a different life challenge; because they saw it as a vocation; and because of the experience of having had their own baby.

The gap between how they hoped their lives as midwives would be, and their experience less than two years later, is stark. What they are articulating with these words is the experience of hope turning into powerlessness. Unsurprisingly, in the descriptions of their practice, the women they are looking after have become invisible, separated from them by the structures in which they find themselves.

If this is the experience of midwives, it is inevitable that women who are being cared for by them will get a pretty shabby deal. There must be hundreds of thousands of women experiencing powerlessness in maternity hospitals throughout the country: some are having their babies and others are low-paid shift workers who carry high levels of responsibility for what happens, yet have little influence on it.

Scene one

If we are to break this cycle, it is crucial that any method we employ to tackle it does not replicate midwives' experience of alienation. Paulo Freire is an educationalist who wrote *Pedagogy of the Oppressed*, on which much of the Theatre of the Oppressed is based. He wrote:

The very structure of [the oppressed group's] thoughts has been conditioned by the contradictions of the ... situation by which they were shaped ... Their perception of themselves as oppressed is impaired by their submersion in the reality of oppression.

By using Theatre of the Oppressed, what we explore is midwives' own perceptions of their reality, without imposing meaning on it. The suggestions – bladders, medicine, guidelines – that are part of the process of building the picture are not judged as right or wrong, as nobody can say that about another's experience. But what begins to happen is that people bring an analytical recognition to the process. In building the picture, and by externalising the structures, a process of deconstruction takes place: 'It was good to actually see so many pressures on [the midwife] and how she felt and behaved', said one participant.

The session starts with a show – a series of scenes showing aspects of life as an NHS midwife – and the audience keys into what is happening quickly. The material they are watching is, after all, their story, gleaned from researching the views and experiences of midwives. Even the process of watching it can make it appear strange. The environment seems to have less power when the invisible bits are held up to view. Certainly, feelings of isolation are broken down as the shared image emerges: 'It made me realise it wasn't just me', said one participant. What is also shared is a sense of wanting it to be different: wanting the pressures to change or disappear.

Waiting to be rescued, for things to change, however, does little to empower midwives. But because this is theatre we can give everyone a magic wand to make it better. This generates an 'if only' wish list: if only we were paid more; if only there were more staff, and so on. What is also being mobilised, however, in waving the magic wand is a political analysis of the structures, values and conditions of a midwifery ethos – and this is both shared and visible.

Scene two

For change to occur, someone has to take responsibility for it. In mainstream midwifery culture, there are many places where such responsibility could lie. There are also places outside the mainstream, where strong models of midwifery care abound. Independent practice has arisen around a recognition that childbearing women need to be the agents of their experience and, in order to enable that, midwives need to work outside structures of oppression. Within the structures it can be harder, and the solutions need to be more collective. There is an important step, however, in taking responsibility for ourselves, wherever we find ourselves within the structure.

So, in a Progress workshop, building on the shared recognition and analysis we move into looking at the individual's behaviour. A scene is shown – at the desk in a delivery suite, or a booking interview at a busy clinic, or in a delivery room – where things just don't go right. Everyone wants it to be different, so everyone has a go. The actors take instructions from the audience as to how to change what their characters do: they are kept on their toes as they improvise suggestions and then modifications to those suggestions. Sometimes the observers don't simply want to watch: they want to come into the scenario themselves to try to affect the outcome. They often comment on how much easier it is to tell someone else to do it differently than it is to have a go themselves! This is clinical life as it is, with an opportunity to stop, reflect and restart to try to do it better. By literally coming into the scene, people can practise ways of making it better and evaluate what they have done, with the luxury of a roomful of colleagues to discuss it with. The scene is replayed: midwives behave differently, and the ensuing change can be discussed and appraised. It isn't necessarily easy: important principles are activated in discussing where to take the scene next. Crucially, unlike many of the conversations on delivery suites about how somebody else could or should do something better, this is people trying it out for themselves. They are engaging at a personal level with the problem and taking personal responsibility for change.

The Practising Midwife 2003; 6(11): 26–28

Epilogue

This is not an exercise in quick fixes. We do not aim to facilitate, but rather (to use Boal's word) 'difficultate'. We believe that midwifery structures are complex, often hidden and frequently unhelpful to midwives and women. We also believe that a process that helps to improve aspects of midwifery culture will benefit women. It appears that, by using Theatre of the Oppressed, midwives are able to look at what is considered 'normal' and 'routine' in different ways. Midwifery culture both shapes and is shaped by our beliefs, attitudes and behaviour.

Working effectively with midwives to increase awareness and insight, and allowing the safe practice of new ways of being, is critical to stopping some of the most damaging aspects of our behaviour and culture. Things can only get better!

The numbers game

Nicki Pusey

As a newly enrolled student midwife just starting out on my first placement, everything I encountered was new: the variety of families I met; the differing hopes and aspirations of the women; each oddly shaped bump to be palpated; the thrill I felt every time I eventually found the fetal heart with a sonic-aid, and later the way I felt triumphant when I located it with a Pinard stethoscope. I particularly remember the way I felt whenever I was left alone with a woman in labour – fully expecting her to have a baby 'just like that'!

I've since learnt that it wasn't my lack of personal experience of labouring (I've had three caesarean sections). Other students who have laboured, some of them often, also felt a rising panic when confronted by an agitated and red-faced woman.

These women were quite often primigravidae, who arrived on the labour ward huffing and puffing and who placed themselves in the care of the midwives, only to find that their labours slowed or that their baby was in an occipito posterior position. This would then lead to hours of discomfort, a growing desperation and the eventual recourse to epidural anaesthesia with or without the addition of synthetic hormonal preparations to augment the slow progress of their labours.

Very often as a student I would attend these women, hoping to witness a normal birth and, later, to be able to claim the birth of their baby as one of the elusive and magical 40 required for students' experience by European statute.

There are days when women come on to the labour ward already in the process of pushing their baby out, whom you guide into a room, for whom you don a pair of gloves and for whom you simply catch the baby to prevent it from falling on to the cold and inhospitable floor, following up with respectful, hands-off provision of care, tea and toast. If you're very lucky you may care for two or even three women like this in a day. This is intrapartum midwifery at its best. And, as a student, it teaches the valuable lesson that birth is normal, and that midwives are there only to guard against a deviation from the normal.

There are other days when the staff arrive on the labour ward to be greeted by a handover that describes 'the primip in room 2, 3 cm, 2:10, baby OP, mum not coping, baby OK at the moment, have tried a bath, feeding her, breathing with her, she's now asking for an epidural'. Now that I am beginning my second year, I no longer leap at the chance to care for these women, and if I do it is often with a heavy heart that circumstances may dictate that this particular woman will not be accounted for in my 'Book of Numbers'.

Because that is how midwifery looks now – a succession of potential numbers.

I love the days when I can practise in the way that I am taught (by the university and by the many fantastic mentors I have had), and the way that I feel is right for these women. But on other days my heart sinks – knowing that I might spend 12 or more hours supporting a woman in her labour, which then ends with an instrumental delivery.

There is nowhere in statute that this experience is recognised – and let's face it, it is this sort of midwifery support that is perhaps hardest to learn. After all, when things are going well women don't actually need midwives to do very much except watch and wait.

So perhaps it is time to get rid of the prerequisite to have 40 'hands-on deliveries', and shift to requirements that better reflect the nature of caring for women – time spent with women in labour, time spent supporting breastfeeding, time spent on antenatal education and pre-pregnancy health promotion. We already learn these skills, yet they are not recognised as an intrinsic part of a midwife's role. But if they were, wouldn't the outcomes of labour, breastfeeding and infant health be better. Or am I just naive?

The Practising Midwife 2003; 6(10): 41

Kicking out the oboes

Suzanne Colson

Last month, I was invited to lecture a group of midwives from the French Midwifery Syndicat in Paris about the public health aspects of breastfeeding. You can imagine my surprise when their General Secretary, Francine Dauphin, handed me the 'Symphonic rationale' below.

I had thought that frustration with a service that often undermines midwives was a problem unique to the UK and other English-speaking countries. During the past 15 years, I have often believed that the French midwifery grass was greener. What an eye-opener! Our French sisters seem to encounter the same kinds of management problems.

Not only did the following parody make me laugh about our common predicament (even though it is not really funny), it also enabled discussion about other French/UK comparisons, highlighting similarities around how midwives can best deliver care.

Mothers and babies have similar needs the world over. We discussed, in particular, how postnatal care is a second-class citizen and how politics and hospital management often use marketing models and business rationale to guide decisions, thus undermining holistic care and resulting in real constraints to the midwifery remit to promote health. We compared notes and discussed the public health potential of small family birthing centres.

This open and frank exchange of ideas resulted in a joint decision to organise a bi-centre bilingual conference (Paris/Canterbury) in the near future about the public health role and effectiveness of small family birthing centres.

Symphonic rationale

(translated from the French and adapted by Suzanne Colson)
The head of midwifery at St Elsewhere NHS Trust had a concert ticket for Schubert's Unfinished Symphony. Because she was unable to attend, she gave her ticket to her friend and colleague – the trust finance officer. The next day, the head of midwifery asked her colleague if she had enjoyed the concert. Instead of the usual mundane response, 'Yes, it was brilliant. Thank you for the ticket', she was surprised to receive a typed memorandum with the following points:

Subject: Comments on Schubert's Unfinished Symphony. Date: Last Monday

1. I enjoyed the concert. However, it seems to me that there were some long moments during which the oboes had nothing to do. I recommend that their number is reduced and their work redistributed among everyone in the orchestra to avoid these long moments of inactivity.

2. The 12 first violinists played exactly the same note. This is redundant and costs a fortune in salaries. I recommend that the number of violinists be reduced throughout the string section. When the music needs to be louder, surely a good-quality amplifier would be more cost-effective.

3. A considerable amount of energy was spent playing the quavers. This is demanding and excessive. I recommend that the quavers be replaced with crotchets. This will halve the energy output and will also reduce costs because we will be able to replace the expensive professional players with cheaper apprentices.

4. It seems to be a waste of precious resources to have the brass instruments play a passage that has already been played by the violins. If these redundant parts were eliminated, the overall length of the concert could easily be reduced to two hours and 20 minutes maximum.

5. Along the same lines, the second movement is very slow. This is an unjustifiable waste of time. Today, no enterprise can afford such a reduction in team production and turnover. It would appear that the orchestra leader is responsible for this reduced pace and his post should be made redundant without delay.

Conclusion: Please note that if Schubert had been more attentive to the above points, he would have had ample time to finish his symphony.

Is this cost-effectiveness gone mad?

The Practising Midwife 2003; 6(9): 40

You can take a horse to water...

When it comes to breastfeeding, midwives should be guided by the mother and her instincts

In my relatively short time as a qualified midwife I have always found breastfeeding a difficult area, particularly in the early days of the neonate, when different health care professionals offer what seem to be widely conflicting advice, especially when a healthy term infant is reluctant to go to the breast.

I am committed to breastfeeding, attend study days and always try to be as proactive as possible but, when starting a community post, this was the area that worried me. The old adage, 'you can take a horse to water but you can't make it drink', hung over me.

Recently I had an empowering experience. Juliet and Bill had just had their first baby – a large, term male after a long labour that had culminated in a ventouse delivery. I first saw Juliet on day 3. She had been breastfeeding since the birth and was keen to continue but she felt that the baby, although latching on adequately, had a poor suck. My heart sank and I started thinking of horses. However, I observed a feed and could see nothing wrong, so I reassured her that all looked well, that the colostrum he was getting must be adequate for his needs and that when her milk came in the problem would be resolved.

On my return the next morning nothing had changed. The baby would latch on but suck poorly for a few minutes, then go to sleep – and the milk was not yet in. The baby was pink, alert and urinating, so we discussed methods of trying to make him more interested at the breast, including expressing a couple of drops of milk onto the nipple. Despite Juliet's best efforts and my verbal guidance, no milk was forthcoming and Juliet again said she could feel no change in her breasts. Again, I reassured her, thinking that it would surely arrive later that day, and the baby was fine. When I rang for an update later on, Juliet was pleased to tell me that the baby was sucking much more enthusiastically, so I felt the crisis was over and all would be well.

Next morning, on day 5, I found Juliet and Bill were even more anxious as the milk had still not arrived, her breasts were soft and there was no change. Again, on examination, the baby was a good colour, alert and would settle fairly easily after having been to the breast. My insecurities were rising fast, but I really did not want to destroy Juliet's confidence by suggesting formula top-up feeds, so I tried to apply all that I had been taught. I reassured Juliet that she could trust her body to supply the milk and discussed how well the baby appeared. Juliet then informed me that both her mother and sister had had a similar situation, with milk not arriving until day 5. This information gave me great comfort, and after more reassurances all round (for my benefit as well!), I left.

I did not see the family for the next two days; a colleague visited in the interim and so I did not know what to expect. It was therefore wonderful to find Juliet overflowing with milk and an expertly sucking baby. It turned out that the milk had not actually come in until day 6!

However, Juliet had been very distressed that my colleague had discussed the option of top-up feeds. She said that she felt her capabilities as a mother were being questioned and that she 'wasn't up to the job'. She felt her confidence could not have dealt with such a blow; fortunately, the milk arrived in time to prevent this from occurring.

On reflection, I feel I have learnt a great deal from this experience: that nature must be trusted where all is normal, that I knew more than I thought I did and that if you take a horse to water it will drink – eventually!

The Practising Midwife 2003; 6(8): 39

Pushing the boundaries: independence in the NHS

Lynn Walcott

Catherine was already more than halfway into her second pregnancy when she contacted me about having independent care. Her first baby had been born in the local large obstetric unit with NHS midwives some five years previously. On paper, a relatively 'normal' birth belied the intensive and difficult experience Catherine recalled.

Her main reason for looking for independent care was that she wanted a known and trusted midwife to help her avoid a repeat of the difficulty she experienced in her first labour achieving the type of delivery she constantly requested.

Catherine's first birth had been marred by constant 'discussions' declining the 'offered' interventions that the midwives felt necessary. A long, latent first stage spent on an antenatal ward was followed by a rapid, active first stage, then a transfer to the labour ward when in transition and subsequently a slow second stage with some possible fetal distress apparent.

During this, Catherine reiterated repeatedly her desire to achieve vaginal birth without augmentation, epidural or assisted delivery – all were recommended on several occasions. Hearing her story, and later reading the hospital notes, I marvelled at Catherine's strength and conviction, both about what she desired and also about what was best for her baby. Her husband, Mark, was wonderfully supportive both with that first experience and with Catherine's intentions second time around.

Factors that were to complicate planning, but which did not impact directly on the actual birth experience (and are therefore not discussed in this article), were: being under a consultant obstetrician as the pregnancy had occurred following fertility treatment; a scan identifying a possible problem with the baby; and the potential of NHS midwives being involved as I did not yet have an independent partner.

Catherine wanted to give birth in hospital right from the beginning, and did not see why natural birth could

not be achieved in this environment. As with many midwives, I kept an open mind, believing that Catherine might change her mind about going to hospital if labour progressed quickly; I reassured her that I would have everything available should this be the case. However, as I got to know Catherine, it became apparent that once she made up her mind, that was it! So I resigned myself to a hospital birth.

Since becoming independent I have acquired honorary contracts in four hospitals, and this means that many of my enquiries from women are for planned hospital births. Regardless of my own belief system about birth, I have found that as a midwife I wish to support women's informed choices and, unlike the NHS, I have no desire to direct those choices. I feel very strongly that the NHS does not support informed choice in maternity care, which I hope to illustrate if I ever get round to finishing my study for my degree – 'Informed choice within the NHS: a flawed concept'.

Catherine's labour began, as so often with multiparous women, one night after arranging for her other child to be with grandparents. Worry-free, Catherine could labour peacefully. I was called following spontaneous rupture of membranes (SROM) at half past midnight, but there were no contractions so I suggested that we all rest and that Catherine should ring me when she was having regular contractions. Less than 30 minutes later she rang again – she was having period-like pains every four minutes. I offered to attend, as I was 45 minutes away and sensed that Catherine needed me to be present to ensure that there was no lingering anxiety and that labour could progress peacefully.

On my arrival, Catherine was obviously relaxed and not yet in established labour. I informed the local labour ward at the obstetric unit that we would call when ready to come in. Within an hour and a half, through observing Catherine, I felt that the labour had established. When the next two contractions brought some rectal pressure, I suggested that transfer to hospital was now or never – especially as Catherine indicated that she would have attended the labour ward some time ago had she not already had a midwife with her!

We arrived at the hospital at 4.05 a.m. and settled into the pool room, where the staff had kindly prepared the pool. The coordinator and I had not met before, and my usual anxieties as to what kind of support I would receive began to set in.

I have had a variety of experiences, ranging from complete indifference to enthusiastic practical support. One of the initial concerns delivery coordinators often raise is how I assess progress in labour. Of course, in hospital, dilatation is used as the main indicator, and if one does not use this system conflict may occur.

I had transferred in with Catherine just before transition, using my own observations of contractions and behaviour. How do you write this down on the board? I informed the coordinator, 'S', that I felt that Catherine was approaching full dilatation, and that I would only come out of the room again if there were problems and I required assistance. S was a little surprised, but did not comment, and I did my usual trick of cocooning myself with 'my woman', desperately hoping that S would trust my judgement and not be one of those anxious types constantly knocking on the door! I have actually experienced a labour ward sister knock on my door every 10 minutes in second stage to ask, 'Have you had a baby yet?'.

Once back in the pool room, I settled into my usual mode, trying to be unobtrusive with necessary monitoring of fetal and maternal well-being. I was expecting second stage within the hour after a period of mobilisation to get the contractions going again. Catherine was in the pool, and I was looking forward to a beautiful, uncomplicated catch, having recently experienced two difficult first labours both needing obstetric assistance.

At half past six, Catherine announced that she felt 'suddenly awake'. The sun had just risen, and as she began to feel odd pushing/pulling sensations I recognised that second stage was beginning, transition having been the lull in contractions on arrival in hospital.

Through the next hour, the contractions became erratic, both in strength and frequency, and as they virtually came to a halt I started to get a little concerned. Something wasn't quite right. Here was a 'multip' with a baby in the LOA position, certainly fully dilated, nothing palpable abdominally, and yet the baby was not falling out!

Catherine was a little bit confused too, but tired and relaxed, so I suggested tucking up for a nap in the bed. Both mother and baby were fine, and in the absence of any specific concerns I felt that action was not necessary.

I informed S of our plan to take an hour or so of rest, and if contractions had not returned to have a vaginal examination (VE) to help assess the situation and allow decisions to be made.

S was more comfortable now that I had intimated that I was intending to perform a VE; conversely, I was less comfortable, as I only do VEs these days when I think that something is not quite right. She also asked if I was considering augmentation with syntocinon. I already knew Catherine's determination to avoid all interventions unless absolutely necessary, and informed S that we would be trying other methods to increase uterine activity.

Just as the hour was coming to an end, contractions started again. Catherine was happy for me to do a VE so that she could decide what to do next. My findings were to confuse me further. Far from discovering some odd presentation or internal impediment, I found the ideal situation – no cervix, cephalic presentation, +2 to spines, LOA position. This baby could be seen just by parting the labia, and yet was not falling out!

I racked my brains – what on earth could the hold-up be? I recalled the notes on Catherine's first delivery. It had been a slow advance once the vertex was visible, even for a 'primip'. I was beginning to think that Catherine must have some particular type or shape of pelvis that was the problem. Again, the baby and mother were fine. I discussed my findings with Catherine and offered augmentation, epidural and ventouse – or at least obstetric opinion – but she declined as there was no emergency and she was determined to push the baby out herself. Once again I informed the coordinator, and once more she accepted my judgement and plans. We were going to mobilise and try some directed pushing while upright.

Within half an hour, the vertex was visible, but it was still to be almost an hour before birth. During this painfully (literally) slow advance, Catherine put everything she had into birthing her baby. Her husband was vital, both in his verbal support and physically, as Catherine hung on to her man's neck, squatting during each expulsion. The directed pushing seemed to help, as the pushes gradually became more spontaneous.

I now had a new concern as I had a perfect view of everything. I watched in complete awe as the anal dilation increased and increased more than I had ever believed possible, while Catherine also complained of acute pain in the rectal area.

Oh no, I thought, I'm going to see a horrendous third degree tear, or worse! But the perineum was stretching beautifully and the head was crowning – there seemed no point in initiating any other action or assistance now. The head delivered, very slowly, LOA. Then there was an agonising four-minute wait until the next contraction, and 'the problem' was revealed.

This was no simple compound presentation. The right hand was clutching the nape of the neck, with the elbow beneath the chin. Just try that now – taking your right hand past your chin, then your left ear, and holding on to the back of your neck. Imagine this baby coming through the pelvis... Far from having a problem pelvis, Catherine had an extremely roomy pelvis to have enabled this baby to have been born at all.

I had seen only a slight 'nick' on the perineum, blood loss was minimal and Catherine had a beautiful baby boy who cried lustily. Phew!

How foolish, though, to think that it was all over. Of course, both I and the coordinator were relieved. 'Del' was written on the board in big letters! But, as we all know, a mother's work is not finished yet – the placenta still had to be born.

Catherine wanted to do this stage herself too, although I would have been happy to manage things actively following such a slow second stage. But Catherine was not bleeding and so, over an hour later, following a breastfeed, she attempted to push the placenta out. As there was no sign of separation, I recommended catheterisation, as Catherine was not able to pass urine. This was successful – some 500 ml of clear urine – but by now Catherine wanted everything over with, so opted for active management.

Following syntometrine IM, I initiated cord-controlled traction. The cord was friable, and I resisted snapping it completely as on examination it actually appeared to be velhementus. Again we tried maternal effort, as the uterus was well contracted. I could see the placenta at the introitus now, but was not convinced that it had completely separated.

Throughout the third stage Catherine had reiterated that she did not want obstetric interference, so I knew that I would just have to try and get the placenta out. In the end, a combination of maternal effort, fundal pressure and massage, with traction on the placenta that was visible, did the trick – almost three hours after birth! Finally, we could all relax.

The first stage was calculated as six hours, the second three hours and 55 minutes, and the third two hours and 53 minutes. Catherine, a 'multip', had achieved what she wanted, safely, within an NHS hospital. She had avoided syntocinon augmentation, epidural, assisted delivery and manual removal of the placenta.

This experience really stretched me, mainly because it was taking place within an NHS hospital. Many independent midwives regularly push boundaries – in the home environment. The strength of this woman – along with a coordinator who allowed me to practise autonomously – had enabled me to push the boundaries imposed by delivery suite guidelines.

I could not have done this alone. Only when women are strong can midwives be strong.

Catherine's story

After the birth of my first baby I felt I had learnt a lot that would make it easier and less traumatic second time round. My first birth had been long and drawn out. I spent a great deal of time lying on my back wearing a monitor, and I experienced back pain that seemed unrelated to the normal birthing process. I also saw a number of midwives during labour, and have no idea of the name of the midwife who delivered my son.

I remained convinced that natural birth was the best thing for both mother and child. With this in mind, and the added complication of recent recovery from a back problem (I feared an epidural could make the problem worse), I hired an independent midwife.

I felt much calmer once in the care of Lynn. She understood my medical history, my views on natural birth and I was a person – not a number. I looked forward to her antenatal visits and so did my four-year-old, who could listen to the baby's heartbeat and learn what everything in Lynn's bag did! The perfect birth beckoned. First stage of labour was just as I had hoped. I had contractions almost as soon as my waters broke. There was the reassurance of Lynn giving her judgement of when to transfer to hospital. It was not the slow process it had been first time round. The birthing pool was available at the hospital, everything was going well and I was looking forward to second stage.

I remembered pushing not being as painful as first stage – a sort of productive pain unlike any other pain. This was not at all how second stage felt this time, and I was quite confused about what I was feeling. There was constant pressure on my back passage and I was convinced I needed to go to the loo. I took a while to understand this was how pushing was going to be this time. I tried the birthing pool – and was not comfortable. I tried lying over the top of the bed and pushing – and was not comfortable. Squatting on the floor seemed the easiest way to get things moving. My poor husband was almost pinned to the side of the bed as I clung to him and pushed.

It hurt and seemed to take forever. Although I was offered pain relief and told I could have ventouse or other help, it never crossed my mind to use it. I was just too focused on what I was doing. It felt like I was going to split open, but only when I pushed that hard did the baby move.

About 10 minutes before John was born I suddenly thought I had made an error of judgement and that he would never be born naturally because I couldn't go on for much longer. Then he arrived and cried loud and strong – it was all worth it.

We sat on the floor of the birthing room – dad, mum and baby together – mistakenly thinking the pain was all over. Delivering the placenta had been quick and relatively easy last time. John and I sat together on the floor for an hour – no placenta arrived. I was tired and uncomfortable, and so asked for the umbilical cord to be cut so that I could sit on the bed. Still the placenta would not come out.

Now that John had arrived safely and was sleeping peacefully I wanted a shower and a rest, so I asked for the injection. I thought that with the injection there would be no more pushing; the placenta could just be pulled out. It didn't work – the cord was coming away from the placenta when Lynn pulled.

It was looking increasingly likely that intervention would be necessary, and having managed so far I definitely did not want an epidural at this stage. Lynn explained that it would be medically necessary unless the placenta was out within half an hour, but we could try pushing while she manipulated my stomach.

At this stage I was having trouble controlling my muscles because I had already pushed so hard to give birth to John. However, the thought of the epidural concentrated my effort, and with a lot of help from Lynn the placenta was expelled. A few stitches and it was all over.

In retrospect it was a very scary experience. I would describe the birth as a well-managed trauma. Without Lynn and my husband I could not have coped, and I think it would have left an emotional scar for life.

Acknowledgements

I would like to thank Catherine and Mark Bassom for their permission and help in preparing this article.

The Practising Midwife 2003; 6(7): 24–27

Pushed to the limit

Rosie Kacary

In 1995 I left three children under the age of five at home to embark on a midwifery training course. I did this not because I hated motherhood but because I felt compelled to improve women's experiences of pregnancy and childbirth. Much of my training left a lot to be desired, but it gave me the requisite qualification and reaffirmed my belief that the vast majority of women would have a much better time if they were cared for in their own homes by a midwife they knew and trusted.

I served my apprenticeship in a local hospital and, just as soon as anyone would have me, found my dream job as a community midwife. Now my real work could begin. I could start forming proper relationships with women and their families and have the opportunity to influence the kind of care they received. I could sleep soundly in my bed knowing I had done a good job.

Like the majority of my colleagues, I am dedicated, committed and very passionate about the work I do. The NHS only survives at all due to the goodwill of its staff, and I have more than most!

So why, after a mere four and a half years, has the NHS caused me such extreme frustration that I am on the point of resigning? Surely I am precisely the kind of highly motivated, enthusiastic midwife it so desperately needs to retain?

I have no fear of change if it is change for the better, but when managers railroad through the most enormous changes which don't appear to be research-based and which have huge implications, not just for women but also for grassroots clinical midwives like me, no matter how hard I try I cannot view the proposals in a positive light.

When my manager sends me a memo telling me I must advise women to expect a maximum of a 24-hour hospital stay, that I may make only three postnatal visits and that an audit tool is being devised to look at any discrepancies in the number of visits I have done, there is a clear implication that if I deviate from this norm my wrist will be slapped.

When I am told I have to give up as many fixed commitments during my working week as possible, such as parentcraft classes and antenatal clinics – the very forums where friendships are forged and relationships cemented – so that I am free to be sent to the main delivery suite to work, I want to scream.

When I am told I can no longer offer an early labour assessment overnight – the exact time when women most need this service – I just want to weep. Where is my autonomy, my ability to manage my own time and my own caseload, and look after women properly, the way they deserve?

I appreciate that there are times when there are too many women in labour and too few midwives to look after them. This is clearly a problem. On paper, at least, providing a fully integrated service must seem like the golden goose. For once, you can staff need rather than areas. But, in my opinion, it will cause far more problems than it solves, not least because it fails to take into account the strengths and weaknesses of individual midwives. It requires us all to be equally competent and equally happy working in any environment at any given moment. Sadly this is not the case.

My own strengths lie in forging close relationships with women, in finding out the things that are important to them, and then doing my utmost to help them achieve it. I cannot provide this level of care to women I meet for the first time in labour. My job satisfaction depends on knowing my women. Other midwives are excellent at high-dependency care. They no more want to spend a day in the community than I want to spend one in theatres. Both skills are equally valid and equally as vital. The truth is that the skills are different and some of us enjoy one thing more than another. To attempt to make us all expert at everything is insanity. It will result only in nothing being very good and those of us who strive for excellence feeling dejected, frustrated and ultimately leaving a profession we entered with such high aspirations and idealism. But perhaps mediocrity is what the NHS does best.

Midwives like me aren't prepared to settle for second best. If we can't do the job properly, then we'd rather not do it at all. Particularly this job. It's too important and it matters too much not to get it right. If the NHS continues to drive away midwives like me, then it really is in trouble. Retaining good staff has nothing to do with money; it's much more fundamental than that. If the exodus is going to stop, somebody really needs to listen.

The Practising Midwife 2003; 6(6): 42

My birth story

Andrea Wolahan's joyful home water birth, with an additional perspective from independent midwife Virginia Howes

Andrea Wolahan, Virginia Howes

I woke up on the morning of my estimated due date with period-like pains, similar to those I had had the week before. I didn't think too much of them as they had come and gone last time with no progress. I made a trip to the bathroom and found that I had spotted a bit of brown blood – I wondered whether this could be a show, but it didn't really look like a mucus plug so I decided this could mean anything from labour being imminent to it starting next week! I seemed to need to empty my bladder a lot over the next hour – did that mean that the baby had moved down further? My husband decided to put off leaving for work for another hour to see whether anything speeded up, but in the end we decided it would be silly for him not to set off for work. Things seemed to be slowing down rather than going anywhere.

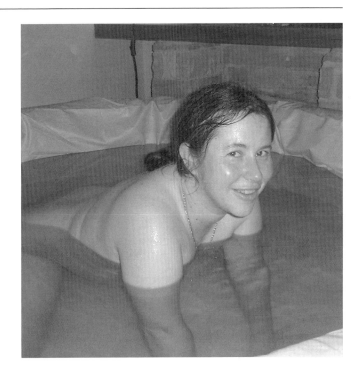

I stayed in bed for a while to get some rest and then got up to get on with the day and tried not to think about things. Whether it was a nesting instinct, or something similar, I don't know, but I decided to clean the house out, bedrooms, toilets and so on, just in case something did happen. I was still getting period-like pains, but nothing that I couldn't ignore or that were any regular distance apart.

I finished cleaning the house, had some lunch, and decided to sit down and watch a film for the afternoon. I was still getting period-like pains at this point but not really with any regularity. I hadn't attempted to time anything at this point. I was still spotting brown blood and this was beginning to worry me at this point, so I decided to give my independent midwife, Virginia Howes, a call. It was now around 4 p.m. I wasn't really thinking anything was imminent at this stage but thought that it would be good to put her in mind that labour might be starting in the next day or so. I also wanted some reassurance about the bleeding, as I thought a show just came and went and wouldn't have been there all day long. Virginia was interested that things appeared to be starting but neither of us was

worried that anything was going to happen immediately. Virginia was not concerned about the bleeding, which reassured me. I mentioned that my bowels had been loose the night before and we wondered whether this might mean things were about to happen.

I started to feel I should time the contractions, just to see how close they actually were. They didn't seem to be that regular and were lasting from 30 to 40 seconds. However, by 5 p.m. things had started to pick up quite a bit and it felt like the contractions were coming every five minutes or so, still lasting around 40 seconds. I decided to call my husband, who works in London, at about 5.30 p.m. just to see when he would be coming home and, I suppose, to give him a bit of a hint that I would like to see him sooner rather than later. He asked me how often the contractions were coming and whether I had spoken to Virginia again. I didn't really want to tell him how often, given that I knew that at five minutes they were really a lot closer! He made me promise to phone Virginia again before his train got in at 6.35 p.m. For some reason I still felt the birth wasn't necessarily going to happen for ages and had felt a bit silly ringing Virginia again so soon. I promised that I would call Virginia and rang her at 6.10 p.m. I could still talk quite normally through a contraction, which surprised me, as off the phone I think I had found it harder to speak.

Virginia reassured me that even if I did get to second stage before she arrived I would have quite a while to spare (she was an hour's drive away). She said I should ring her again when contractions were five minutes or so apart and were lasting around a minute. I agreed to do that as it made sense that, if she arrived at our house tonight, we might not need her till the following day and then she would be tired.

My husband arrived home at around 7 p.m. I went to the toilet again at 7.10 p.m. and this time I definitely lost my mucus plug with a slight tinge of blood in it. The brown spotting seemed to have subsided by this time. We started timing the contractions, with me shouting 'yes' when one began and 'no' or 'gone' when the contraction had finished. I found it quite hard to determine when one had actually finished, as they seemed to fade away rather than just stop. They now seemed to be lasting anything from 30 to 60 seconds and were varying from three minutes apart to five minutes. They were more regular but still not in a set pattern. At this point I mentioned to my husband that we didn't have the pavlova that Virginia had always joked with me that she wanted for my labour. My husband asked if I wanted him to pop up to Waitrose for one and we decided that he should, with me continuing to time the contractions in his absence. It was now just after 7.30 p.m. and contractions were coming roughly every two to three minutes and lasting from 30 to 55 seconds. I still felt able to cope with them really well and it didn't panic me that I would be on my own for a brief period. I still didn't really think things were going to happen that quickly. However, I was finding it incredibly difficult to sit down on anything, including my birth ball, and found that the only way I could cope was by standing and rotating/swaying my hips with each contraction and using my breathing. I also tried to relax the muscles around my cervix with the contraction, as I had heard that that would help.

In my husband's absence I decided to cook some cheese on toast, one of my favourites. I did two slices but only managed to eat half of one slice; my appetite wasn't quite what I thought it was! My husband came back and we carried on timing the contractions together; they were still wavering at two to three minutes apart and lasting for just over a minute. We sat down to watch *Holby City*. I couldn't concentrate and we had to turn if off! At this point my husband decided that we should call Virginia again as things were definitely picking up. Virginia suggested that we go for a walk for an hour. I was dubious that I could manage an hour so we settled on a half-hour walk. We left for our walk in the dark and luckily didn't bump into any neighbours. We walked along the flat rather than up the hills; it is quite hilly in our area. I was now finding it really annoying if my husband talked to me during a contraction and eventually I told him so. I just found that I couldn't answer him and had to concentrate entirely on the contraction. I could still walk through a contraction, but most of the time found it easier to just stop and sway my hips a bit and breathe through it. I felt like I was going to be sick a couple of times but just had that taste in my mouth; I was never actually sick.

We came back to the house. Virginia rang to say that she was on her way anyway and suggested that we start to fill the pool. It was now around 9.30 p.m. and we started to time contractions again.

I was feeling really frustrated: I wanted to get things out from my labour bag in the upstairs bedroom but was finding it really hard to get there and take things out with the contractions. I managed to find myself a fruit and nut bar, which I only half ate. Virginia rang again to tell us that she was nearly with us. I asked my husband to find my bag with my aromatherapy oils in and we put on some rose oil in a vaporiser. We carried on timing the contractions until about 11 p.m., when Virginia arrived. She apologised that she had not arrived sooner; I hadn't even realised that it had taken her longer than the usual hour! Apparently there had been a pile-up on the M25 and she had been stuck in the traffic. She had rung the police to tell them that she was a midwife attending a woman in labour and they had told her to use the hard shoulder with hazards flashing. The police then escorted her off the motorway.

The pool had taken a bit longer to fill than when we had had a dummy run at the weekend. We had been quite glad of the practice run, as on emptying the pool we had flooded the kitchen – an undiscovered overflow pipe in the kitchen sink that we now know about! Virginia checked my pulse and blood pressure and the baby's heart rate; thankfully she didn't suggest any vaginal examination. It was really difficult for me to lie on my back, so she carried out her checks as quickly as possible. All was normal and she told me I could get into the pool. I got in and waited, at her suggestion, for a contraction to begin so that I could get under the level of the water and see what pain relief it gave. I didn't really notice much difference in the pain but it did feel good to

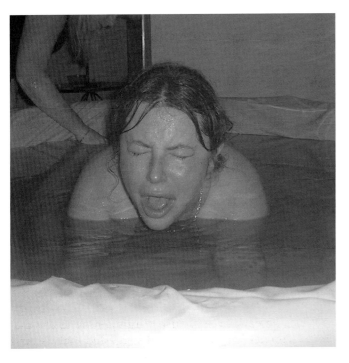
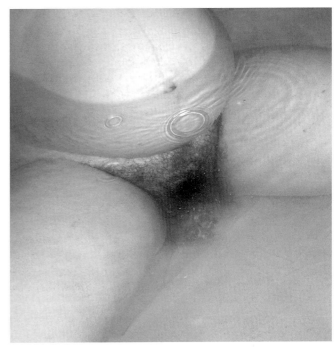
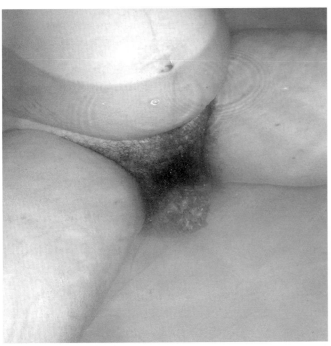
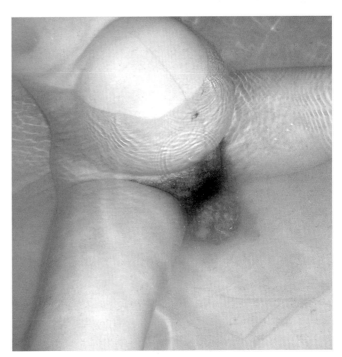

have the water all around me, quite comforting. The water temperature was 36 degrees at this point. Virginia suggested that I get on all fours and get into moving with the contractions so that it was automatic. The contractions continued to come thick and fast but I was no longer timing them at this point. They did seem to be even more frequent though than before. I was really surprised that each contraction now seemed to end in my lower back, which I had assumed only happened with a posterior presentation. At one point I felt an involuntary pushing-down sensation, which I noted but ignored really as it felt too early to be pushing. I had planned lots of music that I wanted to have on for the birth but it didn't really seem to be necessary or needed when the time came – we put on one CD, Peter Gabriel's 20 Greatest, and then forgot about the music.

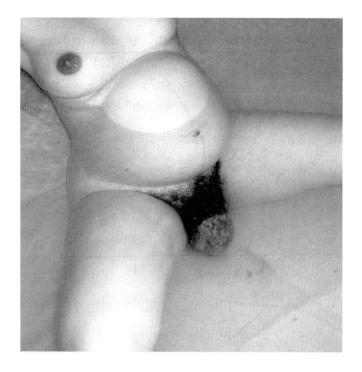

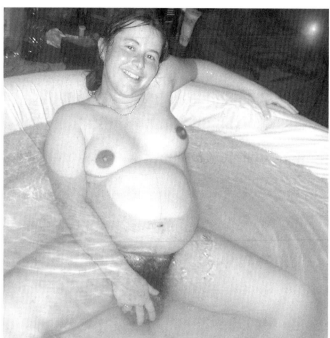

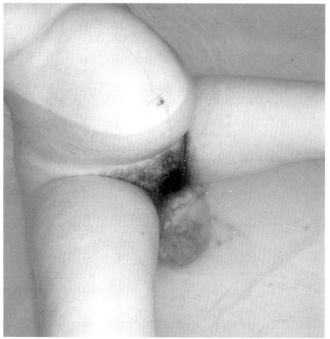

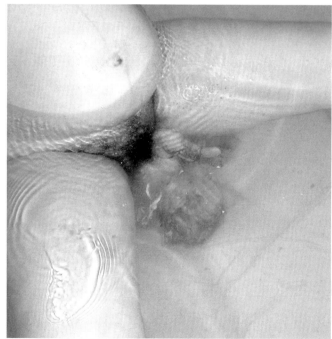

At 11.50 p.m. I felt my waters go, a feeling I will always remember, a pop and sudden gush into the pool waters. Virginia checked the fetal heart rate, which was fine at 147 b.p.m. Soon after my waters breaking I felt that I wanted to push. Virginia said that that was okay to do, which I hadn't been sure about as I remembered you shouldn't really push until confirmed fully dilated. I found that I was calm and felt fine between contractions and just knew that I had to concentrate and go with the contractions when they came. I found that I could deal with the pushing by yelling through the contractions as I pushed, something I didn't quite anticipate I would do before the event. I don't think I felt any real panic about the labour though at any point! Virginia checked the fetal heart again at 0.10, 0.20 and 0.30 a.m., and it was still fine. Both my husband and Virginia were by this point taking lots of pictures.

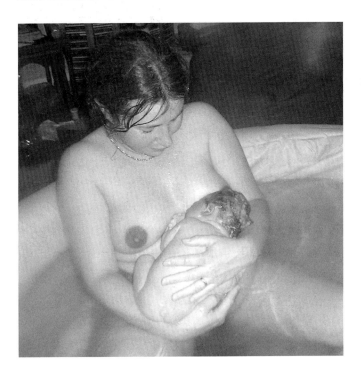
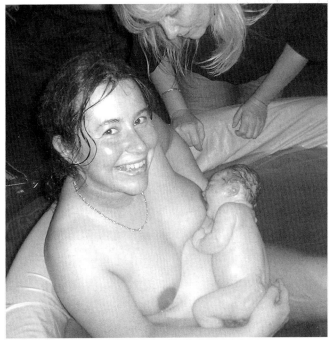

The head was now beginning to crown. I had been pushing for a while, thinking that the baby was making no progress at all, as I expected to be able to feel more tension as she came down the birth canal than I actually did. Virginia suggested that I move to sit on the edge of the pool step for the birth. As the head crowned I wondered whether the head was going to be able to come out without me tearing badly. Virginia encouraged me to feel the head, which I could slightly feel. I carried on pushing with the contractions and yelling my head off and suddenly the head came out. I was able to sit and wait for the next contraction with my hand feeling my baby's head, which was marvellous. The shoulders were born into the water with the next contraction. Not as painful a sensation as the head being born but definitely an experience, as I could feel the baby twist round to bring one shoulder out after the other. My husband had been prepared by Virginia to catch the baby, which he did, although she tried to slip out of his hands in the water. He brought her up to me saying 'it's a girl'. She spluttered for a few seconds and then howled; it was 0.48 a.m. in the morning and my daughter was born. She was beautiful and plump, with lots of brown hair covered in mucus. It was really amazing to see her at last and I was particularly fascinated by her little feet and hands, on which she seemed to have really long fingers and toes. The cord was quite short and we could just about get her to my breast whilst waiting for the placenta to arrive. She had an initial feed whilst we waited for another contraction and then looked around to see her new surroundings; she was very alert. The contractions didn't

seem to start up again as they had before, not in the same way anyway. Virginia suggested that I stand up and try to push down and I felt something shift within me. The placenta was then delivered into the pool at 1.20 a.m. with a small amount of blood, which Virginia estimated to be about 300 ml. Once the placenta had been delivered my husband cut the cord and Virginia tied it with dental floss. I was then helped out of the pool with my baby for both of us to be wrapped up. Virginia checked me to see whether there was any tearing that required suturing. We decided that as I had only a small tear that this could be left alone. The Apgar scores were recorded for my daughter as 10/1 and 10/5. She had arrived with a grand weight of 8 lb 2 oz and measured 52 centimetres in length.

I definitely didn't think a first labour would be as quick as it was for me, eight hours and 20 minutes from start of active labour to end of third stage. I really think that it helped that I was upright and active for most of the day and that I really wasn't worried at any time during the labour, which must have meant that I relaxed a fair bit. Hiring an independent midwife was definitely the right way for my husband and I to have gone as we had total confidence in Virginia on the day and it was so good to have someone helping us that we knew and trusted. I have come out of it feeling that I had exactly the birth I wanted, even though I couldn't quite foresee in advance how it would be on the day as it was my first birth. I was really hoping that I would be able to avoid any drugs and possibly even the gas and air, and am really glad that in the end all I needed was my breathing and the water. I am still waiting to find the perfect recipe to cook the placenta stored in the freezer though.

The midwife's story

Andrea knew what she wanted from the very beginning: a normal home birth with as little interference as possible. She was well read on the subject; in fact, I was very surprised at her depth of knowledge about the whole pregnancy and birth process. Her choice of 'homework' reading during the pregnancy was midwifery texts! She was always smiling and I nicknamed her 'giggler'.

When the day arrived for the birth Andrea rang me at about 4 p.m. to say that she had had a show that morning. With her baby as active as ever and her feeling fine, I assured her that all was well and that labour could well be imminent or be a week away. A couple of hours later she called again to say that she was having contractions but that they were irregular in duration and strength. I explained that contractions may take a while to become regular and asked her to keep me informed.

A while later I spoke to Laurence, Andrea's husband, who appeared relaxed but quite sure things were happening! I advised them to go for a walk to keep things going and to while away a bit of time. The last thing I wanted was for Andrea to lose all that wonderful positivity that had sailed her through the pregnancy. At about 9 p.m. I decided that, although her frequent phone calls were telling me she was coping well, I felt in her heart she wanted me there, even though she had not verbalised it. I called to inform them I was on my way and set off to do the usual one-hour journey.

When I was almost there, to my horror, I got stuck in a queue behind a motorway accident. I telephoned Andrea from the car to say I was almost there but I was really trying to gauge whether or not I should take action over the delay: from her puffing and panting I decided that the answer to that was a definite 'yes'. I telephoned the Metropolitan police, who were very obliging and escorted me off the motorway. I arrived at Andrea's a few minutes later to find the contractions very regular now, approximately every three to five minutes, and Andrea was pacing. This amazing woman was still giggling!

I checked all vital signs for Andrea and her baby, and all was well. Laurence offered me the chance to go and get some sleep but I declined, saying that I didn't think this was going to be a long haul from this point.

Andrea got into the pool and remained on all fours for about an hour until she informed me that her membranes had ruptured. Although no visual evidence of this was apparent, with her being in the pool, I had no reason not to be fully confident in her diagnosis. A short while later Andrea began to make loud expulsive noises and signs of full dilatation were very obvious. At no point did I think a vaginal examination was necessary. I listened in to baby at regular intervals. It was not long before the baby was crowning and at this point I suggested to Andrea that she might like to turn around in order that her baby was born in front of her. While I like to 'suggest' as little as possible where positions are concerned, I always think it is nicer for women when they are in the pool not to have to be struggling to turn around and lift their legs over the cord when their babies are born under water. In this instance it was exactly the right thing to do, as the umbilical cord was very short and only just long enough for baby to reach the breast.

Andrea gave birth to Erin with ease. She was in control, she was smiling and interacting with her baby when only her head was born. When she finally pushed her completely out, Laurence lifted her to the surface while I took pictures. Andrea stayed in the water to birth her placenta and her blood loss and perineal damage was minimal. The baby fed like a dream and I left them all snuggled up in bed a couple of hours later. I had done almost nothing at all except observe and be the photographer, and yet I left the house knowing I had truly fulfilled my role as this amazing woman's midwife.

Photographs taken by Laurence Wolahan and Virginia Howes.

The Practising Midwife 2003; 6(1): 12–19

A Wise Birth revisited

Penny Armstrong

In late 1988, during a Pennsylvania snowstorm, Sheryl Feldman and I sat by a fire and formulated the questions we wanted to answer in *A Wise Birth*. We had witnessed the ease with which women in the Amish and Mennonite cultures birthed at home. What perplexed us was why this ease did not necessarily accompany the births of the well-informed, articulate, and in-charge women of modern American culture.

I recently had the occasion to re-read sections of *A Wise Birth*. I was struck by how relevant our observations were to the challenges I find as I return to practice, after 10 years of teaching. My work at our tertiary care center, the community hospital, and the birthing center leave me with the same questions I had at that time and a lot of the same conclusions.

I did not expect a major cultural shift in maternity care in that amount of time, but neither did I expect to find that we continue to institutionalize in-hospitality. It surprises me that the decisive and analytical women, who are changing so many other aspects of American culture, have not taken on birth. Somehow, they have failed to name the neglect in maternity care in this country and to recognize that we continue to set up a deeply wounding and difficult passage for them.

In *A Wise Birth*, we observed that as a culture:

We do not woo women into giving birth. We do not trail our fingertips on the beds we have made up, anticipating their coming … We do not touch them, rejoice in them, admire them, laugh with them, or stand by them.

… Given the responsibilities of the mother, it is odd that we cripple the power that comes with birth. It is curious that we do not know to give human warmth, which attenuates pain. It is unthinkable that we, wanting human life to go on, cut wound, sap, and scar the women who do the work …

… She does not accuse us – those of us who failed to be generous to her, to name her strengths, to nourish her, to give to her … She does not notice the absence of humility, awe, and caring among us; instead she absorbs the neglect, the

nonanswers, the damage, and the responsibility. She criticizes herself and she lives with the memory of the experience and the judgment she makes of herself as a mother …
(Armstrong & Feldman, 1990)

As I once again tune my ear to the talk of birth, I hear colleagues say that the wounding is increasingly due to the choices the women and their partners make; it is they who are colluding in the disruption of the natural processes by demanding interventions. As midwives we are trained to be sensitive to birthing families' wishes. So we are torn; do we give them what they ask for knowing it is more likely to lead to a loss of power, a dampening of the experience, or to wounding, scaring, and an especially challenging transition to parenthood?

As this professional debate continues, it is shaded differently than it was even a decade ago. We seem to be putting more responsibility for the cascading interventions and accompanying loss of power on the birthing women and less on the obstetric culture of which we are a part. As midwives we can still say, proudly, that we do woo women into giving birth. But are we doing all that we can in the face of the cultural imperatives that so profoundly affect our birthing environments?

In *A Wise Birth* we observed that the quality of a birth arises, in good part, out of the culture from which it came. As midwives, we can choose to believe that we are trapped by cultural determinism and that we have no choice but to ride the waves that continue to erode the power that women can bring to, and exercise during, their birthing experiences.

But we must challenge ourselves to remember that culture is created by individual acts. For midwives, that may mean the intervention we acquiesce to even when we know it is not needed, or the birth we do not allow to unwind at its own pace because of office pressures. It may mean the policy work that we avoid even though we know the decisions will affect our birthing environments. Or maybe it means failing to understand and respect the use of alternatives and old-time skills. Or, most troubling of all, it may mean blaming women for not finding their own way through a birthing culture beset with negative birth messages, lack of generational support, and unrealistic expectations for the new mother.

As we try to understand how our culture shapes birthing women, we also must continuously examine our own contributions to the birthing culture. We must stand back and observe ourselves with the keenness, kindness, and toughness we usually reserve for our clients. It takes discipline to be able to spot the decisions, actions, or nonactions, which lead us into collusion with practices that fail to promote health – both within the birth experience and in the transformation to parenthood. Failing to exercise that discipline is a violation of the trust that has been passed down to us by virtue of the ancient and honorable title, midwife.

REFERENCES

Armstrong P, Feldman S. 1990. A Wise Birth. William Morrow, New York

Journal of Midwifery and Women's Health 2002; 47(3): VIII

Compare and contrast: three births in one day

Anne Adamson

Sonia's story

Three o'clock in the morning and my pager awakens me. I squint at it blearily and see the name of a woman expecting her fifth baby. I phone her quickly. She speaks to me in slightly breathless tones, obviously having just completed a contraction, and I say I will get to her home a.s.a.p. My husband says sleepily, from the comfort of our bed, that he will make me a cup of tea, but I tell him there's no time.

I page my colleague, Kate, and ask her to set off at the same time as me. She has further to come and I'm afraid she'll miss the birth – although she's liable to miss it anyway, because this is the most radical and independent woman I think I have ever cared for, and among other things, she doesn't want another midwife to be present when she gives birth. We reached a compromise some weeks ago about the presence of another midwife and Kate knows she may have to sit in the car outside when she arrives! It's nothing personal – this is just the way Sonia wants to do things.

Driving along the blissfully empty roads on the convoluted route to Sonia's, I am excited at the prospect of how Sonia will handle this labour and birth. I am used to sitting on my hands in normal labour and watching things unfold, but it is comparatively unusual to attend a woman so completely sure of herself and her baby. Sonia has had four previous normal deliveries (four delightful boys whom she home-schools, ranging in age from nine to 18 months). Her three eldest sons were born at home in Australia with an independent midwife. Her fourth was born in a hospital in Belgium.

Sonia booked late with us and, as she had had no scans during her pregnancies and did not know the date of her last period, I worked out a rough delivery date from fundal height and the size of the baby. She has always been able to tell me precisely how the baby was lying before I palpated her, and had palpated a heartbeat

before I booked her. I always listened to the fetal heart with my Pinard, as Sonia did not want her baby exposed to any ultrasound.

Drawing up outside Sonia and Geoff's, the door has been left ajar and I unload my equipment from the boot and creep inside, not wanting to wake the boys. Sonia grins broadly at me from where she is reclining in an armchair between contractions and Geoff greets me. The video camera is already set up in their small living room. There is very little room for manoeuvre, what with the three-piece suite, a large cupboard, a desk and the inflatable birthing pool, but somehow we all manage to squeeze in. During contractions, Sonia drops into a squat and holds onto some stepladders for support. She used the birthing pool before I arrived, but doesn't want to get back in yet. Kate arrives not long after me and is ensconced in the office outside in the garage with tea and biscuits – just as well it's a mild night!

I 'set up' unobtrusively, but Sonia, who never misses a trick, despite being in heavy labour, notices my baby oxygen and declares we won't need it. I expect she is right – she usually is!

Sonia recites some Biblical verses to herself as the contractions increase in their intensity. She and Geoff have a strong Christian faith and Sonia says it is largely because of what she believes that she has such complete confidence. I keep a low profile and busy myself writing notes in the connecting room, only disturbing the flow of the labour to 'listen in'. However, Sonia asks me to join them and likes to have me near when she goes to the nearby lavatory. She tells me two of her boys were born when she was on the loo and she wants me there to catch this one!

Sure enough, less than two hours after my arrival, Sonia gives birth to her fifth son sitting on the toilet. I hear her waters plop into the toilet with a mighty 'plosh' and, within seconds, they are followed by the baby's head. I support the head, and ask Sonia to push down onto my shoulders as I kneel in front of her so that she can stand for the birth of the body. Then she sits down again to hold him in her arms. He roars lustily, and Vince, the second eldest, age 7, arrives on the scene to gaze silently at his newborn brother with awe, whilst Geoff films the scene from the doorway. What a moment! I'm not sure who is the most thrilled – the parents or me! I feel I am the learner here. Although I have always asserted that I have learned almost everything I know from the mothers and their babies and, as a result, have constantly had to adjust my practice, this woman, this birth, this family have completely humbled me. I realise that not only will I have to mentally overhaul my midwifery practice – I will also have to overhaul my life!

Within 10 minutes of the birth, Sonia declares she would like a bath. However, the cord is still pulsating, so it's not time to cut it yet, but this does not deter Sonia, who simply hares up the stairs with the baby still attached, me following closely, and gets into the bath which Geoff has just run for her. Then it's downstairs again to recline once more on the armchair, as although the three eldest boys are now all wide awake, James, who shares his parents' room, sleeps on, and Sonia is afraid of disturbing him. Sonia gets afterpains and stands up periodically to try and deliver her placenta into a bowl. It eventually comes, about 45 minutes after the birth, delivered by Sonia in her usual neat and tidy style! (Geoff declined to cut the cord earlier, declaring he'd done that several times now and didn't really feel the need to do it again, so Vince volunteered.) The boys have lots of questions for me in the kitchen, where I check the placenta. Brett wonders whether the placenta is part of 'mummy's private parts' that have somehow come away, but I reassure him!

Kate has been let in by now, and has an interesting time getting to know Sonia, Geoff and the boys, as she did not meet them antenatally. Most of the clearing up has been done and at 6.45 a.m. I depart for our Birth Centre some miles away to assist Jayne at another delivery, leaving Kate to finish at Sonia's.

Hiromi's story

There are striking contrasts between Sonia and Hiromi, and it is these huge variations in the women we care for and their previous birth experiences which make midwifery such a fascinating profession and which stretch us to our full capacity. It takes me an hour to reach the Birth Centre as traffic is already beginning to build up and I have ample opportunity to reflect on this as I drive along.

Hiromi booked with Jayne at 16 weeks. This was her third pregnancy. She had a very early miscarriage between her first birth, two and a half years previously, and her current pregnancy. After a normal pregnancy with her first child and spontaneous labour at term, Hiromi had an emergency caesarean section for apparent 'fetal distress' at 8 cm dilatation. A subsequent pelvimetry had shown the pelvis to be of adequate proportions. Hiromi and her husband, Paul, had found the labour and birth very frightening and Hiromi felt dehumanised by what had happened to her at the hospital. The couple now sought to avoid a similar situation arising and Hiromi was keen to have this baby vaginally.

This couple had needed an enormous amount of reassurance from both their midwives because of their past experience. This involved obtaining their previous notes and going through them meticulously together so that Hiromi and Paul had more understanding of what had occurred. It also involved their exploring the possibility of using the hospital's new 'low-tech' facility – but Hiromi did not fit the necessary criteria, having had a previous section. Accompanying them at 36 weeks for a hospital antenatal visit to see Hiromi's consultant obstetrician finally convinced Hiromi that she did not want to have another baby there. Paul, however, remained a little sceptical and sought additional reassurance, so we put him in touch with two women who had recently had vaginal deliveries after previous caesareans who were happy to talk to him.

Hiromi had paged Jayne at 3.30 a.m. this morning as I was on my way to Sonia's labour. Jayne and I had communicated about what to do in the event that I was still at Sonia's when Jayne needed me to assist with Hiromi, but we had learnt from experience that these things usually work out! We decided to 'play it by ear' for the time being and see how the two labours progressed. Jayne met Hiromi and Paul at the Birth Centre at six o'clock and asked me to attend not long after.

I arrive at 7.45 a.m. Hiromi is in the pool in the downstairs birthing room and is contracting strongly and frequently. She is coping excellently with loving support from Paul and lots of encouragement from Jayne. At 8.10, Jayne examines Hiromi in the pool and finds her to be nearly fully dilated, with bulging membranes and the head at plus one station.

At 9.40 Jayne performs another quick vaginal examination in the pool as Hiromi is feeling impatient and tired, and thinks she might need an epidural. As she is fully dilated, Jayne explains to Hiromi that it is too late for this, but thinks a change of scene may help, so Hiromi gets on all fours on the birthing mat for a short while, where she pushes spontaneously from time to time. Jayne suggests a walk into the living room, where I put lots of inco pads on the floor and sofa, and Hiromi kneels on the sofa and looks out of the window into the garden between contractions. Hiromi is soon pushing spontaneously with every contraction, whilst Paul spoons honey into her mouth to give her an energy boost! Hiromi feels she isn't making progress – we all assure her that she is.

By 11 o'clock, we are all back in the birthing room, where Hiromi tries the birthing stool, but finds it uncomfortable. She returns to a kneeling posture. Paul continues plying Hiromi with honey and is very supportive and loving. Hiromi pushes well with each contraction. She has a short spell seated on the loo, as the upright posture adopted and the lack of pressure on the perineal area make it an ideal position, then she returns to her favourite kneeling posture on the birthing mat. At 11.43, Jayne can just see the vertex advancing and receding, and encourages Hiromi. Hiromi agrees to give the birthing stool another try, with Paul seated behind her on the sofa to support her back. This position seems to really help, and a lot more of the baby's head is visible. It is getting very exciting – and Jayne offers to show Hiromi how well she is doing with the aid of a mirror, but Hiromi says she doesn't want to see it! However, Paul does, and is pleased to see we aren't kidding him on!

Hiromi finds the intensity of the baby's head on the stretching perineum too much, and has another 10–15 minutes back on her knees, finally trying a supported squatting position with her back against Paul as he sits on the sofa. By 12.18 the head is almost crowning – Hiromi cries out that it is 'very painful!' and Jayne comforts her and says it will soon all be over. At 12.24 Hiromi and Paul are rewarded with the birth of a beautiful son (3650 g), who is almost born in the caul. After a physiological third stage and the cord cut by Paul, the placenta follows at 12.50.

An hour later, everyone (including the midwives, who are having a well-earned break in the living room, well within earshot of the birthing room) is tucking into a big cooked breakfast. (I haven't found many women and their partners refuse this after all that hard work!)

I compare the differences between the two labours and births I have been privileged to attend today. One baby born to a very experienced mother with complete faith in God, herself and the miraculous workings of her body; the other mother, undermined and emotionally raw from her first labour and birth, feeling her way through this very different, new experience and unsure how it will all end. In many ways, the intensity of undrugged vaginal delivery when a woman has had a previous caesarean is more of a shock to the mother than it is to a first-time mother. On the previous occasion, she was subjected to a major surgical intervention in the stark surroundings of an operating theatre filled with personnel, most of whom she had never met. This is set against the backdrop of

what has passed before, which may have been terrifying in itself. Now she finds herself in a dimly lit, cosy birthing room devoid of almost anything technological, with just her husband and two known and trusted midwives, undergoing an experience shared by millions of women all over the world, but which is also utterly unique to her.

Angela's story

But it's not all over yet for me! I am in the unique position today of attending three births in 24 hours. However, this last one is an elective caesarean section, so I am not actually required to be 'hands on'. The operation was actually scheduled to take place tomorrow, but has had to be brought forward as Angela was mildly contracting when she visited the consultant obstetrician this evening.

I leave the Birth Centre at 3.30 p.m. and arrive home at four-ish. Angela and her husband, Gavin, are not seeing the obstetrician until later in the day, but Angela pages me to say she is having mild contractions. I suggest she puts on her TENS and keeps the appointment, since first labours usually take their time, so there is little possibility of her having to have a caesarean in the midst of strong labour.

The diversity amongst women never ceases to amaze me, but I feel as though I am going from one extreme to the other today. Angela and Gavin could not be more different in their approach and feelings about labour and birth than Sonia and Geoff – with Hiromi and Paul floating somewhere in between!

This is Angela's first baby. She booked at 14 weeks and had an uncomplicated pregnancy. However, she reached 42 weeks with no sign of labour approaching, so I arranged a scan for her at the couple's request. All was well on the scan, but the obstetrician thought the baby was at least 10 lb – which surprised him, since it did not palpate as being that size. He advised elective caesarean section.

I visited Angela and Gavin the day after to discuss options with them, but they had been getting increasingly anxious as the days had gone by, even though it is common for the women in Angela's family to go two to three weeks 'overdue'. The pronouncement that the baby was big had further increased their anxiety, and they decided they would like Angela to undergo a caesarean.

That was two days ago, as it had taken that time to find an obstetrician with a 'space', since the obstetrician who did the scan did not have any vacancies, and here was Angela starting to labour at long last, at 42 + 3! However, there was no way Angela was going to contemplate having this baby vaginally, so having seen the obstetrician, she paged me later in the evening to say the caesarean was scheduled to take place at 10 o'clock that night.

Having had a lovely soak in the bath and eaten dinner, I set off on the long drive to the hospital where Angela was to have her caesarean, which was one I had not been to before. I found Angela and Gavin on the Labour Ward waiting to be seen by the anaesthetist and looking rather anxious. Angela had her TENS on and was experiencing mild contractions, and Gavin was already in his 'greens'.

By 9.40 we are all in theatre, and Angela is having her epidural inserted. 'Knife to skin' at 9.55, and at 10.04 p.m. a 4800 g baby boy is born! I get lots of good photographs as he is born and afterwards. He is certainly letting us know he is around, and screams lustily. His parents are pleased but dazed, of course.

An hour or so later I am heading home and gratefully fall into bed almost 24 hours after I vacated it. I doubt I could've planned such a day if I'd tried – three completely different births in three completely different settings with three completely different couples!

The Practising Midwife 2003; 6(2): 17–19

The Un-Peel Report

Gill Walton

I was visiting relatives over Christmas. As is usual on arrival I was offered a drink … tea, coffee, hot chocolate, sherry, wine, brandy, whiskey and even Ovaltine! I opted for coffee, and then more choice … filtered, instant, decaf, caffeinated, cappuccino – wow! I settled boringly for decaf. Then the next barrage of choices … milk? … skimmed, semi-skimmed, whole, Coffeemate … sugar, Canderel, brown, cubed … mug, cup, coffee cup! You get the picture, I'm sure.

How life has changed! Tea or coffee, milk and sugar – simple, we all knew where we were. Choices for childbirth are the same. Place of birth … hospital, birth centre (integrated or stand alone), midwife, independent, GP, consultant? Then choices in labour! Epidural, spinal, TNS, entonox, pethidine, water, acupuncture … birthing ball, stool, sitting, standing, squatting! If women access the Internet there are even more choices to confuse the issue!

Before the Peel Report (1970), choice was home or hospital, with gas and air and a spot of pethidine if you were lucky! 'Changing Childbirth' (Department of Health, 1992) advocated choice for women and control over that choice, but have we gone too far? Women face a barrage of choices in 2003, starting at the first contact with the midwife, where it is usual to ask where they want to have their baby, heavily weighted to hospital! How do midwives have the time and the enthusiasm to explain all the choices? How do we give informed choice and promote normality? Maybe we need to rethink our approach to offering choice.

Let us start with the choice of place of birth. Understanding and really feeling how it is to be a midwife happened to me when I attended my first home birth. I finally understood the complex relationship between the ability of the woman's body to labour and give birth and the power of the quiet and confident support from a midwife. I have fortunately spent the rest of my midwifery career being confident of home birth

and encouraging my midwifery colleagues to be the same. However, my persuasion of midwives to support home birth is not enough. I know that with the current home birth rate being as low as 1% in some areas, midwives do not get the experience of being with a woman at a home birth. This is essential if they are going to support women's choice and believe in that choice. Persuading women is even harder, as the majority of women think that having a baby at home is just not normal!

How can we change this and make it normal and accepted by women and midwives to have a baby at home? One way would be to ensure that midwives believe that home birth is safe. They need support and experience in caring for women in an uncomplicated labour in a home setting. They need access to the evidence for home birth, in bucketloads! I believe that every student should attend at least five home births in their training and every midwife at a home birth must have a student or another midwife who hasn't attended a home birth with her. That's a start! Women need to see and feel our confidence in home birth.

Like many services, in Reading we have implemented early labour assessment at home in the hope of helping women experience at least some part of their labour in a home setting. The choice to stay at home for birth can even be made in labour. But it is still not enough. Let's be totally radical! What if we adopted an 'opt out' approach to choice of place of birth, as we currently do in some services with HIV testing. Women with uncomplicated pregnancies would be offered 'opt out' home birth – a policy for all women to have a home birth unless they choose not to. The weight of the information and the enthusiasm would start with home, moving to other options after debate and discussion about the pros and cons of home birth.

Choices for labour could be given in the same vein, with non-pharmacological methods being the 'opt out' –

then we could stop advertising a 24-hour epidural service! That certainly would be a good move. One of my colleagues was telling me that the statistics for her unit show that if women in normal labour have an epidural, they only have a 30% chance of a normal birth.

We could even go as far as 'opt out' mobilisation and remove the beds – the list is endless. Women can have choice, of course, but the choices and information are added as they opt out.

The Peel Report in 1970 recommended hospital birth on the grounds of safety (no evidence!). The Un-Peel Report in 2003 recommends home birth on the grounds of safety (plenty of evidence!). 'Opt out' home birth has to be the future in our quest to reclaim the empowering and positive experience of birth. We must make a concerted effort to normalise birth and help women and midwives believe in the fact that most women can labour and give birth without intervention, and that can happen at home.

Now back to the relatives – when they come to me offering that drink, it's easy: 'opt out' wine ... we don't usually get any further!

The Practising Midwife 2003; 6(2): 4

Goodbye, and thanks

Jane Bowler

Well, I've said goodbye to *The Practising Midwife*, after four enjoyable years as Managing Editor. Taking on the journal was a challenge, especially since I was a complete stranger to the world of midwifery, I have never had a baby (nulliparous!) and I'd rarely come within nappy-sniffing distance of one.

School sex education may have put paid to the chances of me ever going into labour. The first film (the one with the sex) was bad enough; the mechanics of it all came as a bolt out of the blue to me. But the second film was the clincher – a flickering cine film shown to us in twos and threes in a tiny dark room, featuring a woman screaming the place down, with her feet in stirrups and a cameraman zooming in on her privates (which looked as if they were about to burst). No thanks, not for me.

By dint of reading every word of *The Practising Midwife* every month, I soon learned quite a lot about what midwives do. Having attended my first RCM conference, I flippantly reported back to my co-worker Gwilym (a designer who, after four years on the journal, remains admirably calm when faced with pics of naked women and their bits) that midwives fell into two breeds: fat, friendly ones and thin, scary ones. Looking back, I have changed my opinion – slightly!

Midwifery is a profession in crisis, a profession under siege. This has had the effect of making midwives pretty defensive. Reading the news pages of *The Practising Midwife* every month, I got the message again and again: midwives are persecuted, underpaid, stressed out and dropping like flies. They're fighting tooth and nail to preserve their right to help women give birth to babies, against the doctors and nurses who, between them, have got the high-skill, high-tech and the low-skill, low-paid bits of midwifery covered, and who are rapidly closing up the gap in the middle. (And one of the most disturbing prospects I've come across is the possibility that independent midwives in the UK will be forced to stop being with women because they cannot afford soaring insurance costs.)

There's a kind of desperation in midwives' determination to prove their worth, with endless qualifications and research projects. Now, I'm still an outsider, but a lot of it seems to be taking a hammer to crack a nut. I've learned that labouring women generally don't like to be interfered with, that women attending antenatal clinics don't like to be prodded without at least a few friendly words of introduction, and that women (and men) attending antenatal classes don't like being patronised. Hurray!

I've learned that a good birthing environment is like a warm, safe nest where a woman feels in control – or rather, where she feels safe enough to not be in control, to stop intellectualising or worrying about doing the right thing, and can relax into a deeper mental state, letting her body do the natural thing. Key concepts for me were Judith Ockenden's (2001) point that a couple would find it difficult to make love in the kind of hospital conditions typically offered to the labouring woman, and Esther Culpin's (2003) report that Michel Odent, who attended her home birth, seemed to gather all the information he needed about her labour by silently watching and listening to her.

To return (with apologies) to the fat and thin midwives, I now feel able to refine my point of view. Some midwives are engaged in a fight to prove their worth by producing research and evidence on which to build guidelines for practice. And I take the point, ably put by Belinda Phipps (2002), that, in a world where facts and figures are the new gods, midwifery will struggle to be taken seriously unless it speaks the same language.

However, other midwives are looking to the distant past, and to other cultures for inspiration. These are the gentle, intuitive women who became midwives because they love women and babies, and are enthralled and grateful to be in on the miracle of birth.

Some of the happiest midwives I've come across are those who have stopped fighting the system and are working on the fringe – like the American ones who just do what they can to offer an alternative to the technological norm.

I've also learned a bit about babies in the past four years. My nephew James was born with multiple disabilities, and lived for just three months in the SCBU at Hammersmith Hospital. His disabilities were completely unexpected, and one midwife burst into tears at his birth – a dreadful, spontaneous reaction that we will never forget. We'll also always remember the caring and committed SCBU staff who cared for James and his family. I learned a lot – about ventilators, syringe drivers, milk banks and tube feeding. About the risks in life, learning to face death, and about the importance of being with people, of simply being human, at the extremes of the beginning and end of life.

REFERENCES

Culpin E. 2003. Home breech birth. The Practising Midwife, 6(1): 10–11

Ockenden J. 2001. The hormonal dance of labour. The Practising Midwife, 4(6): 16–17

Phipps B. 2002. Normal birth – does it matter? The Practising Midwife, 5(2): 23–24

The Practising Midwife 2003; 6(5): 42

Competition details

To enter the competition discussed in the Introduction to this book, please send a postcard, letter or email to:

Natalie Friend
Elsevier
32 Jamestown Road
London
NW1 7BY
England
n.friend@elsevier.com

Your postcard/letter/email should include your responses to the questions in Section 5 and your contact details, so that we can get in touch if you are a winner, and/or so that we can ask your permission if we decide to explore the idea of publishing responses in any form in the future.

The closing date for this competition is 31st December 2006. Five winners will be drawn randomly from all responses received by this date, and the five winners of the £100 Elsevier book vouchers will be notified in January 2007.

By providing your details, you consent to signing up to the Elsevier mailing list and eAlert service. This service provides you with quarterly emails about the latest books, journals and exhibitions in midwifery. The personal information that you provide will be used by Elsevier Limited, 32 Jamestown Road, London, NW1 7BY. It will be used to service your registration, to improve our website and online service and, with your permission, will be used by Elsevier Limited to inform you about relevant services and products. The information will not be sold or shared with third parties. To unsubscribe to eAlert, please visit:

http://intl.elsevierhealth.com/ealert

We will not use your response or name in any future articles or books on this topic without contacting you first to ask for permission.

Good luck!

Index

Notes

Page numbers suffixed by 'b' indicate boxed material: page numbers suffixed by 't' indicate material in tables: page numbers suffixed by 'f' indicate figures.

A

Abbreviated Scale for the Assessment of Psychosocial Status in Pregnancy, 61
access
  'Better Birth Environment' survey, 13
  midwife-managed units, 4
acid–base balance, 146
  acidosis, 146–147
    metabolic component, 147
  blood gases, 145
  buffers, 146
acidosis *see* acid–base balance
acute clinical situations, normal (physiological) birth, 30
admission criteria, midwife-managed unit, 3, 3b, 7
adolescent mothers, 210–221
  age effects, 213
  antenatal care, 219–220
  concealment of pregnancy, 213
  education, 212
  emotional expectations, 214
  father, role of, 212, 213
  Government policy, 211
  interconnecting dimensions, 212–214, 212f
  maturity
    immaturity *vs.*, 212–213, 214, 216
    Levinson's stages of adulthood, 217b
    perceived, 213
  motherhood, meaning of, 211–212
  older teenagers, 216–221
    attitudes to sexuality, 218–219
    misplaced labelling, 217–218
    negative aspects, 218–219
    terminology, 216–217, 217t
  postnatal education, 220
  pregnancy reasons, 210, 212–213, 219
  relationships, 212, 214

  responsibility, 214
  return to education, 213
  sex education, 210–211
  as a social problem, 210
  stigmatisation, 212
  study, 211–214
    aims, 211
    data collection, 211
    ethical considerations, 211
    focus group interviews, 211–212
    results, 212–214
    sample, 211
    setting, 211
  support, need for, 212, 214
  trends, 210
  truancy, 213
adrenaline, 204–205
Advanced Life Support in Obstetrics (ALSO) course, 171
advertising, body image, 90
anaemia
  delayed cord clamping effects, 115, 121
  immediate umbilical cord clamping, 122
anaerobic metabolism, fetal energy production, 146
animals
  immediate umbilical cord clamping, 122–123
  'pasmo,' 153–154
antenatal care
  adolescent mothers, 219–220
  birth positions, 150–151
  disabled mothers, 222
  guidelines, 59
  Lichfield Victoria Maternity Unit, 162
  West Wiltshire Primary Care Trust birth centres, 168
antenatal record (*Mutterpass*), 59, 60b, 61
Apgar score, blood gases, 145
approval seeking, body image, 90
aromatherapy, birth centres, 162, 168
arterial blood sample, blood gases, 147, 147t
Association for Improvements in the Maternity Services (AIMS), 96
attendance, breastfeeding support groups, reasons for, 102, 102t
autonomy, 18–28

  antecedents and consequences, 19–20, 20b
  barriers to, 23–24, 24–25
  characteristics of, 19–20, 20b
  concept analysis, 19–20
  conceptual framework, 20, 21f
  desire for, 25–26
  exercise of choice, 18–19
  'freedom,' 20
  importance of, 18
  'independence,' 20
  interpretation, 20
  practice structure *vs.*, 23
  reduced frequency prenatal visits, 74
  study into, 20–24
    barriers to autonomy, 23–24
    data collection/analysis, 22
    educational effects, 24
    ethics, 20–21
    facilitators of, 23
    findings, 18
    implications for practice, 18
    professional position, perceptions of, 24
    recruitment, 20–21
    sample, 18, 21–22, 22t
    understanding of autonomy, 22–23

B

baby, breastfeeding position, 191
'babymoon,' 203–205
base deficit (BDecf), 146t, 147
base excess (BE), 146t, 147
Beck Depression Inventory-II (BDI-II), 180, 181–182
behavioural effects, delayed cord clamping, 122
Belize, working in, personal experience, 48–54
beta-endorphin, 204
'Better Birth Environment' survey, 10–13
  access to facilities, 13
  design, 10–11
  helpful aspects, 11
  personal interactions, importance of, 11
  place of birth, 11, 12t
    home births, 12
    hospitals, 13
    midwife-led units, 12

sucking ketosis, 198
support groups *see* breastfeeding
support groups
Breastfeeding Best Start project,
191–196
design, 194
elimination of 'practice' effect,
195–196
implications for practice, 196
launch of, 193
participants, 194
procedure, 194–195
scoring system, 195
trainers, 195
breastfeeding support groups
attendance reasons, 102, 102t
contact about, 102, 102t
efficacy, 103
evaluation, 100–105
demographics, 104
findings, 101–103
questionnaires, 101
intervention acceptability, 104
member demographics, 101, 101t,
102t, 104
perceived advantages, 103, 103t
acceptability, 104
breech birth
home birth, 139–140
normal (physiological) birth,
137–138
personal experience, 137–138,
139–140
buffers, acid–base balance, 146

C

caesarian section
attitudes to, 10
delayed cord clamping, 119
on demand, 15–17
legal aspects, 15–16
risks, 16
'standards of care,' 16
elective *see* elective caesarian
section
inappropriate reasons, 15
increase in, 10
reasons for, 15–16, 15t
psychological distress, 16
risks, 16t
capillary leak syndrome, delayed
cord clamping, 119
cardiac output, dextrose infusion
effects, 142

cardiopulmonary effects, delayed
cord clamping, 115, 121–122
cardiovascular effects, breastfeeding,
199
care satisfaction, midwife-managed
unit, 6, 6t
Cartwright, Ann, 96
CESDI (Confidential Enquiry into
Stillbirths and Deaths in Infancy)
emergency situation requirements,
172
MMU case study, 4
Changing Childbirth (DoH, 1993), 9
birth centres, 166
continuity of care, 7
childhood obesity, breastfeeding, 199
choice of labour, personal
experience, 255–256
'churching,' 204
clonazepam, postpartum
depression, 183, 184
commitment, breastfeeding, 84–85
communication
ethnic minorities, 35, 36
post-traumatic maternity, 226
complementary and alternative
medicine (CAM)
Lichfield Victoria Maternity Unit,
162
West Wiltshire Primary Care
Trust birth centres, 168
concealment of pregnancy,
adolescent mothers, 213
concentration, during pregnancy, 87
concept analysis, autonomy, 19–20
confounding factors, delayed cord
clamping studies, 118–119
consultant units, Lichfield Victoria
Maternity Unit, cooperation with,
162
continuity of care
Changing Childbirth (DoH, 1993), 7
midwife-managed unit, 5, 7
transfers in labour, 169
cord blood analysis *see* blood gases
cost-effectiveness
reduced frequency prenatal
visits, 75
reduced frequency prenatal
visits, descriptive study, 74
'symphonic rationale,' 234–235
culture
body image, 90
postnatal care, 203

D

data analysis/collection
adolescent mothers study, 211
autonomy study, 22
breastfeeding study, 80
delayed cord clamping studies,
117
midwife-managed unit studies, 4
reduced frequency prenatal visit
studies, 72–73
definite choice, breastfeeding, 81–82
dehydration, during labour, 142
delayed cord clamping, 115
benefits, 121–122
anaemia effects, 115, 121
behavioural effects, 122
blood volume effects, 115,
115f
breastfeeding duration, 122
cardiopulmonary effects,
115, 121–122
gut circulation, 122
haematology, 121
blood volume measurements, 119
capillary leak syndrome, 119
delivery methods/speed, 119
disadvantages, 119–121
hyperbilirubinaemia, 115,
120–121
hyperviscocity, 120
polycythaemia, 115,
119–120
tachypnea, 115, 121
level infant is held, 118
oxytocic drug use, 119
physiologic effects, 118, 118t
practice implications, 123
research implications, 123
studies, 116–122
confounding factors,
118–119
data analysis, 117
interventions, 116
outcome measures, 116–117
search strategies, 116
selection criteria, 116
study descriptions, 117
uterine contractions, 119
vaginal *vs.* caesarian birth, 119
demographics
breastfeeding, 79, 80–81
breastfeeding support groups,
101, 101t, 102t, 104